GIVING BREASTMILK

BODY ETHICS AND CONTEMPORARY BREASTFEEDING PRACTICE

Published by:
Demeter Press
140 Holland Street West
P. O. Box 13022
Bradford, ON
L3Z 2Y5
Tel: (905) 775-5215
Email: info@demeterpress.org
Website: www.demeterpress.org

Demeter Press logo based on Skulptur "Demeter" by Maria-Luise Bodirsky
<www.keramik-atelier.bodirsky.edu>

Cover Art: © Trustees of the British Museum. Used with permission.
Cover Design/Interior Design: Luciana Ricciutelli

Printed and Bound in Canada

Library and Archives Canada Cataloguing in Publication

Giving breastmilk : body ethics and contemporary breastfeeding practices / edited by Rhonda Shaw and Alison Bartlett.

Includes bibliographical references.
ISBN 978-0-9866671-0-7

1. Breast milk. 2. Breastfeeding--Moral and ethical aspects. 3. Breastfeeding--Political aspects. I. Bartlett, Alison, 1961- II. Shaw, Rhonda

RJ216.G59 2010 649'.33 C2010-904505-X

GIVING BREASTMILK
BODY ETHICS AND CONTEMPORARY BREASTFEEDING PRACTICE

Edited by
Rhonda Shaw and Alison Bartlett

DEMETER
TORONTO, CANADA

Table of Contents

II. SHARING MILK

III. MILK POLITICS

IV. MILK THEORY

Mapping the Ethics and Politics of Contemporary Breastmilk Exchange

An Introduction

ALISON BARTLETT AND RHONDA SHAW

IT IS IMPOSSIBLE TO think of social life without considering how it is held together by gift-exchange practices, yet breastmilk exchange is virtually absent in the literature on body gifting and tissue economies. The current volume seeks to redress this gap. In different ways, each chapter in the volume takes up the idea that breastfeeding is not just an aspect of maternal being or a bio-genetic relation between a mother and an infant, but an ethical relation that defines a particular form of give and take between two or more human beings, as well as work that women do. To this end, the volume collects some of the most recent and interesting study being carried out on and around the topic of breastmilk, and is positioned as part of an esteemed lineage of mostly feminist but always women-centred writing on breastfeeding since the 1980s. This writing is distinct from how-to books on breastfeeding as it is primarily interested in questions of ethics and epistemology, philosophy and politics of breastmilk, and their effect on practice.

Reviewing that body of work over the past two decades, it seems to clearly fall into two categories: historical studies and cultural analyses, both fundamentally concerned with the controversies established between breastfeeding and infant formula politics. The work of Valerie Fildes and Rima Apple emerged almost simultaneously, with Fildes' *Breasts, Bottles and Babies: a History of Infant Feeding* published in the United Kingdom in 1986 while Apple's *Mothers and Medicine: a Social History of Infant Feeding, 1890–1950* was released in 1987 from the United States. Both of these histories highlight the shifts in infant feeding and their inextricable social contexts. The work of two biological anthropologists, Patricia Stuart-Macadam and Katherine A. Dettwyler, generated a groundbreaking collection of essays dedicated to giving a more holistic view of breastfeeding by providing cross-cultural, biocultural and evolutionary perspectives, in their 1995 volume *Breastfeeding: Biocultural Perspectives*. While their collection pivots on the diversity of cultural practices, it also warns in the introduction of "the perils of ignoring the 'bio' factor of the biocultural equation" (1), reminding us that change in social behaviour can have commensurate effects on biology. An increasing curiosity for the apparently displaced practice of wet-nursing was rewarded with Janet Golden writing *A Social History of Wet Nursing in America: From Breast to Bottle*, published in 2001.

The emergent literature on the cultural politics of breastfeeding must also be located in the mid- to late-1980s, with Maureen Minchin's Australian publication *Breastfeeding Matters* (1985) being highly influential during this period when she was involved in establishing certification for Lactation Consultants. Gabrielle Palmer's seething critique of the effects of formula companies marketing in the developing world in *The Politics of Breastfeeding* was released in 1988. Almost simultaneously across the Atlantic, Penny Van Esterik's pivotal work, *Beyond the Breast-Bottle Controversy* was published a year later in 1989, arguing that the infant formula case makes transparent the unsatisfactory relations of women and their bodies to issues of economics, technology, medicine, and labour conditions. These issues emerged again the late 1990s in *Milk, Money, and Madness: The Culture and Politics of Breastfeeding* by Naomi Baumslag and Dia L. Michels (1995), and then with Linda Blum's *At the Breast: Ideologies of Breastfeeding and Motherhood in the Contemporary United States* (1999). The United States seems to have been a particularly intense site of critique, as its breastfeeding practices wane statistically even while activism becomes increasingly public with 'lactivist' and online protests becoming more frequent. Bernice Hausman's *Mothers' Milk: Breastfeeding Controversies in American Culture* in 2003, however, expands the range of controversy to include the public anxiety of breastmilk carrying viruses amongst other forms of dis-ease. Expanding the intellectual possibilities of the topic is also evident in recent work from the southern hemisphere. Fiona Giles' *Fresh Milk: the Secret Life of Breasts* (2003) offers a range of arguably subcultural but definitely marginalised narratives about breastmilk and its uses. Giles is especially interested in the adult use of milk, for medication or pleasure, and its capacities for queering the substance and its intellectual approaches. Alison Bartlett's 2005 *Breastwork: Rethinking Breastfeeding* reads breastfeeding across a range of discursive media to propose a shift in thinking about breastfeeding from the values of modernity to postmodernity in order to address contemporary values. It's also important to note that this 'breasted' body of work on infant feeding is part of a considerable corpus of writing on motherhood, maternity and reproduction over the same era and longer, many of which include breastfeeding.

As this summary moves across a bookshelf of two decades of work, it becomes clear that the foundational work of historicising and critiquing existing social ideologies of capitalism, consumerism and patriarchy has been—and continues to be—necessary and important. It also becomes evident that a new set of intellectual discussions is beginning to emerge that extends on that foundational work, and much of this can be seen in the work presented at conferences and in journals. A 2004 issue of *Australian Feminist Studies,* for example, samples work on breastfeeding subjects in fiction, economics, race relations, queer theory, psychoanalysis and philosophy (see Bartlett and Giles), and since then breastfeeding has been extended to issues of pedagogy and geography, amongst other fields (Davidson and Langan; Noxolo et al). *Giving Breastmilk* seeks to bring together a range of this emerging work that is paving new intellectual ground and includes contributions from new researchers as well as those who are well-established in the field. Given the enormous response to the call for papers for this volume, with over 50 abstract submissions, excluding invited contributions, we can confidently say that it samples only a fraction of the fascinating research currently being undertaken.

The chapters in this volume easily fall into a number of categories, but we've chosen to cluster them according to the ways in which milk affects knowledge and praxis, through making and sharing milk and politics and theory. Each section highlights the fact that the place of breastmilk in culture and politics is never neutral, always contested. This is evident in the first section of the volume, "Making Milk," where the authors turn their attention to what mothers say about producing and giving breastmilk. The effect of reading so many interview excerpts in this section is a reminder of the differences between giving breastmilk and writing about it, but also of the productive relation between the two in the generation of new knowledge and discursive domains. The first chapter of the volume introduces Cindy Stearns' latest research on the breast pump. Privileging mothers' experience in her interviews with women Stearns asks why they pump, and how they experience it, noting fair amounts of frustration and diminished achievement in comparison to giving milk directly from the breast, but pride in the effort of those who would pump rather than buy formula. Language is repeatedly identified as crucial to understandings and practices of giving breastmilk. In their chapter, Copelton et al. draw on the established literature of infant feeding as ideological when they conduct focus groups to document mothers' understanding of infant feeding whether breastmilk or formula. They notice that all women are cognisant of the well-publicised advantages of breastmilk, and can make those arguments to support whatever kind of feeding they elect to practice. In their words, "mothers engage in ideological work to cope with the disjuncture between the dominant cultural logic that breast is best and women's own varied beliefs and experiences of infant feeding." Annette Beasley is also interested in the promotional message that breast is best, and her proceeding study involves analysing journals available to New Zealand midwives for their infant feeding content directed at midwifery professionals. Beasley identifies themes around breastfeeding practice, barriers and support, and education and promotion, as well as accompanying product advertising for breast pumps and formula in some journals. If this sounds contradictory, then Monica Campo's chapter is also interested in the tensions of breastfeeding, specifically around women's conflicting ideals of sexuality, maternity and self. Her chapter on the lactating body uses women's descriptions of how they feel about their bodies to identify clusters of conflict mothers constantly monitor and negotiate in maintaining their maternal identity, especially in relation to sexuality and the public/private divide. The final chapter in this section aptly reminds us of how much breastmilk is appreciated. Karleen Gribble's innovative research here reports what speaking Australian breastfed infants have to say about breastmilk, to which they respond with answers like *happy and cuddly, warm and snugly, milk is yummy*. Gribble provides arguments to counter the contentiousness of long-term breastfeeding, by characterising breastmilk for these infants as normal, as delicious food, as comfort, care and intimacy. This chapter brings together a number of the themes of this volume around the positive benefits of giving breastmilk, but in a frame that avoids the usual medicalised and moral discourses. Instead pleasure and fulfilment for giver and receiver are emphasised.

The following section groups together research on "Sharing Milk." It seems that the idea of sharing milk, not necessarily with your own baby, is gaining increasing purchase for curious researchers and practitioners alike. Rhonda Shaw picks up this work, through the ethics of human milk banking in the initial chapter of this section. Shaw draws attention to the pros and cons of human milk donation and how views of embodiment, identity, community, and generosity shape the debate between those who argue for the commercialisation of breastmilk and those who promote the donation of human breastmilk as an altruistic act. Although public health campaigns currently stress non-remunerative breastmilk donation, Shaw questions the straightforward equation of altruism and the pure gift with donation in this domain. More debate around human breastmilk donation is needed, she argues, especially now that milk banks, in which lactating mothers give their milk for the benefit of others, are on the increase again. The recent reemergence of milk banks around the globe is the subject of Naomi Bromberg Bar-Yam's chapter, which begins with a report on the newly established community milk bank in the Boston area by a group of committed volunteers. Bar-Yam's tale is instructive in charting some of the ethical and practical considerations that arise in setting up such an extraordinary service, but is also inspirational in narrating the efforts of a small group of people dedicated to making the project work within a network of institutional imperatives. Tanya Cassidy on the other hand, is on the receiving end of a community milk bank as her baby is provided with donor milk in Ireland, and she describes her sense of an "invisible community based on a unique and invaluable form of giving" in this cash-less economy. Her chapter, "Comparing Sharing and Banking," joins with Abdullahi El-Tom to tell the story of his mother generously breastfeeding a neighbour's contemporaneously born son in the Sudan, thus creating kinship between Abdullahi and Mohamed as milk brothers. The exigencies of Ireland and the Sudan decades apart and the relations established between families and strangers are brought together in this chapter through Malinowski's concept of the gift to consider the relative merits of anonymity and familiarity for donors and recipients. Staying with the theme of donated milk but shifting this time to New Zealand, Carol Bartle's chapter turns our attention to neonatal intensive care settings. Noting the low rate of exclusive breastfeeding for babies born over 37 weeks, Bartle's qualitative research examines the ways in which breastmilk is made, given, measured, and regarded in NICU by talking to mothers and staff at the unit. Connecting with some of the issues Cindy Stearns raises in her chapter on pumping milk, Bartle's research records the efforts of women to ensure a supply of breastmilk for their premature babies. Staff responses and anxieties however are revealing in accounting for what Bartle calls the 'subterranean' practice of using donor breastmilk by mothers who must negotiate medical regulations and normative practices in order to avoid the use of formula feeding. These three articles on widely divergent aspects of donor milk are testament to the diversity of practices, both formal and informal, that circulate milk for sharing. Taking these practices now to Canada, Tasnim Nathoo and Aleck Ostry provide a history of wet-nursing, milk banks and black markets from the early twentieth century to today. They identify the ways in which breastmilk is yoked to rhetoric of nationhood, and cycles between being considered commodity and charity over the century. In contrast to Cassidy and El-Tom's chapter, they identify the thriving cashed-up economies in which milk is currently being exchanged. Nathoo and Ostry's chapter placed here is a useful reminder that infant feeding is always embedded in social and political contexts.

The chapters that begin the next section on "Milk Politics" draw attention to the positioning of breastmilk as both cure and poison. The section begins with an invocation by Penny Van Esterik on the current debates around HIV/AIDS infection and prevention through breastmilk. In a self-confessed 'raw' but productively passionate piece of writing, Van Esterik reports on the cross-dialogues held in and between two conferences in Toronto in 2006, with a follow-up conference in 2008 updating the issues at stake. The investments in knowledge and cultural mis/understandings are writ large in this play of perception and power between the 'global north' and the 'global south', as well as the overdetermined impact of gender, and Van Esterik concludes by listing directions for future gendered and situated research needed to make informed policy decisions. Jennifer Reich then turns our attention to more specific issues of class and race in her chapter on how child protective services in the United States interpret breastfeeding and maternal love for their clients. Taking the cases of two young white mothers charged with possession of drugs, Reich demonstrates the varying meanings of breastfeeding and the varying toxic dangers of breastmilk to the court of law in which they appeared: one woman was forced to wean her baby after it was removed from her custody while the other was allowed to continue breastfeeding. In contrast, Reich comments on her own invisibility as a lactating researcher whose practices were not subject to the regulative gaze of the same courthouse as she entered each morning to follow the cases. Following the theme of milk as an imagined carrier of both moral and biological dangers, Bernice Hausman revisits the 2002 West Nile Virus scare in the United States which was often and incorrectly reported as being transmitted through breastfeeding. Hausman draws on the way 'risk' is culturally codified to argue that fears of such infection "demonstrate typically American fears of microbial dangers that threaten North America from afar," as well as a "deep ambivalence about women's capacities to nourish their children outside of medical scrutiny." In making this compelling argument, she concludes that breastmilk itself is regarded as risky. If milk is one of the flows, movements and energies that constitute our habitat, as philosopher Elizabeth Grosz argues of cities, then breastmilk is surely one of those flows, and its proximity to toxicity in this section of essays registers the fears and phobias of the culture about which each author writes. The work in this section draws attention to the capacity of breastmilk to be widely interpreted, bearing multiple and even opposing meanings in similar circumstances, and therefore bringing distinct differences to the construction of knowledge, policy and politics.

The final section on "Milk Theory" demonstrates the ways in which specific intellectual theories have the capacity to reanimate discussions and practices of giving breastmilk, as breastmilk might also have the potential to affect theoretical paradigms. Indeed, the fact that philosophy, psychoanalysis and social theory are brought to bear on this cluster of chapters suggests that these scholars have taken breastmilk to work, in affecting their thinking. Karen McBride-Henry and Rhonda Shaw present a study of breastfeeding women in New Zealand using the methodology and analysis of reflective lifeworld research, which combines existential and interpretive phenomenology. Heidegger's concept of care is mobilised to read breastfeeding as a productive response to the 'call to care' he identifies as exemplifying an authentic mode of solicitude or being-with another that characterises how women in this study saw their mother-infant relationships. Keren Epstein-Gilboa continues this interest in human relations in her chapter on breastfeeding envy as obstructionist. Following Melanie Klein, she proposes that the (individual and collective) psychic mechanisms of unresolved envy manifesting in "simultaneous hate and love" can be applied to breastfeeding when it is praised but also interfered with and even destroyed through "feelings of contempt for and debasement of adored nursing objects." Thus, unresolved envy of breastfeeding objects can affect women's breastfeeding practices individually and collectively through institutional systems. This politically thought-provoking approach is followed by Alison Bartlett's consideration of what to do about time: its loss, its language, and its liminality. Breastfeeding is often understood as profoundly time-consuming, untimed and makes mothers time-poor in a world that champions productivity and efficiency. Bartlett argues that breastfeeding changes our perception and habitation of time, and even poses a radical intervention into commonly held assumptions about linear time. So this chapter considers some alternative approaches to time as eternal, reciprocal, and even addictive, in order to argue for the restoration of women's agency in living 'milk' time. Agency also features in the final chapter of the volume by Fiona Giles, who reminds us of lactation's often overlooked but potent place in regimes of filmic and visual representation. Giles' chapter analyses the 2001 film *Visitor Q*, directed by Takashi Miike. The film features a mother of grown-up children whose discovery that she can still lactate is given such significance that it induces a reconciliation of the (dysfunctional and estranged) family. Her milk is prolific, flooding the kitchen in an excess of production and pleasure, and the film climaxes with her joyfully suckling her husband and grown daughter at each breast. Giles traces an ethical relation of embodied gifting through the theories of Mauss, Derrida and Diprose to argue for a new conception of lactation as an act of self care, rather than a gift that depletes or even reciprocates. Through the mechanism of this film, she proposes that lactation "provides an analogy for the gift of connection which benefits both parties," effectively removing breastfeeding from the realm of self-sacrifice to recover the mother's agency.

In sum, the diverse work collected in *Giving Breastmilk* attests to the potency of the topic of breastfeeding and breastmilk sharing and the moral imaginations of its contributors to give serious attention to women's investment in the health and well-being of others through breastmilk exchange. We trust this will continue, and that your reading of it generates more new thinking.

REFERENCES

Apple, Rima. *Mothers and Medicine: A Social History of Infant Feeding, 1890-1950.* Wisconsin Publications in the History of Science and Medicine, Number 7. Madison: University of Wisconsin Press, 1987.

Bartlett, Alison. *Breastwork: Rethinking Breastfeeding.* Sydney: University of New South Wales Press, 2005.

Bartlett, Alison and Fiona Giles, guest eds. *Australian Feminist Studies* 19.45 (2004): 269-271.

Baumslag, Naomi and Dia L. Michels. *Milk, Money, and Madness: The Culture and Politics of Breastfeeding.* Westport, Conn.: Bergin & Garvey, 1995.

Blum, Linda M. *At the Breast: Ideologies of Breastfeeding and Motherhood in the Contemporary United States.* Boston: Beacon Press, 1999.

Davidson, Deborah, Debra Langan. "The Breastfeeding Incident: Teaching and Learning Through Transgression." *Studies in Higher Education* 31.4 (2006): 439-52.

Fildes, Valerie. *Breasts, Bottles and Babies: a History of Infant Feeding.* Edinburgh: Edinburgh University Press, 1986.

Giles, Fiona. *Fresh Milk: the Secret Life of Breasts.* Sydney: Allen & Unwin, 2003.

Golden, Janet. *A Social History of Wet Nursing in America: From Breast to Bottle.* Cambridge: Cambridge University Press, 2001.

Grosz, Elizabeth. *Space, Bodies and Perversion: Essays on the Politics of Bodies.* Sydney: Allen & Unwin, 1995.

Hausman, Bernice L. *Mothers' Milk: Breastfeeding Controversies in American Culture.* New York: Routledge, 2003.

Minchin, Maureen. *Breastfeeding Matters: What We Need to Know About Infant Feeding.* Alfredton, Vic: Alma Books, 1998.

Noxolo, Pat, Parvati Raghuram, and Clare Madge. "'Geography is Pregnant'

and 'Geography's Milk is Flowing': Metaphors for a Postcolonial Discipline?" *Society and Space* 26.1 (2008): 146-68.
Palmer, Gabrielle. *The Politics of Breastfeeding.* London: Pandora, 1988.
Stuart-Macadam, Patricia and Katherine Dettwyler, eds. *Breastfeeding: Biocultural Perspectives.* New York: Aldine de Gruyter, 1995.
Van Esterik, Penny. *Beyond the Breast-Bottle Controversy.* New Brunswick, NJ: Rutgers University Press, 1989.

I. MAKING MILK

The Breast Pump

CINDY STEARNS

WHILE OFTEN UNACKNOWLEDGED AS such, breastfeeding is time consuming and labor intensive work that only women can perform and it is work that is sometimes perceived by women as demanding and without relief. The breast pump is of obvious potential value to women because it enables mothers to provide breastmilk for their child while being apart from them for a variety of possible reasons. However, the promised benefit of pumping comes with potential costs, including the work of pumping and the symbolic and constructed meanings of performing motherhood with a pump.

Like breastfeeding, pumping breastmilk is a decision that women make in an environment of societal expectations concerning appropriate maternal behavior. Here I describe and analyze in-depth interviews with breastfeeding mothers who reflect on their experiences and feelings concerning their use of the breast pump, the value of breastmilk, and the criteria for good motherhood. In providing the perspectives of breastfeeding mothers, this paper augments philosophical and cultural discussions of the breast pump (Bartlett; Hausman; Kukla) as well as the empirical studies of women's use of the breast pump (Avishai; Blum; Gatrell).

METHODS

In-depth, open-ended interviews were completed with 66 women in Northern California. The interviews were completed in two stages: 51 were interviewed from 1996-1998 (Stearns); and in an effort to explore additional issues and explore themes in more depth, 15 additional women were interviewed from 2005-2006.[1] The interviews were almost always conducted in women's homes and typically lasted between one and two hours. Interviews were tape recorded and transcribed.

A snowball sample was utilized with attention to developing a sample diverse in terms of age, race, sexual orientation, and ability. Strategic contacts were made with the government-subsidized Women, Infants, and Children (WIC) program, mothers' clubs, a teen parenting program, breastfeeding classes, and lactation consultants and all of these contacts recruited participants. The participants ranged in age from 18 to 42. The participants ranged in social class from poor to wealthy. Four mothers characterized themselves as having a disability and receiving disability benefits. Two mothers described themselves as lesbians and the rest as heterosexual (most were married and living with their partner). One interview was conducted in Spanish and all others were in English. The racial demographics reflect the primarily white county where the research was conducted. Eighty-one percent of the sample identified as white/Caucasian, eleven percent identified as Hispanic/Latina, six percent identified as American Indian/Native American, and two percent did not identify their race. In all, the women had breastfed a total of 108 different children. The weaning ages ranged from a few weeks to seven years. Fifty-nine percent (n=39) of the sample reported using a breast pump.

WHY DO WOMEN PUMP?

The existing social science research on breast pumps is limited in quantity and tends to focus primarily on working mothers and the questions of how and why they utilize pumps to facilitate paid employment (Avishai; Blum; Gatrell). Both Avishai and Gatrell interview working women employed as professionals and/or managers about their breastfeeding experiences and find that using the pump to facilitate working outside the home is fraught with difficulty, including worries about leaking breastmilk and/or pumping and storing breastmilk while they are at work. For example, three of Gatrell's sample of twenty mothers in the U.K. "ceased breastfeeding due to anxiety at the prospect of managing their lactating bodies in the workplace" (398). Another three of Gatrell's participants ended breastfeeding within one month of returning to work as a result of their continuing struggles to find private space to breastfeed and store milk in their workplaces. Blum's discussion of pumping is also mostly focused on the workplace, although her analysis is embedded in a wider-ranging exploration of race, class, motherhood and breastfeeding ideologies in the U.S. Blum finds that for working class mothers, the breast pump was a "major, even definitional, part of the experience" of breastfeeding and that using the pump at work was viewed as highly problematic due to workplace constraints and/or unease with lack of privacy in pumping and storing milk (134). None of the working class black women and only a few of the working class white women who "told successful breastfeeding stories were willing to negotiate breastfeeding when they went back to work" (167). Blum notes that the research participant who had the "most positive experience using breast pumps on the job" was a white, working class woman who had "one of the highest status jobs" (135).

In this paper I add to the insights of these empirical studies on pumping by exploring women's ideas about and experiences with pumping both within and outside of the workplace. The women in this study used the pump to accommodate paid employment outside the home as well as for many other reasons. Many women used the pump to enable short time periods away from their child for leisure activities and/or errands. Mothers also utilized a pump to continue producing breastmilk when the physical act of breastfeeding directly to a child was not possible (e.g, poor latch, maternal use of short-term medication, engorgement, maternal surgery, infant illness, etc.), to enable overnight and longer vacations away from their child, to allow their non-nursing partner to gain the experience of feeding the child, to provide a store of milk for emergencies, and/or when they didn't want to breastfeed in public.

The question of why women choose to pump is more complex than the pragmatic criteria outlined above. In several of the above situations, women could avoid pumping and provide prepared infant formula. While a woman who is away from home regularly for extended periods of time could not maintain her milk supply with formula substitutions, many mothers who are gone on an occasional basis could use infant formula and still maintain a breastfeeding relationship and an adequate supply of milk. Some mothers did in fact substitute with occasional bottles of formula, however others were adamant about never providing formula and only allowing their child to have their breastmilk. Given that formula is arguably easier and more convenient for women as compared to the work of pumping, it becomes important to look closely at the social context for idealizing and pursuing exclusive breastfeeding.

In this study, the women who pumped and had a goal of exclusive breastmilk articulate a strong belief in the superior value of their breastmilk as compared to infant formula substitutes. For these women, the troubles of pumping (outlined below) are the price one pays to produce what they valued as the best infant food possible. In line with this thinking, the justification for pumping almost always draws upon a narrative of the superiority of the "natural" milk that only a mother's body can produce. The following are examples of how women invoke the natural in describing the superior value of the breastmilk product that they produce at the pump:

> *For me personally I just feel it's the most natural thing for a mother to do, the most healthy way of, of feeding a child, a baby, a child.* (Jane, white, age 20, WIC recipient, not working)

> *Well, basically I was just convinced that it was the best thing, you know, nutritionally without a doubt and emotionally for the baby and the mom. You know, I think it's just natural and beneficial to the relationship and certainly, you know, the best nutrition for their immune system and all of that.* (Beth, white, age 41, middle class, not working)

> *For me it is just a natural thing to do – to nurse your child and to form attachment. And it's really a wonderful way to form the bonds with your child. It was something that I wanted to do for a long time and I knew that*

> *I would.... It was never a question, for me it was a natural fit.* (laughing) (Melanie, white, age 35, lower middle class, working full-time)

> *Well I just also think that it's such a natural thing, I mean, all animals do it. And to think a baby, I mean, that's what they want to do I would think. I mean in nature, with animals I don't really see the moms walking up to them and trying to stick their breasts into the baby animal's mouth. The animal, the babies know to do that. So somewhere, I mean I would think that a human child would know to do that and to, to not, to not do that, it seems just not, it just goes against nature. I've always been one to try and follow what nature says. I don't know.* (Jill, white, age 31, lower middle class, working part-time)

> *Economics was the first thing. It was the cheapest route to go. It seemed like the natural thing to do. There was never really any question that I wouldn't.* (Francine, age 35, lower class, full-time student)

> *'Cause it's natural and I don't really trust formulas either.* (Maria, white, age 18, WIC recipient, not working)

The natural narrative is consistent in all the women's explanations for pumping. However, the narrative of natural rarely stands alone but is instead buttressed by other reasons for utilizing breastmilk rather than formula, some ideological and some practical. As evidenced in the above quotes, women believe breastmilk is more natural because it is nutritionally superior, emotionally beneficial to the baby and mother, facilitates attachment, and is also innately what female bodies and human infants are "intended" to do given their human instincts and physical bodies. On the practical side, some women described the economic value in breastmilk as its use means that dollars are saved when infant formula does not need to be purchased.[2] A few other women mentioned distrusting and rejecting formula because of its association with the corporate practices of infant formula companies.

The belief in the natural and superior value of breastmilk is created and supported by the medical, public health, and popular assertion that "breast is best" which is now well known. Public health campaigns promoting breastfeeding in the U.S. are widespread and increasing numbers of women are initiating breastfeeding in recent years. In fact, almost all of the women interviewed in the second wave of this study were fairly adamant about the superiority of breastmilk over infant formula. As compared to the women in the first phase, they were more likely to pump and more likely to have a goal of exclusive breastfeeding.

The strong social and cultural value placed on breastmilk and breastfeeding means that breastfeeding is now essential to a woman's performance as a mother. Murphy suggests that by "deciding to formula feed, the woman exposes herself to the charge that she is a 'poor mother' who places her own needs, preferences or convenience over her baby's welfare. By contrast, the 'good mother' is deemed to be one who prioritizes her child's needs even (or perhaps especially) where this entails personal inconvenience or distress" (187-188). Lee's recent study of mothers in Great Britain provides clear evidence of this. She describes women's despair when they can't breastfeed and must turn instead to formula and concludes "(h)ow good a mother a woman is has come to be measured by whether she breastfeeds" (1088).

Women who breastfeed thus can lay claim to "better" or "superior" mothering by providing their "natural" product to their children via pumping. The naming and advertising for breast pumps plays upon this idea of a personalized product that enhances or sustains women's natural product. Popular brands include the Ameda Purely Yours Breast Pump with Backpack and Dr. Brown's Natural Flow Electric Breast Pump. Many of these pumps come with "natural feeding" bottles. Taken together, all of these products, from breastmilk to pumps to backpacks to bottles, are commodities that are created and consumed in support of women's efforts to perform as good mothers and to be seen as good mothers.

THE EXPERIENCE OF PUMPING

Pumping, like breastfeeding, is learned and requires some knowledge and experience for women to perform it correctly and effectively. Expressing milk in itself does not require a pump and two women in the study became skilled at hand expressing their milk, although this was an infrequent rather than routine means of extracting milk. Most women made use of manual or electric pumps.

Some women learned how to use the pump in the hospital when their newborn had difficulty with breastfeeding. These women used hospital-grade electric pumps and had some instruction from hospital staff on how to go about using them. Most women first used a pump after their child was an established nurser. Learning to use a pump for these women involved a more active process of information seeking. Women most often turned to friends, breastfeeding handbooks, lactation consultants, WIC, and La Leche League for information on how to go about pumping.

Mothers expressed a fair amount of frustration with pumping. Pumping was hard to do for some with the quality of the pump often being seen as the reason. Many women wanted better, more expensive pumps than they could afford. For most women, the gold standard of pumping is the double electric model as this pump was believed to provide a lot of milk very quickly compared to other methods. Norma (Latina, age 37, middle class, not working) describes why she chose a more expensive pump:

> *It was the top of the line kind of thing but shoot, you know. I looked at some of the hand pumps and I said this will not work for me. I am not patient.*

> *I just want this to be done, fill up that bottle and she can have it later and that worked out fine actually since she nursed for nine months.*

Not all women could afford to purchase or rent the more expensive pumps and this was a source of dissatisfaction. As one mother noted, "All I have is this crummy, battery-operating thing." Interestingly, women who received benefits from WIC were more likely to have access to these pumps because they were often provided for free to encourage breastfeeding.

Pumping was usually perceived as time consuming and inconvenient. An important component of effective pumping is fitting in the activity along with the direct breastfeeding of a child. Producing milk for storage beyond regular production was often taxing. Women found certain times of day (usually the early morning) produce more milk, but this has to be worked around the baby who may also want to be fed at the same time.

The work involved in pumping meant that some women felt frustrated at the "price" they had to pay to have some time away from their child. Margo, a 21 year old white woman who was not working, describes her feelings about using the pump to gain a little free time for herself:

> *I was so discouraged that this was how I was gonna have more time to myself. I had to sit here while everybody sleeps, to get myself up just to pump in the morning, you know, I could just have that extra hour of sleep.... I was very discouraged.*

A stay-at-home mother describes her work to produce enough to cover her absence for a short vacation:

> *For some reason I don't love pumping. I went to a wedding in San Diego when M (older child) was this age and I had to pump for a month before I left because she was only drinking milk—she was four months—I had to pump for a month to have enough. But it worked and I would rather pump a bottle and go and not have to worry.* (Gail, white, age 35, lower-middle class, not working)

Pumping seems to be a kind of emotional insurance for Gail as upon further questioning she said that she did not think formula would actually harm her child. However, leaving breastmilk rather than formula behind allowed this full-time stay-at-home mother to make a claim to a worry free trip.

Women who worked outside the home had to pump more frequently and had to pump away from the privacy and convenience of home. These women shared many of the same challenges as the 15 middle class, working women studied by Avishai who experienced pumping as "a labor-intensive, time-consuming, challenging, and stressful enterprise" (143). Explicit accommodation (e.g., lactation stations) for pumping was not available to any of the women in the study. A few mothers pumped in the car at lunch. A law professor pumped in her car on the freeway while driving her one hour commute. A first grade teacher locked her classroom door at lunch and pumped and ate her own lunch, noting that she became "stir crazy" not being able to even go to the teacher's lounge.

Pumping at work can be time consuming, inconvenient, exhausting and potentially embarrassing. A mother who worked for a newspaper pumped at the sink in the multi-user bathroom and cringed at the fellow employees who looked at her strangely and described her frustrations:

> *It was very embarrassing and ... difficult to pump because of course when you're pumping you really need to relax otherwise the milk doesn't come and it's like for nothing ... I probably used my whole break pumping, so 30 minutes.* (Sue, white, age 40, middle class, working part-time)

Jill describes working as a stylist in a hair salon and using the back room to pump, causing awkwardness with her male boss:

> *You know the people at work were really good. If I have to go into the back room and pump and, you know, they're very supportive and they give me privacy or, you know, or they're accepting of it. C (her boss) just gets to the point where he just doesn't come in the back room. I mean he's married and he had 2 daughters and his wife has breastfed, 'cause I asked him one day, did N not breastfeed? Oh yeah and I said, you seem so uncomfortable with it. And it's not like I go into the back room and whip my shirt off, I mean I'm very discrete about it because I care about his feelings too and, and I'm not the type of person that just says, well this is a totally natural thing and I'm going to breastfeed my child and I don't care who's around and, I don't feel that way at all, because I know that a lot of people are uncomfortable with it.*

Women who worked outside the home had the most to say about pumping and much of their discourse was complaint. They were unhappy with the lack of privacy in pumping, the lack of down time at work (no breaks or lunches without pumping), the difficulty in being able to relax and produce milk quickly, the loud (and publicly revealing) sound of the pump, and the physical exhaustion.

FROM INTERACTION TO MEASURED COMMODITY

Pumping changes ideas about breastmilk. When placed in a bottle for all to see, breastmilk can be evaluated on a number of dimensions. While breastmilk is often viewed as "liquid gold" it is also a commodity of potential embarrassment. Fiona Dykes describes how women contend with "the dualism between breastmilk being portrayed as natural, pure, and life giving fluid" and also as "akin to other body secretions and as representative of the uncontrolled, chaotic, dangerous and polluting female body" (91). An example of these competing notions is apparent in one woman's description of her own mother's discomfort with handling a just-pumped bottle of breastmilk:

> *When I was back in New Jersey, uh, she (her mother) knew that nutritionally it was the best thing for the baby and she would watch Zee (her son) so I would pump here and there and there was one time I handed her some milk and she was like "Ew it's still warm" and you know, threw it back on the counter and was really grossed out by it, really grossed out by it.* (Chelsea, white, age 27, lower middle class, not working)

Similarly, some mothers described that they were careful to keep expressed milk hidden at work so that nobody would be offended.

Breastmilk also can be evaluated in terms of quantity and this was a common theme. How much milk should a woman produce through pumping? How long should it take her to produce that much? How much milk must she leave behind for her child to be satisfied? As a consequence of pumping, women start to measure their output and view themselves as "suppliers" of a valuable, storable commodity. Their ability to supply, the amount of time it takes them to produce certain amounts of milk all become relevant to their evaluation of their mothering work. Furthermore, women describe themselves as producers in the context of pumping. Their success isn't measured by a satisfied baby but instead by a net weight measured in ounces. As Martha (white, age 37, middle income, not working) describes her worry about feeding her large male baby—"when you are nursing, it is hard to tell. When you are pumping, you know how much you are producing." Sue (white, age 36, lower class) went back to work for three days a week when her daughter was eight weeks old. She describes her low production through pumping and the exhaustion that resulted:

> *It was horrible. I was horrible. And um, she um, but I expressed little, I mean I'd only get, I'd net four ounces, was a lot to get. It was more like 2 ounces at a time and, um she'd go though the day on that little bit of milk and never, and then nurse all night long and all evening. We had a family bed. I think that's why I'm still tired!* (laughing)

Often the mothers who pursued exclusive breastfeeding expressed a strong sense of urgency concerning production and supply so that they could avoid the use of infant formula. Like many mothers, Sue was having trouble pumping enough milk and expressed her anxiety: "that was the thing; I mean I was so nervous about keeping on top of it." Nadia (Native American, age 30, working class, part-time student, part-time school bus driver) describes her efforts to increase production, including going to La Leche League meetings but reported that they didn't help her because she still "couldn't get her milk to come out any faster."

A few mothers were able to produce a lot of milk easily and this was often a source of pride. One woman noted, after a lot of early struggles with production and pumping, that she became an abundant producer and her husband described with pride "you're producing enough milk to feed Ethiopia!"

THE VALUABLE COMMODITY AND THE COMPENSATORY PRODUCER

The goal of exclusive breastfeeding is in fact one that few in this study achieved. Several of these mothers endured a good deal of inconvenience related to the time and physical requirements of pumping. Some of these mothers' work at pumping might be viewed as heroic. However, no matter how much time, energy, and diligence pumping requires, it's an activity that is framed as second best—as a compensation for something better.

Dorothy's story of pumping and breastfeeding is an example of this phenomenon. Dorothy is a 41 year old, white, single mother who had saved enough money through her job as a fire fighter to take a year's leave to be at home with her child. Her daughter was born a week late and by c-section on a Friday in a hospital and they returned home on a Monday. While her daughter had breastfed successfully in the hospital, it became clear to Dorothy that something was not right at home. Her baby was nursing constantly but not swallowing and Dorothy did not sleep for days after returning home. She called friends and then a lactation consultant who determined that the baby "wasn't latching right, she was just gumming, she wasn't sucking, which wasn't stimulating my milk to come in." In order to stimulate her milk, Dorothy was advised to begin a regimen of pumping every two hours followed by feeding. In order to avoid nipple confusion she would feed her daughter with a supplemental feeding system (a system of tubing connecting to a milk source) and using her finger would feed her as much breastmilk as possible.[3] Although she pumped frequently, supply was slow to build up and Dorothy occasionally gave "her formula with finger feeding so she would you know, get something to eat. I felt horrible." Dorothy eventually established mostly direct nursing with her child at about six weeks of age, but in those early weeks of almost no sleep became extremely exhausted and described herself as emotionally traumatized:

> *I mean you just feel like a bad mom. I can't give my child food. I am bad. I am a horrible mother . . . I remember I was just sitting in the rocking chair when it was in this room and bawling, just bawling, pumping and bawling, and looking up and wondering what is the lesson I am supposed to be learning? I don't know what it is. I don't know what my lesson is. I am not getting it.*

Dorothy recounted the details of her struggle to breastfeed as a single mother of her first child, living alone with occasional help from long-distance family, with great emotion and detail. Although Dorothy is a female firefighter in a large city, not an easy career path for a woman who began that work in the early 1990's, she compares her work as a firefighter with pumping and notes "I used to say that going to the fire academy was the most difficult thing I had done in my life, but that was until this."

Dorothy's challenges are more pronounced than most moms, but several others in this study also went to great lengths to pump and provide their child with breastmilk rather than formula. This hard, physical work, like many of the physical challenges of breastfeeding, often goes unnoticed by public health officials and researchers (Kelleher). Despite all of these efforts, mothers typically viewed their mothering through pumping as second best. Dorothy, for example, describes that she never felt like a "normal mom" when she was pumping.

Rebecca Kukla's observation that "pumping and express feeding is positioned by a wide majority of health sources as an inherently marginal and suboptimal feeding practice" is relevant to how the women perceive pumping (160). In women's discussions they often frame pumping and providing breastmilk as being a good effort, but never the best effort. Carol, a white, 30 year old, lower-middle class, stay at home mother, describes a common view in the study and in contemporary conversations about mothers who go back to work but continue to pump:

> *I know there are women who go back to work that are pumping and ... I think breastfeeding is really the best thing and for a woman to go to the trouble of pumping at work I just think, you know, good for you. I mean at least, yeah I think breast is best and it'd be nice for the baby to have your breast but at least you're still very concerned about its nutrition.*

Clearly, the implication in her discussion is that pumped milk is second best but nonetheless the best that a working mother might be able to do. In this sense, pumped breastmilk has intrinsic social value as a signifier of good mothering. It is a compensatory act with significant meaning in the work of mothering. When women can't meet the ideals of intensive mothering described in depth by Sharon Hays, at the least they can provide the product of their nature as mothers.[4] In doing so they can elevate their status as compared to formula-using mothers and come closer to the ideal of the always physically available ideal mother.

MOTHERING THROUGH AND WITH THE PUMP

Barbara Katz Rothman suggests that breastfeeding should be viewed as a process and a relationship rather than a product. She writes breastfeeding "has come to mean the production, transmission, and ingestion of breast*milk.* The focus on the milk, the *product,* changed our understanding of the *process*. Suckling or nursing became breastfeeding, getting the milk made and transported into the baby" (82). For Rothman this is another revealing example of how women's bodies are commodified and breastmilk becomes a product that stands apart from the mother.

In this study it is clear that breastmilk is in fact a commodity with high value in the construction of the good mother. Providing exclusive breastmilk to a child is the gold standard of one of the most promoted and idealized contemporary mothering practices, breastfeeding. The use of the word "exclusive" as the ideal practice of breastfeeding is itself revealing concerning how breastmilk is being constructed as an extremely valuable commodity, as is its popular moniker "liquid gold."

Exclusive breastmilk, like other experiential commodities such as exclusive hotels, restaurants and clubs, is a privileged commodity provided only to those who have the resources to access it. Performing exclusive breastfeeding is, in this sense, a "class" act which signifies to others a superior maternal performance, one that requires a commitment to culturally dominant mothering ideals, a good and expensive breast pump, hard work, and time among other things. Nonetheless, pumping (whether an exclusive or partial food source) is not ideal mothering, and its performance is always secondary to hands-on (or breasts-on!) mothering. Pumping does help along the mothering project, however as it often functions as a means through which women publicly compensate their children for not being present to feed them directly. It is a symbol and a practice used to construct the compensatory mother, who is culturally positioned as at least better than the mother who does not pump at all and far superior to the mother who provides formula.

The School of Social Sciences and the Research, Scholarship, and Creative Activity Program (RSCAP) at Sonoma State University provided important financial support for this project. I am grateful to the participants and my student research assistants (Sandi Davis, Ellen Heimann-Sullivan, Colleen Rodriguez and Alicia Diaz Said) for help with this project.

[1]In terms of the comparability of women's experience in the two stages, breastfeeding rates increased during this time period and the variety and availability of breast pumps seems to have grown alongside that trend. It is possible that more women in the general population were pumping in the second stage of the study compared to when the study first began. However, there is a lack of data on the prevalence of the use of the breast pump in the U.S. today or historically (Labiner-Wolf et al., 2008). Therefore, a more precise understanding of trends in the use of breast pump and how these trends might affect the interpretation of the data discussed here is not possible.

[2]This does not mean, however, that breastmilk is "free" as there is the labor

value of the producer mother, although this is typically not acknowledged.
[3]Finger feeding is the preferred method in the early weeks. Professionals believe that it avoids confusion between mother's nipple and an artificial nipple ("nipple confusion"). The latter requires less work for babies and there is a concern that babies will prefer the bottle and reject the breast if a bottle is offered in the first weeks.
[4]Hays insightfully describes the dominant ideology of intensive mothering in her study of mothers in the U.S. Intensive mothering requires a fully engaged mother who is the primary caretaker and assumes ultimate responsibility for the constant nurturing of her child's optimal physical, social, and emotional development.

REFERENCES

Avishai, Orit. "At the Pump." *Journal of the Association for Research on Mothering* 6 (2004): 139-149.

Bartlett, Alison. *Breastwork: Rethinking Breastfeeding*. Sydney: UNSW Press, 2005.

Blum, Linda M. *At the Breast: Ideologies of Breastfeeding and Mothering in the Contemporary United States*. Boston: Beacon Press, 1999.

Dykes, Fiona. "Resisting the Gaze: The Subversive Nature of Breastfeeding." *Exploring The Dirty Side of Women's Health*. Ed. Mavis Kirkham. New York: Routledge, 2007. 87-100.

Gatrell, Caroline Jane. "Secrets and Lies: Breastfeeding and Professional Work." *Social Science and Medicine* 65 (2007): 393-404.

Hausman, Bernice L. *Mother's Milk: Breastfeeding Controversies in American Culture*. New York: Routledge, 2003.

Hays, Sharon. *The Cultural Contradictions of Motherhood*. New Haven: Yale University Press, 1996.

Kelleher, Christa M. "The Physical Challenges of Early Breastfeeding." *Social Science and Medicine* 63 (2006): 2727-2738.

Kukla, Rebecca. *Mass Hysteria: Medicine, Culture and Mother's Bodies*. Lanham, MD: Rowman and Littlefield, 2005.

Labiner-Wolfe, Judith, Sara Fein, Katherine Shealy and Cunlin Wang. "Prevalence of Breast-Milk Expression and Associated Factors." *Pediatrics* 122 (2008): S63-S68.

Lee, Ellie. "Health, Morality, and Infant Feeding: British Mothers' Experiences of Formula Milk Use in the Early Weeks." *Sociology of Health and Illness* 29 (2007): 1075-1090.

Murphy, Elizabeth. "'Breast is Best': Infant feeding decisions and maternal deviance." *Sociology of Health and Illness* 21 (1999): 187-208.

Rothman, Barbara Katz. "Laboring Now: Current Cultural Constructions of Pregnancy, Birth, and Mothering." *Laboring On: Birth In Transition in the United States*. Ed. Wendy Simons, Barbara Katz Rothman, and Bari Meltzer

Norman. New York: Routledge, 2007.
Stearns, Cindy. "Breastfeeding and the Good Maternal Body." *Gender & Society* 13 (1999): 308-325.
Stearns, Cindy. "The Work of Breastfeeding." *Women's Studies Quarterly*. 37 (2009): 63-80.

The Ideological Work of Infant Feeding

DENISE A. COPELTON, REBECCA MCGEE, ANDREW COCO,
ISIS SHANBAKY AND TIMOTHY RILEY

BREASTFEEDING HAS BECOME A crucial component of the ideology of intensive mothering, with maternalist and medical organizations now widely endorsing it. According to Stephanie Knaak, breastfeeding is both "a medical gold standard for infant feeding and a moral gold standard for mothering" (197). In the United States, La Leche League (LLL) was instrumental in equating good mothering with breastfeeding since the 1950s, and shifting the medical community's belief in the superiority of formula feeding to the view that breast is best (Blum 63). By 1978 the American Academy of Pediatrics (AAP) recommended exclusive breastfeeding for the first four to six months, and today AAP promotes breastfeeding for the first twelve months, with exclusive breastfeeding for the first six (496). All contemporary mothers are expected to *try* to achieve this intensive good mother ideal.

However, according to the National Center for Health Statistics (NCHS), older and more highly educated women are more likely to breastfeed than younger and less educated women. Hispanic mothers are more likely than other racial-ethnic groups to breastfeed and to breastfeed longer (NCHS 158). If breastfeeding is widely endorsed by the medical community, why do so few U.S. mothers breastfeed, and why for such short durations? Clearly, women are not positioned equally to achieve this breastfeeding ideal.

Public health research promotes a positive view of breastfeeding informed by medical "'facts' that women need to be informed about and convinced of" (Wall, 593). They cast breastfeeding in positive terms and construe formula feeding negatively as noncompliance. In a recent survey, Amal K. Mitra, Amal J. Khoury, Agnes W. Hinton and Cathy Carothers (68) measured breastfeeding knowledge based on agreement with statements such as "Breastfeeding develops a strong bond between mother and baby" and "Breastfeeding at night is easier than bottle feeding." Quantitative measures like these presume one correct view of breastfeeding and cannot explore meanings that fall beyond the survey's scope. However, to understand women's infant feeding decisions we answer Peter Conrad's (150-1) call for a patient-centered perspective focused on the meanings of medical recommendations in people's everyday lives. We also follow Cindy Stearns in the previous chapter of this volume to ask: what *meanings* do mothers attribute to their infant feeding practices?

In her examination of the ideology of intensive mothering, Sharon Hays compares the experiences of working and stay-at-home mothers. The "mommy wars" pits stay-at-home moms against working supermoms. Supermoms are derided for not engaging in full-time mothering, while stay-at-home moms are derided for not having careers and failing to contribute to society in culturally recognized ways (i.e., through *paid* work).[1] A recent addition to these "mommy wars" is the competing cultural images of breastfeeding and formula feeding mothers. Bolstered by medical ideologies espoused by health professionals, and maternalist ideologies supported by LLL, the belief that breast is best sometimes positions breastfeeding mothers against formula feeding ones (Blum 85-90). For example, a recent U.S. public service campaign emphasized that "Babies were born to be breastfed" (USDHHS), and a feminist economist recently declared that "artificial feeding is the tobacco of the twenty-first century" (Smith 377). Such pronouncements of the naturalness and unassailable health benefits of breastfeeding depict formula feeding mothers as both unnatural and an imminent threat to infant health. How, then, do mothers respond to the breast is best mantra?

Elizabeth Murphy examined women's anticipatory and retrospective accounts of infant feeding decisions, arguing that such decisions are morally charged ("Breast" 187-8). Following from C. Wright Mills' (906) work on "vocabularies of motive," Murphy investigated pregnant women's motive talk as an "interactional strategy" that permitted women to view breastfeeding as optimal, and yet deviate from the mandate to breastfeed ("Anticipatory" 130). Virginia Schmied and Deborah Lupton found that although many women subscribe to the breast is best ideology, their experiences of infant feeding differ and those who view breastfeeding as promoting mother-infant bonding may feel guilty if their experiences fall short of the ideal (246). Christa Kelleher found that often mothers were surprised by the negative physical aspects of early breastfeeding, including sore nipples, mastitis, and leaking, which caused some women to cease breastfeeding or supplement with formula (2730-35).

We found that mothers engage in ideological work to cope with the disjuncture between the dominant cultural logic that breast is best and women's own varied beliefs and experiences of infant feeding. This entails "select[ing] among the cultural logics at their disposal in order to develop some correspondence between what they believe and what they actually do" (Hays 133). For example, Hays found that stay-at-home and supermoms generate a list of reasons why staying home or working makes them better mothers. Central to both groups' narratives is the belief that good mothering is child-centered, expert-guided, labor-intensive and financially expensive—in short, that good mothering is necessarily intensive: "[r]ather than taking divergent paths, as one might expect, *both* groups attempt to resolve their feelings of inadequacy by returning to the logic of the ideology of intensive mothering" (Hays 134).

Like Hays, we found that the *meanings* of breastfeeding and formula feeding are similar for women engaging in both. Both formula feeding and breastfeeding participants affirmed the maternalist and medical ideologies that point to four key advantages of breastfeeding: health benefits, convenience, financial advantages, and promotion of mother-infant bonding. However, formula feeding mothers also challenged these ideologies by attributing these characteristics to the act of infant feeding generally. Both breastfeeding and formula feeding mothers highlighted the health benefits of their chosen method, emphasized its convenience, maintained that their method was economical, and insisted that it promoted parent-infant bonding. We show that the ideological work of infant feeding enables women to support the cultural logic that breast is best, despite some women's choice to formula feed.

METHODS

We conducted four focus groups with pregnant women, first-time mothers, and women with children from prior pregnancies. All participants had either given birth within the past year or were expecting to do so within three months. Two focus groups were comprised of formula feeding mothers and two of breastfeeding mothers, totaling 15 and 13 women respectively. According to Pam Carter (73), because many women combine formula and breastfeeding, the distinction between these two groups masks the tremendous overlap between them. Thus, we allowed participants to classify themselves as formula feeding or breastfeeding mothers based on their current or intended (for pregnant participants) feeding method. Our resulting sample of 28 women consisted of 16 Latinas, ten whites, one Asian and one Egyptian. Respondents ranged from 18 to 33 years old, and varied by marital status, educational attainment, and employment. Mothers were recruited by prenatal care nurses with whom they had previous contact and good rapport. To ensure confidentiality, we use pseudonyms for all participants. As an incentive to participate, women were given $25 gift certificates redeemable at a local mall, offered free child care during the focus group session, and given taxi vouchers.

All participants were receiving prenatal and obstetrical care from the Family Health Service at Lancaster General Hospital in Lancaster, Pennsylvania and participating in Healthy Beginnings Plus (HBP), a state-funded program offering prenatal and postpartum services to low-income women eligible for Medicaid. Women with family incomes up to 185 percent of federal poverty guidelines are eligible for HBP, which aims to meet women's medical and psychosocial needs by providing specialized courses on childbirth, exercise, smoking-cessation, nutrition, parenting, and breastfeeding. Participants are assigned a physician who provides complete prenatal, delivery, and infant care; a nurse coordinator who offers a variety of counseling and educational programs; and a counselor who assists with transportation, housing, and other needs during pregnancy and postpartum.

The HBP program director, a non-Hispanic white, and another staff member who was African American, both registered nurses trained in focus group facilitation, conducted the focus groups between April and June 2005 in English at the HBP clinic. Moderators followed a semi-structured interview guide, with questions on participants' intentions and experiences of, attitudes toward, and assessments of the advantages and disadvantages of breastfeeding and formula feeding. Because focus groups are "social spaces in which participants construct the 'patient's view' by sharing, acquiring, and contesting knowledge" (Lehoux, Poland, and Daudelin 2092), moderators encouraged dialogue among participants. Since peer influence and support are important determinants of women's infant feeding practices, the group nature of the interviews encouraged participation and contributed to the ease with which most respondents discussed their experiences. Group rapport was evident by participants' light-hearted banter and high participation levels. Consensus was evident by participants' frequent nods and verbal agreement, and when these were absent, moderators attempted to assess agreement by soliciting divergent opinions.[2]

Focus groups were videotaped and transcribed. We analyzed the transcripts using the inductive approach described by Anselm Strauss and Juliet Corbin, coding key themes as they emerged. Consistent with the collectivist orientation of focus group research and the methods of analysis described by David Morgen, we based our results on collective sentiments shared within the group.

FINDINGS

Because breastfeeding is now a pivotal element in intensive mothering, breastfeeding and formula feeding mothers engage in ideological work to construct their infant feeding method as logical and optimal. Contrary to public health research, which assumes that formula feeding mothers lack sufficient knowledge about the benefits of breastfeeding, we found like Annette Beasley in this volume that formula feeding mothers actively engage the breast is best discourse promulgated in medical and maternalist ideologies.

ENGAGING THE BREAST IS BEST DISCOURSE

Both breastfeeding and formula feeding women were aware of the four benefits of breastfeeding as previously mentioned: health benefits, convenience, financial or economical benefits, and ability to promote bonding. Breastfeeding mothers cited these as significant factors in their decision to breastfeed. Hasina summarized her reasons for breastfeeding, which include three of the four frequently touted benefits of breastfeeding:

> *I think maybe because it's the most natural thing to do. It's good for you, good for your baby ... It doesn't cost anything. It's always ready. You don't have to have a bunch of bottles.*

While not completely discounting these benefits, formula feeding mothers viewed these as deriving from *the process* of infant feeding rather than the method. They maintained that formula feeding had its own health benefits, was easier and more convenient than breastfeeding, was economical, and promoted mother-infant *and* father-infant bonding. Formula feeding mothers offered rejoinders to the breast is best mantra which questioned the advantages of breastfeeding, but nevertheless affirmed the four key qualities used to support it.

THE HEALTH BENEFITS OF BREASTFEEDING

Health and well-being were central themes in women's infant feeding narratives. Both breastfeeding and formula feeding groups noted that breastfeeding is considered the healthier option. For example, the first breastfeeding group underscored the health benefits of breastfeeding:

> Mercedes: *I have noticed that they don't lose no weight at all, because she didn't lose anything and she's so strong that I don't believe it. Like she pushes herself and she's already doing stuff that I have seen some other babies at older ages are starting to do, and it's just amazing.*
>
> Marisol: *Yeah, she actually lifted half of her body and then she went back down.*
>
> Gabriella: *Yeah, I saw her.... And actually when I was pregnant, I was reading a lot of magazines and stuff. I used to get* American Baby, *and I was reading that if you breastfeed, the kid's brain starts developing earlier and everything. And I noticed that with my daughter because she started walking at the age of nine months and started crawling when she was like six months. And she's a very smart baby.... So that's mostly what encouraged me besides my mother-in-law, was the magazine that I was reading while I was pregnant.*

Women in the breastfeeding groups offered personal accounts attesting to the health benefits of breastfeeding. Breastfeeding mothers cited numerous sources of support for their decision, including women's and baby magazines, friends and family members, teachers, social workers, physicians, nurses, and other health care workers (see also Copelton 142-45). Hasina remarked:

> *My friend, she's a nurse at the women and babies hospital, and she said that babies who breastfeed during the first year, they say that's good, because their brain development and such.*

Clearly, as Marisol noted: "It is out that breastfeeding's good." Women hear this repeatedly from a variety of sources.

The formula feeding focus groups also discussed the health benefits of breastfeeding. Teresa noted: "I heard breastfeeding is just way more healthy for them ... it would be better for them." Teresa's tone is almost apologetic, and she implies that breastfeeding *would be better*, if she had adopted it. Yet, formula feeding mothers also were quick to mention drawbacks of breastfeeding:

> Isabella: *My cousin, she just had a baby and she breastfeeds it, but the baby grows too quick when you're breastfeeding. They don't, they don't look like a baby. They grow too big and too fat too quick.*
>
> Teresa: *It's healthy, that's why. It's healthier.*

While Isabella and other formula feeding women affirmed the health benefits of breastfeeding, they also emphasized certain consequences as negative—the infant grows too fast and no longer resembles a baby. By constructing these as drawbacks rather than proof of health benefits, formula-feeding mothers reduced the cognitive dissonance created by engaging in formula feeding while simultaneously viewing breastfeeding as the healthier option.

The second formula feeding group acknowledged a danger of bottle-feeding:

> Teresa: *I know that people say it's bad, propping the bottles up in bed. I heard that's not good and a lot of people do it. That's one thing that I know is not good at all, but yet they could throw up, spit up and choke.*
>
> Arlene: *They can get ear infections.*
>
> Isabella: *What you mean, prop the bottle?*
>
> Teresa: *They prop the bottle ... just leave their baby lying there ... and they can suck air up.*

The group narratives differed somewhat between the first and second formula feeding groups. Whereas the second group highlighted the health risks of propping bottles, the second highlighted what they viewed as health benefits of bottle feeding. They believed that being able to strategically position the baby during bottle feeding helps to *prevent* ear infections.

> Karen: *I'm a control freak so for me [formula feeding] allowed me to control the position which I think played a part in preventing ear infections.*
>
> Moderator: *Can you talk more about that, what you meant by control?*
>
> Karen: *Yeah. As opposed to my baby's down here [feeding at my breast], and there are different positions to breastfeeding. You know, their tubes*

are tilted the way ours are so a lot of the fluid gets in there and it causes more ear infections as opposed to bottle feeding, you can adjust the position and have them in a more semi-upright position. And I found that after the switch [to formula feeding], she had less ear infections. It made a big difference in my book.

Part of Karen's rationale for continued bottle feeding includes her perception that her daughter suffered fewer ear infections compared to when she breastfed her. In turning the health benefits of breastfeeding into disadvantages or by disavowing the documented health benefits, formula feeding mothers relied on personal experience to support and counter the health rationale for breastfeeding. Importantly, formula feeders do not entirely discount the health benefits of breastfeeding. They are supportive, but they view the health "benefits" of breastfeeding as highly contextual.

BREASTFEEDING AS CONVENIENT

Convenience was a common theme in the breastfeeding focus groups, with multiple participants in both breastfeeding groups highlighting the ease of night feedings:

Hasina: *It's always ready. You don't have to have a bunch of bottles to mess with.*

Gabriella: *Yeah, you're sleepy, just can--*

Mercedes: *Even when you're lying down, you can just rest … in the bed and … say there you go.*

Hasina: *And it's always at the right temperature. It's just everything together.*

Mercedes: *For me it's more convenient, the breastfeeding, especially at night time, than the bottle, because she's asleep. She's sleeping with me right now and it's like right there. I don't have to actually get off the bed because I will just do it right there. And it's so easy.*

When asked to name the best part of breastfeeding, Rosaria explained,

Carrying less bottles. You just get up and go. You have the milk every time, right there and then.

Breastfeeding mothers stressed not having to clean or warm bottles day or night as breastfeeding's main convenience. Breastfeeding women viewed the time required to prepare formula for each feeding as an extra burden rendered unnecessary through breastfeeding.

Formula feeding groups also recognized the potential convenience of breastfeeding, especially at night:

> Marta: *You don't have to get up in the middle of the night. You just [motions as if uncovering breast] shesh [everyone laughs].*

Yet, there was disagreement about which infant feeding method was most convenient. Unlike breastfeeding groups, which depicted breastfeeding as more convenient, formula feeding groups expressed greater diversity of opinion. The convenience of breastfeeding was something they "read about" or "heard about," though many were skeptical. Frequently, their own experiences or those of friends and family members belied the supposed ease of breastfeeding, and, at times, formula feeding offered its own distinct conveniences:

> Benita: *Bottle feeding is much easier. You have more time, like while the baby's drinking the bottle, you can do other things and still keep an eye on them.*

> Michelle: *That's what I've been confused about because some people say breastfeeding is easier and I found it hard to understand when people think that. Stay-at-home moms maybe it'd be more convenient [to breastfeed], you didn't have to make a bottle in the middle of the night, but I found it more convenient [to formula feed].*

Often formula feeding mothers tied the convenience of formula feeding to the difficulty of breastfeeding at work or school:

> Isabella: *I had my son when I was young so I had to go to school. So, I mean, it was hard even like to pump. So it was easier just to give him the formula and that's it.*

Karen agreed that formula feeding was more convenient, but discounted the role of work:

> *[Working] didn't play the biggest part because I know working mothers that do breastfeed ... they can juggle both, and if you want to do it you can.*

Clearly, there was disagreement about the relative ease of breastfeeding for working women.

Michelle attempted breastfeeding in the hospital with her first child but intended to formula feed her second. Breastfeeding was "more time consuming" because of the difficulty of getting the baby to latch on and the slow rate of milk production. She construed the extra time (relative to formula feeding) necessary to breastfeed to be an additional burden that formula feeding rendered unnecessary:

> Michelle: *I just think I underestimated it, thought it was going to be easier ... and I wasn't producing a lot of milk ... and ... became kinda leery about it ... I realized going to work and school that it was easier to do the bottle feeding. And with this one, now that I have a four-year-old, I think I'm ultimately going to take the route of bottle feeding.*

As HBP clients, most of our participants had sustained contact throughout their pregnancy with nurses, social workers, and lactation consultants who stressed the importance and ease of breastfeeding. This persuaded some women that breastfeeding was the healthier and more convenient choice. Ironically, these pro-breastfeeding contacts made some mothers less likely to breastfeed because they "underestimated" the physical difficulties they might encounter.

Other women remarked similarly that the time necessary to breastfeed was simply too precious given other pressing parenting duties.

> Arlene: *It takes a while to get it started, and I had a three-year-old so I was too busy [to continue breastfeeding].*

> Anne: *If you have like another kid to take care of and you're real busy, you can still do what you have to do and [bottle]feed at the same time. You don't have to sit down and like take that time to [breastfeed].*

In these instances, bottlefeeding, not breastfeeding, became a time-saving convenience.

BREASTFEEDING AS ECONOMICAL

Both breastfeeding and formula-feeding women complained about the cost of formula. Breastfeeding mothers were especially likely to underscore the low cost of breastfeeding as a significant motivator.

> Soledad: *It's way cheaper!*

> Rosaria: *You spend less money. It's way cheaper!*

Implicit in breastfeeding mothers' narratives is a cost comparison with formula feeding. While both groups agreed that breastfeeding is more economical, the financial equation is complex. Because all participants were eligible for Medicaid, they also typically qualified for the Special Supplemental Nutrition Program for Women, Infants, and Children (WIC), which provides vouchers which can be used to purchase formula and other approved foods. The formula available depends on which manufacturer has an exclusive contract with the issuing state. Because this may not be a mother's preferred brand, some purchase additional formula, which they mix with the free formula. In addition, the amount of formula women receive can be insufficient, so those who choose formula feeding must often supplement the free formula:

> Victoria: *Formula is pretty expensive.*
>
> Others: *Yeah.*
>
> Moderator: *Did WIC help with formula?*
>
> Victoria: *They don't give you enough.*
>
> Others: *Yeah.*
>
> Anne: *They never gave us enough, so we just went out and bought a really good canned milk that didn't last us two weeks.*
>
> Teresa: *WIC did help though because those cans were very, like four dollars, five dollars, so what they help you with—say you had to buy like at least five or six cans until they give you more. So it is a really big help ... You get what you get. It was better than buying it all by yourself.*

While breastfeeding women compared the high retail cost of formula with the low or no cost of breastfeeding, formula feeding women compared the relatively low cost of discounted formula through WIC with the high retail price of formula. Although women self-identified as breastfeeding or formula feeding mothers at the onset of the study, some breastfeeding mothers revealed that they combined breastfeeding with formula feeding. Therefore, breastfeeding was not necessarily zero cost, as women often supplemented breastmilk with formula when milk production was low, when women became ill, or when work or school schedules prevented them from breastfeeding.

BREASTFEEDING AND BONDING

Both breastfeeding and formula feeding mothers were aware of breastfeeding's bonding potential, and breastfeeding mothers affirmed this.

> Alejandra: *When you breast feed a baby, they get closer to you. They look at you all the time when you're breastfeeding. Not like with the bottle, sometimes they just move their head, but when they breastfeed, they just look at you, so you get closer to the baby.*

When asked to discuss what they viewed as the best part of breastfeeding, breastfeeding mothers repeatedly emphasized the one-on-one time with their infant and the closeness this facilitated.

Marisol: *The best thing for me is having her in my arms and seeing her eye contact with me and laughing and connecting with her laugh and smile.*

Hasina: *And to feel her warm heat right next to you there is nothing like it.*

Marisol: *And it's like when they also hold you, it's like…amazing.*

Mercedes: *Yeah.*

Bridgette: *It's something you can do that nobody else, nobody else can do. [Others agree.]*

Breastfeeding mothers' narratives reflect those found in popular discourses that attribute the close bond with an infant to the skin-on-skin contact, body heat, and eye contact of breastfeeding.

Interestingly, formula feeding mothers also highlighted the close bonds they felt with their infants, but attributed these to their own feeding method:

Isabella: *You get more of a bond with them too because you're looking at them face to face constantly.*

Teresa: *The baby gets food and the baby is warm and they get to know your voice better, your face better, they sleep better and everything.*

These comments about formula feeding are remarkably similar to the sentiments expressed by breastfeeding mothers, including body heat and eye contact. Yet, formula feeding groups were aware that these qualities were usually attributed to breastfeeding:

Isabella: *When you breastfeed, they got you. That's what my cousin says. Your heat works at night, your smell, you know, it makes them closer to you, you know?*

Teresa: *Yeah, being together. They know your touch.*

Camelia: *But I know a lot of people that's bottle feeding their baby and they're always with their baby and there's still a bond. You're still going to feel your baby, because it's like they're always crying or they're always touching everything and you've gotta hold them all the time constantly so they're going to have your smell, they're going to hear your voice every day.*

Formula feeding women do not dispute that breastfeeding can promote bonding, but they do dispute that breastfeeding is the *only* way to do so. Instead, they view the process of infant feeding as conveying this benefit—one that both mothers and partners should enjoy equally.

> Carole: *Well, her dad could play a part in it [formula feeding] as well; they had time to bond during that time as well.*

> Karen: *It allowed the father to participate more and bond more.*

Nevertheless, in both formula feeding groups, a counter narrative emerged that centered on the *strain* that unsuccessful breastfeeding can put on mother-child relations.

> Karen: *I tried [breastfeeding] with my son five years ago for about a year and it was more of a stressful time than a bonding time … it just put stress on me 'cause I felt like I wasn't doing a good job with my child because I didn't nurse him, you know … I just thought that breastfeeding the first time around was supposed to be a good experience, but I didn't have that. It felt like it strained the relationship with the baby.*

> Michelle: *I agree with her too. Like I was thinking breastfeeding was going to be like this complete mother/child bonding thing and it was going to be so easy and it wasn't anything like that, and I had a lot of help at the hospital, and it still was frustrating and I felt like being the only one providing any love. I felt me getting frustrated over something like that was not really right so I just wanted to feed her.*

For these women, the actual experience of breastfeeding did not live up to their expectations. Encouraged to view breastfeeding as natural, easy, and convenient, intense frustration ensued when their experiences did not match the ideal. As Michelle notes, merely feeding her baby then became more important than bonding with her.

Women in all the focus groups, both breastfeeding and bottle feeding, complained about the physical aspects of breastfeeding, which some felt impeded mother-infant bonding. They highlighted physical problems such as mastitis, and sore and cracked nipples, but also what several women construed as normal pain.

> Mercedes: *It hurts sometimes because they are so tender…. The first week for me was pretty, um, painful because my nipples were really sore.*

> Thanh: *I've tried to breast feed him for two weeks … and it was like horrible because I was bleeding.*

Belinda: *I gave breast feeding a try, did it for about a month, but it was painful, very painful, you know ... and neither one of us enjoyed having that experience.... There was no fun in that.*

Clearly, some women's experiences of breastfeeding were more difficult and painful than others. Those who experienced difficulties were more likely than those who had an easier time to feel that breastfeeding hindered mother-infant bonding.

CONCLUSION

Breastfeeding and formula feeding mothers draw on the same cultural logic that breast is best when discussing their infant feeding beliefs and practices. The formula feeding mothers in our sample, both white and Hispanic alike, were well-versed in the breast is best discourse and agreed with the medical and maternalist ideologies underpinning it. That formula feeding mothers actively engage the breast is best discourse demonstrates that the personal choice to formula feed is not due to lack of knowledge of the benefits of breastfeeding. Rather, their narratives point to the importance of the social and contextual nature of breastfeeding that is often overlooked in public health research. While they generally agreed with breastfeeding mothers that infant feeding should be healthy, easy, economical, and promote bonding, they maintain that these characteristics apply equally to formula feeding and therefore are not limited to breastfeeding. In drawing on the same sets of issues as breastfeeding mothers, formula feeding mothers engage in ideological work, work to construct their chosen infant feeding method as logical and optimal. These findings point to a similar cultural logic employed by both formula and breastfeeding mothers that is ultimately supportive of breastfeeding despite some women's choice to formula feed.

This research contributes to the sociological and health literatures on the meaning of infant feeding in women's everyday lives. By using qualitative methods to explore working class mothers' infant feeding beliefs and practices, we fill a gap in the existing literature which tends to use quantitative methods to examine more privileged socioeconomic groups. Our findings demonstrate the utility of Murphy's insights regarding the interactional work of infant feeding for understanding U.S. working class women's experiences. Both Murphy's work and our own point similarly to the significance of the ideological and interactional work involved in women's decision-making processes. Finally, like Kelleher's work on early infant feeding, we found that some mothers underestimated the work and time involved in breastfeeding, and were surprised by physical difficulties, which had negative consequences for mother-infant bonding and ultimately for the continuation of breastfeeding.

[1]Feminist scholars argue that mothering is, in fact, socially important work;

yet, the fact that mothering is not paid means that it is often not recognized as work, especially in capitalist societies that equate social value with monetary value. See Waring, *Counting for Nothing*.

[2]See Lehoux, Poland, and Daudelin (2006), Kitzinger (1994), and Morgen (1997) for a discussion of focus group methodology. See Madriz (1998, 2000) for a discussion of the benefits of using focus groups with diverse groups of women.

REFERENCES

American Academy of Pediatrics. Section on Breastfeeding. "Breastfeeding and the Use of Human Milk." *Pediatrics* 115.2 (2005): 496-506.

Blum, Linda. *At the Breast: Ideologies of Breastfeeding and Motherhood in the Contemporary United States.* Boston: Beacon Press, 1999.

Carter, Pam. *Feminism, Breasts, and Breast-Feeding*. London: Macmillan, 1995.

Conrad, Peter. "The Meaning of Medications: Another Look at Compliance." *The Sociology of Health and Illness (7th ed.)*. Ed. Peter Conrad. New York: Worth, 2005. 150-162.

Copelton, Denise. "Pregnancy by the Book: Women's Accommodation and Resistance to Medicalized Pregnancy Practices." Diss. Binghamton University, 2003.

Hays, Sharon. *The Cultural Contradictions of Motherhood*. New Haven, CT: Yale University Press, 1996.

Kelleher, Christa. "The Physical Challenges of Early Breastfeeding." *Social Science & Medicine* 63 (2006): 2727-2738.

Kitzinger, J. "The Methodology of Focus Groups: The Importance of Interaction Among Participants." *Sociology of Health and Illness* 16 (1994): 103-121.

Knaak, Stephanie. "Breast-feeding, Bottle-feeding and Dr. Spock: The Shifting Context of Choice." *Canadian Review of Sociology and Anthropology* 42 (2005): 197-216.

Lehoux, Pascale, Blake Poland, and Genevieve Daudelin. "Focus Group Research and 'the Patient's View'." *Social Science & Medicine* 63 (2006): 2091-2104.

Madriz, Esther. "Using Focus Groups with Lower Socioeconomic Status Latina Women." *Qualitative Inquiry* 4 (1998): 114-128.

Madriz, Esther. "Focus Groups in Feminist Research." *Handbook of Qualitative Research*. Ed. Norman Denzin and Yvonna Lincoln. Thousand Oaks, CA: Sage, 2000. 835-850.

Mills, C. Wright. "Situated Actions and Vocabularies of Motive." *American Sociological Review* 5.6 (1940): 904-913.

Mitra, Amal K., Amal J. Khoury, Agnes W. Hinton & Cathy Carothers. "Predictors of Breastfeeding Intention Among Low-Income Women." *Maternal and Child Health Journal* 8.2 (2004): 65-70.

Morgen, David. *Focus Groups as Qualitative Research.* 2nd ed. Thousand Oaks, CA: Sage, 1997.

Murphy, Elizabeth. "Anticipatory Accounts." *Symbolic Interaction* 27.2 (2004): 129-154.

Murphy, Elizabeth. "'Breast is Best': Infant Feeding Decisions and Maternal Deviance." *Sociology of Health & Illness* 21.2 (1999): 187-208.

National Center for Health Statistics. 2007. *Health, United States, 2007, With Chartbook on Trends in the Health of Americans.* Hyattsville, MD. Available <http://www.cdc.gov/nchs/data/hus/hus07.pdf>. Accessed 2 March 2008.

Schmied, Virginia and Deborah Lupton. "Blurring the Boundaries: Breastfeeding and Maternal Subjectivity." *Sociology of Health & Illness* 23.2 (2001): 234-250.

Smith, Julie. "Mothers' Milk and Markets." *Australian Feminist Studies*, 19.45 (2004): 369-379.

Strauss, Anselm, and Juliet Corbin. *Basics of Qualitative Research.* 3rd ed. Thousand Oaks, CA: 1998.

United States Department of Health and Human Services. "National Breastfeeding Awareness Campaign—Babies were Born to be Breastfed." <http://www.4woman.gov/Breastfeeding/index.cfm?page=Campaign>. Accessed June 16, 2006.

Wall, Glenda. "Moral Constructions of Motherhood in Breastfeeding Discourse." *Gender & Society* 15.4 (2001): 592-610.

Waring, Marilyn. *Counting for Nothing: What Men Value and What Women are Worth.* Toronto: University of Toronto Press, 1999.

"Breast is Best" and Other Messages of Breastfeeding Promotion

ANNETTE BEASLEY

> ...Contemporary societies are subject to great influence from scientific medicine ... warnings about health risks have become common events. People are constantly urged to conduct their everyday lives in order to avoid potential disease or early death. (Lupton 100-101)

IN AN ERA OF evidenced-based strategies of health promotion, the message that "breast is best" dominates public health campaigns designed to encourage women to breastfeed (Shaw 99; Smith 371). Driving such campaigns is the promotion of the scientifically-established health benefits of breastfeeding for infants and their mothers. Generally disregarded by the message that "breast is best" are acknowledgement of breastfeeding behaviours and a mother's decision of whether or not to establish and continue breastfeeding as mediated by social and cultural factors (Van Esterik 146-52; Dettwyler 168; Hausman 277). My interest in messages of breastfeeding promotion arises from earlier research on the experience of breastfeeding among New Zealand women (Beasley), as well as recent involvement as a social researcher in the development of a national strategy to improve breastfeeding rates in this country.[1] Reflecting this interest, this chapter explores the range and orientation of messages on breastfeeding practice, support and promotion conveyed to New Zealand midwives through their professional journals. As trained health professionals, New Zealand midwives are orientated to evidence-based models of best practice, but also adopt a woman-centred model of professional practice founded on the principles of partnership (New Zealand College of Midwives 2007).[2]

BACKGROUND

The development of safe, commercially produced artificial milk precipitated a decline in the rates of breastfeeding throughout much of the industrialised world during the twentieth century (Fildes 101-126). Persuaded by the advantages of the new "scientific" feeding, many "parents followed trustingly where scientific and medical advisors seemed to lead," and opted either to wean early, or not to breastfeed their infants (Minchin 211). In New Zealand, a progressive decline "in the incidence of breast-feeding, with a corresponding increase in artificial feeding" was recorded between 1939 and 1952 (Deem and McGeorge 539). Although a steady increase in the rate of breastfeeding initiation was noted from the mid 1970s onwards, the rates at three and six months continue to fall away sharply (Essex 355-57; NBACNZ 22-23).

By the late 1970s, marketing tactics of the infant formula manufacturers among the world's poorest nations fell under international spotlight. The high infant mortality rate associated with declining breastfeeding rates drew attention to the need to protect at-risk infants from improper use of breastmilk substitutes. Recognition of the adverse impact of artificial feeding on infants of the developing world and concern that the "rates and duration of breastfeeding have historically been lower than ideal" in the industrialised world (Ministry of Health, *The Code in New Zealand* 1), mobilised a succession of international strategies designed to promote and protect breastfeeding. In 1981, the World Health Organisation (WHO) and the United Nations Children's Fund (UNICEF) jointly convened an international meeting to address the issue. A significant outcome was the formulation the International Code of Marketing of Breastmilk Substitutes (The Code). The Code aimed "to contribute to the provision of safe and adequate nutrition for infants" through the protection and promotion of breastfeeding, and "proper use of breast-milk substitutes, when these are necessary" (WHO, *International Code* 8). Member States of the United Nations were urged to implement and monitor compliance in accordance with the principles and aim of The Code.

PUBLIC HEALTH STRATEGIES OF BREASTFEEDING PROMOTION

The language of The Code signalled a new approach to the promotion of breastfeeding, later consolidated through adoption of the Baby Friendly Hospital Initiative (BFHI), (WHO/UNICEF, *Baby Friendly*); Innocenti Declaration (UNICEF); and Global Strategy on Infant and Young Child Feeding (WHO/UNICEF, *Global Strategy*). The Code encouraged governments and health authorities to foster a breastfeeding culture and to provide information and educational materials that clearly identify "the benefits and superiority of breastfeeding" (WHO, *International Code* 10). Member nations were also urged to alert medical professionals and lay populations to "the health hazards of inappropriate foods or feeding methods; and ... unnecessary or improper use of infant formula and other breastmilk substitutes" (10).

Embedded in The Code is the language of risk and benefits, which when applied to the promotion of infant health forged a new discourse on infant feeding. Firmly repositioned within a public health discourse, the promotion of breastfeeding delivers the message that "breast is best." Confronted by a plethora of scientific evidence on the benefits of breastfeeding, mothers are bombarded with information such as: "Breast-milk provides an ideal and natural food for the first months of life" (Aycicek et al. 616). Breastmilk protects infants "from a wide array of illnesses and infections," and "reduces health costs" (Westdahl and Page-Goertz 8). Breastmilk "immunizes" the infant against common infections (Ahmed, Parveen and Island 37), and protects against diarrhoea (Morrow et al 297), and so on.

STRATEGIES OF BREASTFEEDING PROMOTION

Since the mid-1990s, a number of strategies designed to increase the national rates of breastfeeding and duration have been developed within New Zealand. Reflecting international trends, these initiatives are informed by the recognition that increased breastfeeding rates will "contribute positively" to infant and maternal health (particularly, among Maori and Pacific women) through reducing the risk of obesity, and the incidence and impact of cancer, cardiovascular disease and diabetes (Ministry of Health, *A Guide to Action* iii). In line with WHO recommendations, the current goal is to "increase the proportion of infants being exclusively breastfed to six months and the proportion of infants partially breastfed beyond 6 months" (Ministry of Health, "Comprehensive Plan"). Although the impact of social, cultural and economic factors on the decision to initiate and continue breastfeeding are acknowledged, and some policies have been implemented to address specific barriers to breastfeeding, responsibility for the promotion of breastfeeding continues to be regarded as primarily belonging to health promotion.

Generally overlooked by strategies that emphasise the health benefits of breastfeeding are consideration of the mother's personal circumstances and the influence of her socially and culturally informed attitudes and beliefs about infant feeding. A call for a broader approach to breastfeeding promotion is made by Joan Wolf in response to the recent National Breastfeeding Awareness Campaign (NBAC) run in the United States of America. The focus of this campaign on the health risks of not breastfeeding were hard hitting. For example, a series of television advertisements portrayed pregnant women engaged in strenuous sports such as mechanical bull riding. Accompanying each advertisement was the voice-over comment: "You'd never take risks while you're pregnant. Why start when the baby's born?" (597).

Wolf criticises the NBAC for paying "insufficient attention to the psychological, socioeconomic, and political concerns of its intended audience" (595). Reiterating the stance of Penny Van Esterik (146-52), Katherine Dettwyler (168) and Bernice Hausman (277), Wolf points out that breastfeeding holds very different meanings for women from different ethnic and socio-economic backgrounds. Wolf cites the example of Black American women, noting many experience lack of employment security, inappropriate or absent workplace feeding spaces and time flexibility as barriers to breastfeeding. She also draws attention to the legacy of "slavery and race hatred ... marked by forced wet-nursing of white women's children—often to the detriment of their own children" as an additional barrier not easily displaced by messages of health risk (621-22).

Similar criticisms have been levelled at breastfeeding promotional strategies in New Zealand. A recent notable example involved a poster depicting actress Lucy Lawless positioned on the arm of a plush red chair feeding her baby, Judah. Dressed in a white blouse and short black skirt, the pose promotes Lawless' relaxed position as well as her long, fishnet stockinged legs and shiny high-heeled shoes. This image drew a variety of negative responses. For example, concern among Auckland Health Boards that public display of the poster would alienate Pacific people:

> ... it was feared that the "gratuitous" (i.e. uncalled for) display of a woman breastfeeding on the walls of the facilities would make people feel uncomfortable in the premises and deter them from seeking health care. (Shaw 111)

The sexual connotations of the pose were also at odds with the views of Pacific and other ethnic and social groups on "sexuality and motherhood" (Shaw 111). In short, the promotion of "breast is best" via the image of a glamorous, affluent, middle-class white woman breastfeeding appeared to hold as little meaning for many Maori women as did the NBAC campaign for a large number of Black American women.

The limitations of public health policies and promotional strategies on breastfeeding raise questions about the role and influence of health professionals on women's infant feeding decisions and practices. As the key providers of pregnancy and childbirth services within New Zealand, midwives are the health professionals most likely to influence a woman's feeding decisions and early breastfeeding practice. Informing this role is their professional knowledge of breastfeeding practice and awareness of current issues on breastfeeding support and promotion. As an important source of up-to-date professional information on infant feeding, the messages delivered in recent issues of six midwifery journals are now explored.

JOURNAL ANALYSIS

METHODOLOGY

The six journals selected for analysis were chosen because of their availability to New Zealand midwives—three peer reviewed, research orientated journals and three practice-orientated publications. The *New Zealand College of Midwives Journal* (*NZCOMJ*) offers peer-reviewed articles on "midwifery issues ... for a readership of midwives and other people involved in pregnancy and childbearing" (Davies 38). Two issues are published annually in April and October. *Birth* and *Midwifery* are also peer reviewed, research-orientated journals published quarterly by Blackwell and Elsevier respectively. In contrast, two of the three practice-orientated journals—*British Journal of Midwifery* (*BJM*), (MA Healthcare Ltd.) and *The Practising Midwife* (*TPM*), (Elsevier Health

Sciences)—are published monthly. *Midwifery News* is published quarterly for the New Zealand College of Midwives by APN Educational Media (NZ) Ltd. Issues of each journal published between April 2007 and June/July 2005 were selected for analysis. A total of five issues of *NZCOMJ*, eight *Midwifery News*, nine issues of *Birth* and *Midwifery*, and 21 issues of both British practice-orientated journals were examined. To avoid the complications of confounding issues, only items directly focused on breastfeeding were included in the analysis. A total of seventy-four items were identified.

A content analysis was employed to identify the message delivered by each item though examination of key words, findings and orientation of the item (Denzin 242). This technique facilitated provisional classification of the range of issues and their messages under the three general but often overlapping categories of: breastfeeding practice; breastfeeding barriers and support; and breastfeeding education and promotion. The focus of items identified a range of common themes under which each was grouped according to the dominant orientation of the message delivered.

FINDINGS

Eighteen articles and four book reviews were identified in the two British refereed journals. A single book review was the only breastfeeding-related item published in the *NZCOMJ*, aside from breast pump advertisements. Professional notices and employment vacancies were also printed in this journal. Similarly, in addition to research papers, *Birth* publishes book reviews, letters, a calendar of professional events and occasional breast pump advertisements. In contrast, *Midwifery* is almost exclusively dedicated to the publication of research papers and book reviews. The three practice-orientated journals are presented in a magazine-style format. All three provide a wide range of predominantly short items (generally two pages or less) on topics such as: latest research findings and clinical information; policy debates and implementation; news clips; professional issues/viewpoints; and in-service training and conference information and proceedings, in addition to a wide range of maternity and infant feeding product advertisements. Commonly each issue includes advertisements for several brands of breast pumps with the *BJM* alone advertising formula for older infants. Conversely, *TPM* displays a logo depicting a formula can within a barred red circle on the front cover. Underneath the logo is the message, "No formula milk advertisements."

BREASTFEEDING PRACTICE

The thirty-one items focused on issues around breastfeeding practice addressed the themes of breastfeeding policy; clinical practice and management; health professional knowledge; and maternal knowledge, attitudes and practices. Almost of a third of these items focused on policy-related issues, particularly "best practice" outcomes. For example, regular reports and updates on the BFHI and the British Sure Start programme featured in *Midwifery News* and TPM. Presentation of the key findings of a national survey of infant feeding conducted in 2005 attributed an increase in the rate of breastfeeding initiation among lower socio-economic and second-time British mothers to the Baby Friendly initiative (Sachs and Dykes). Conversely, an analysis of electronic birth data recorded in selected American hospitals twenty-four hours before discharge linked poor rates of breastfeeding initiation with inadequate hospital policies and population demographics (Kruse, Feldman-Winter and Rotondo).

Challenging reports of the effectiveness of evidence-based hospital polices was the results of a study of the views of British midwives about baby feeding. "Deviant behaviour," that is, practice strategies "not congruent" with evidence-based baby feeding policy recommendations was identified among hospital midwives. The authors warned that although "the midwifery cultural background is not always conducive to individuals providing care that is woman-centred," breaking the rules is not always acceptable to others in the working environment and risks charges of professional negligence (Faber and Thomson 373).

Other items in this category addressed women's breastfeeding practices within the context of their social and cultural attitudes and beliefs. For example, Amal Omer-Salim, Lars-Ake Persson and Pia Olsson found that Tanzanian women acquired interpreted, selected and organised information about baby-feeding within the context and experience of their daily lives. Elizabeth Simmie's study of the attitudes of Asian and Caucasian mothers identified the need for health professional awareness of the information requirements of different ethnic groups, while Linda Kvist, Bodil Larsson and Marie Hall-Lord found an inadequate level of maternal knowledge about the management of possible complications of breastfeeding.

BREASTFEEDING BARRIERS AND SUPPORT

Strategies and interventions to overcome barriers to breastfeeding initiation and continuation was the focus of a further 29 items. Louise Wallace et al. and Fiona Dykes respectively, emphasised the need for more effective policies to ensure consistent advice is given to mothers in the post-natal wards, and for midwives to be allowed more time to offer mothers emotional support while establishing breastfeeding. Baxter reminded readers that medical interventions may prevent mother and baby togetherness following birth and so impede the initiation of breastfeeding. She called for improved hospital practices to ensure breastfeeding is initiated as soon as possible after delivery, particularly following a caesarean or assisted vaginal delivery. The lack of General Practitioner knowledge and health professional interventions to assist women to breastfeed longer were also identified as barriers to breastfeeding.

Mother/baby togetherness to promote breastfeeding initiation was a notable theme. For example, the benefits of "bio-nurturing" (aka kangaroo care) for "healthy new-born infants ... [who] may safely breastfeed in skin-to-skin contact with their mothers" was promoted by Sheau-Huey Chiu, Gene Anderson and Maria Burkhammer (115). The use of "side car cribs" to assist mothers to maintain closeness with their newborn while in hospital was also promoted.

In addressing the issue of community support for breastfeeding, the success of peer support programmes received the most attention. Fiona McGuiness and Penny Curtis, Rose Woodhill and Helen Stapleton, for example, noted the ability of such programmes to accommodate socio-cultural aspects of breastfeeding practice. Pat Hoddinott, Maretta Chalmers and Roisin Pill identified a reduction in negative experiences of breastfeeding among mothers associated with peer support programmes. These authors also drew attention to the benefits of peer support programmes for volunteers, health professionals and the local community. Finally, a number of news clips identified the need for legislative protection of the right to breastfeed in public in England and Wales, in line with recent changes to Scottish law.

BREASTFEEDING EDUCATION AND PROMOTION

Strategies of breastfeeding education and the need to raise community awareness and support for breastfeeding was a focus of the remaining items. Health risks associated with not breastfeeding was a common theme. For example, Heather Neil argued families need to be informed of "how infant feeding can affect their baby's health and their own, in the long and short term" (37). Alarna Blincoe drew attention to the nutritional benefits of breastfeeding. Readers were also alerted to recent research linking breastfeeding with a lowered risk of Type 2 diabetes in later life. In contrast, Jane Wallsworth cautioned midwives to "be mindful of the choice of words" when encouraging expectant mothers to breastfeed (38). Also addressed was the need to promote community awareness of the benefits of breastfeeding, and the desirability of fostering a breastfeeding culture.

PRODUCT ADVERTISING

Cutting across the themes of breastfeeding practice, barriers and support, and education and promotion were full-page breast pump advertisements in all six journals. The frequency of these advertisements varied from irregular among the research journals, to regular and featuring more than one product brand in the practice journals. With the exception of a couple of advertisements specifically directed at hospital neo-natal facilities, mothers were the target of these advertisements which generally promoted the pumps as an aid to breastfeeding continuance. Typically, maternal comfort and convenience was emphasised through messages such as:

> Natural—feel like real breastfeeding.
> Comfortable—are more gentle than traditional breast pumps.
> Efficient—reduce pumping time thanks to faster "let-down" and maximum milk flow.

In addition to breast pump advertisements, the *BJM* published 52 formula advertisements and 15 company sponsored educational services or events in the 21 issues examined. Characteristically these advertisements delivered messages which compared their brand of formula against the composition of breastmilk through statements such as: "Only breastmilk is better" (Milupa Aptamil); "The closest whey protein to breastmilk," and "Advancing closer to human milk protein" (SMA). Online services for mothers, evidence-based study days and a series of feature articles on related topics such as the infant immune system were also sponsored by formula companies.

REPRESENTATIONS OF BREASTFEEDING

The range and nature of the items on breastfeeding presented in the six midwifery journals highlight a complexity of issues surrounding breastfeeding practice, barriers and support, and promotion. A notable feature of this complexity was contradiction between the messages delivered as demonstrated by the following examples: mothers would choose to breastfeed if they were fully aware of the health benefits of breastfeeding; poor rates of breastfeeding initiation reflect inadequate hospital policies. Breastfeeding is normal and natural; breastfeeding is a socially-learned cultural practice requiring maternal, family and community education. Maternal perceptions and experience affect breastfeeding initiation and duration; individually tailored practice strategies "not congruent" with evidenced-based hospital policy risk professional negligence. Breastfeeding is a community issue; it is the mother's decision whether or not to breastfeed, and so on.

Compounding the contradictory messages delivered by the journals was the inclusion of product advertisements, particularly infant formula advertising in the *BJM*. Although it could be argued that health professionals require access to professional information on artificial baby milk when mothers are unable to breastfeed, the information conveyed by these advertisements is promotional rather than informative. Indeed, because these advertisements target use for older rather than newborn infants they contradict messages addressing the need to increase the rate of breastfeeding duration. The issue of the potential for harm through the inclusion of formula advertisements in health professional journals has been taken up by Magda Sachs who is adamant they "have no place" because they appear to offer solutions for particular problems. Sachs' point is that there are usually other ways to resolve breastfeeding problems (715). She further argues that reliance on advertising solutions to breastfeeding difficulties is a hindrance to the development of health professional skills when supporting breastfeeding continuance.

When considering the overall significance of these six journals and the implications of their messages for New Zealand midwives, an obvious value is that they provide up-to-date international and local research, as well as policy and practice information on breastfeeding. Additionally they offer a forum for communication on current breastfeeding issues and policy developments. More important is the diversity of the messages delivered because they identify multiple representations of breastfeeding. Through drawing attention to the experiential, social and cultural aspects of breastfeeding, these journals complement and extend the narrow public health focus on the health benefits for the mother and infant. Similarly, acknowledgement of multiple representations of breastfeeding calls into question the efficacy of the application of best-practice policies across divergent social, cultural and demographic groups. In short, these journals challenge the inflexibility of breastfeeding policies embedded in "global policies and practices that exist to ensure the protection, promotion and support of breastfeeding *regardless* of [social and] cultural difference" (Schmied, Sheehan and Barclay 50, italics mine). In these ways, the journals examined play an important role in mediating tensions between the evidenced-based model of best practice, and the midwifery ethos of woman-centred professional practice.

[1]The National Breastfeeding Advisory Committee was set up by the Ministry of Health in 2006 to "develop, lead and co-ordinate a national breastfeeding plan aimed at improving New Zealand's breastfeeding rates" (Ministry of Health, *National Breastfeeding Advisory Committee*).

[2]The partnership model of midwifery which underpins the midwifery profession in New Zealand describes the relationship between a woman and her midwife. This relationship "demands…equality within the relationship, with each partner respected for what they bring to the partnership. The health care provider is respected for their professional knowledge and practice skills, and the woman receiving care is respected and valued for her knowledge of herself; and of her individual and unique needs and desires" (Davis 17).

REFERENCES

Ahmed, Shameem, Sadia Parveen, and Ariful Islam, A. "Infant Feeding Practices in Rural Bangladesh: Policy Implications." *Journal of Tropical Pediatrics* 45 (1999): 37-41.

Aycicek, Ali, Ozcan Erel, Abdurrahim Kocyigit, Sahbettin Selek, and Mehmet Demirkol. "Breast-milk Provides Better Antioxidant Power than Does Formula." *Nutrition* 22 (2006): 616-19.

Bailey, Jacqueline. "Modern Parents' Perspectives on Breastfeeding: A Small Study." *British Journal of Midwifery* 15 (2007): 149-52.

Baxter, Jackie. "Women's Experience of Infant Feeding Following Birth by Caesarean Section." *British Journal of Midwifery* 14 (2006): 290-95.

Beasley, Annette. "The Medicalisation of Breastfeeding: Lessons from the Experience of Four First-time Mothers." *Breastfeeding in New Zealand: Practice, Problems and Policy*. Ed. Beasley, Annette, and Andrew Trlin. Palmerston North: Dunmore Press, 1998. 95-110.

Beasley, Annette. "Breastfeeding and the Body Politic." *Women's Studies Journal* 14 (1998): 61-82.

Beasley, Annette. "Introduction." *Breast-feeding in New Zealand: Practice, Problems and Policy*. Ed. Annette Beasley and Andrew Trlin. Palmerston North: Dunmore Press, 1998. 7-13.

Blincoe, Alarna. "Midwives are Ideally Placed to Advise Parents on Optimum Infant Nutrition." *British Journal of Midwifery* 14 (2006): 536-40.

Chiu, Sheau-Huey, Gene Anderson, and Maria Burkhammer. "Newborn Temperature During Skin-to-skin Breastfeeding in Couples Having Breast-feeding Difficulties." *Birth* 32 (2005): 115-21.

Curtis, Penny, Rose Woodhill, and Helen Stapleton. "The Peer-professional Interface in a Community-based, Breast Feeding Peer-support Project." *Midwifery* 23 (2007): 146-56.

Davies, Rhondda. "Journal Guidelines for Contributors." *New Zealand College of Midwives Journal* 36 (2007): 38.

Deem, Helen, and Murray McGeorge. "Breast-feeding." *New Zealand Medical Journal* 57 (1958): 539-56.

Dettwyler, Katherine. "Beauty and the Beast: The Cultural Context of Breast-feeding in the United States." *Breastfeeding. Biocultural Perspectives*. Ed. Patricia Stuart-Macadam and Katherine Dettwyler. New York: Aldine de Gruyter, 1995. 167-216.

Davis, Deborah. "Evidence Based Health Care: Raising Issues from a Midwifery Perspective." *New Zealand College of Midwives Journal* 3 (2005): 14-18.

Denzin, Norman. *Interpretive Ethnography. Ethnographic Practices for the 21st Century.* Thousand Oaks: Sage, 1997.

Dykes, Fiona. "A Critical Ethnographic Study of Encounters Between Midwives and Breast-feeding Women in Postnatal Wards in England." *Midwifery* 21 (2005): 241-52.

Essex, Charles. "Breastfeeding Rates in New Zealand in the First 6 Months and the Reasons for Stopping." *New Zealand Medical Journal* 108 (1995): 355-57.

Fildes, Valerie. "The Culture and Biology of Breastfeeding: An Historical Review of Western Europe." *Breastfeeding: Biocultural Perspectives*. Ed. Patricia Stuart-Macadam and Katherine Dettwyler. New York: Aldine de Gruyter. 101-126.

Furber, Christine, and Ann Thomson. " 'Breaking the Rules' in Baby-feeding Practice in the UK: Deviance and Good Practice?" *Midwifery* 22 (2006): 365-76.

Hausman, Bernice. "The Feminist Politics of Breastfeeding." *Australian Feminist Studies* 19 (2005): 273-85.

Hoddinott, Pat, Maretta Chalmers, and Roisin Pill. "One-to-one or Group-based Peer Support for Breastfeeding? Women's Perceptions of a Breastfeeding Peer Coaching Intervention." *Birth* 33 (2007): 139-46.

Kruse, Lakota, Lori Feldman-Winter, and Florence Rotondo. "Comparing

Sociodemographic and Hospital Influences on Breastfeeding Initiation." *Birth*, 32 (2005): 81-85.

Kvist, Linda, Bodil Larsson, and Marie Hall-Lord. "A Grounded Theory Study of Swedish Women's Experiences of Inflammatory Symptoms of the Breast During Breast Feeding." *Midwifery* 22 (2006): 137-46.

Lupton, Deborah. "Foucault and the Medicalisation Critique." *Foucault, Health and Medicine*. Ed. Petersen, Alan, and Robin Bunton. London: Routledge, 1997. 94-110.

McGuiness, Fiona. "Community Support is Key for Breastfeeding Mothers." Editorial. *British Journal of Midwifery* 14 (2006): 4.

Medela®. "Inspired by Babies—Pioneered by Medela." *The Practising Midwife* 10 (2007).

Minchin, Maureen. *Breastfeeding Matters.* 4th ed. Melbourne: Alma Publications, 1998.

Ministry of Health. "National Breastfeeding Advisory Committee." (n.d.) <http://www.moh.govt.nz/nbac>.

Ministry of Health. *Guidelines for Healthy Breastfeeding Women.* Wellington: Ministry of Health, 1995.

Ministry of Health. *Infant Feeding. Guidelines for New Zealand Health Workers.* Wellington: Ministry of Health, 1997.

Ministry of Health. *Breastfeeding: A Guide to Action.* Wellington: Ministry of Health, 2002.

Ministry of Health. *Implementing and Monitoring the International Code of Marketing of Breast-milk Substitutes in New Zealand: The Code in New Zealand*. Wellington: Ministry of Health, 2007.

Ministry of Health. "Comprehensive Plan to Inform the Design of a National Breastfeeding Promotion Campaign." 2007.

Milupa, Aptamil. "Only Breastmilk is Better—So What's New?" *British Journal of Midwifery* 15 (2007).

Morrow, Ardythe, Guillermo Ruiz-Palacios, Mekibib Altaye, Xi Jiang, Lourdes Guerrero, Jareen Meinzen-Deff, Tibor Farkas, Prasoon Charurrvedi, Larry Pickering, and David Newburg. "Human Milk Oligosaccharides are Associated with Protection Against Diarrhea in Breastfed Infants." *Journal of Pediatrics* 145 (2004): 297-303.

Neil, Heather. "Making Breastfeeding a Reality." *The Practising Midwife* 9 (2006): 37-40.

National Breastfeeding Advisory Committee of New Zealand. *National Strategic Plan of Action for Breastfeeding, 2008-2012*. Wellington: National Breastfeeding Advisory Committee, 2008.

New Zealand Breastfeeding Authority. "Baby Friendly Accredited Hospitals." 2008. <http://www.babyfriendly.org.nz/page.php?13>.

New Zealand College of Midwives. "About the NZCOM." 2007. <www.midwife.org.nz/index.cfm/1,175,438,0,html/About-the-NZCOM>.

Omer-Salim, Amal, Lars-Ake Persson and Pia Olsson. "Whom Can I Rely

On? Mother's Approaches to Support for Feeding: An Interview Study in Suburban Dar es Salaam, Tanzania." *Midwifery* 23 (2007): 172-83.

Sachs, Magda. "Milk Advertising Should not be Allowed in Journals." *British Journal of Midwifery* 13 (2005): 714-15.

Sachs, Magda, and Fiona Dykes. "Infant Feeding Trends: Early Indicators." *The Practising Midwife* 9 (2006): 15-19.

Schmied, Virginia, Athena Sheehan, and Lesley Barclay. "Contemporary Breast-feeding Policy and Practice: Implications for Midwives." *Midwifery* 17 (2001): 44-54.

Shaw, Rhonda. "Performing Breastfeeding: Embodiment, Ethics and the Maternal Subject." *Feminist Review* 78 (2004): 99-116.

Simmie, Elizabeth. "Breastfeeding: Different Ethnic Background, Different Perceptions?" *British Journal of Midwifery* 14 (2006): 20-26.

SMA Nutrition. "We've Changed." *British Journal of Midwifery* 15 (2007).

Smith, Julie. "Mothers' Milk and Markets." *Australian Feminist Studies* 19 (2004): 369-79.

UNICEF. *Innocenti Declaration.* Florence: UNICEF, 1990.

Van Esterik, Penny. *Beyond the Breast-Bottle Controversy.* New Brunswick: Rutgers, 1989.

Wallace, Louise, Orla Dunn, Elizabeth Alder, Sally Inch, Robert Hills and Susan Law. "A Randomised-controlled Trial in England of a Postnatal Midwifery Intervention on Breast-feeding Duration." *Midwifery* 22 (2006): 262-73.

Wallsworth, Jane. "Don't Mention the 'B' Word!" *The Practising Midwife* 8 (2005): 36-40.

Westdahl, Claire, and Sallie Page-Goertz0. "Promotion of Breastfeeding—Beyond the Benefits." *International Journal of Childbirth Education* 21 (2006): 8-16.

Wolf, Joan. "Is Breast Really Best? Risk and Total Motherhood in the National Breastfeeding Awareness Campaign." *Journal of Health Politics, Policy and Law* 32 (2007): 595-636.

World Health Organization (WHO). *International Code of Marketing Breast-milk Substitutes.* Geneva: World Health Organization, 1981.

World Health Organization/UNICEF. *Ten Steps to Successful Breastfeeding.* Geneva: World Health Organisation, 1989.

World Health Organization/UNICEF. *Global Strategy for Infant and Young Child Feeding.* Geneva: World Health Organization, 2003.

The Lactating Body and Conflicting Ideals of Sexuality, Motherhood and Self

MONICA CAMPO

THE EXPERIENCE OF BREASTFEEDING has become a topic of interest among feminist scholars over the last decade; however there are still few qualitative accounts particularly in Australia. As Christa Kelleher points out, much feminist scholarship on this issue has "tended to focus on the historical, ideological, discursive and meaning-making aspects of breastfeeding" (2728) or on macro issues of economy, class and policy (see for example Avishai; Blum; Carter; Dettwyler; Dykes; Maher; Palmer; Stearns; Wall). While feminist discursive analyses of breastfeeding are useful, the breastfeeding experience is not merely a negotiation between various discourses; it also involves women using their bodies in a mammalian and inescapably biological manner. Notwithstanding, some feminist scholarship has addressed the embodied and theoretical aspects of breastfeeding (Bartlett; Britton; Dykes; Giles; Hausman; Shaw; Van Esterik; Young). Within the overt physicality of the breastfeeding experience there are said to be several "paradoxes and dilemmas" raised (Kelleher 2728). The fluidity of the breastfeeding body and the mother/child symbiosis for example, radically challenges mind/body and self/other dualisms, presenting alternatives to the idea of autonomous selfhood in Western societies (Bartlett "Breastfeeding, Bodies" 153; Hausman 276; Shildrick 16; Van Esterik; Young). Fiona Giles also points out that bodily fluids, such as breastmilk, cause social unease, threaten to undermine the social order, and disturb the boundaries between inside and outside: public and private and between the individual and society (1). As Magrit Shildrick argues, the leaks and flows of women's bodies challenge the very basis of the Western logos based on the Cartesian mind/body dualism (43).

On political levels, breastfeeding provides ideal opportunities for arguing the importance of the body in female or specifically maternal subjectivity. While highlighting women's bodily difference can be met with unease within feminism, some theorists argue that emphasising difference shows the way in which dominant models of subjectivity are inherently male-biased although positing as "gender-neutral" (Braidotti; Grosz; Shildrick). Corporeal feminists argue that a focus on the differences reveals modernist accounts of selfhood that are inadequate for theorising female experience. Further, a re-focus on women's bodily differences will enable new and non-dualistic models of subjectivity to emerge, which are more fluid and inclusive (Braidotti; Gatens; Grosz; Shildrick). Breastfeeding, as a political issue for women, should force an acknowledgement of the embodied nature of gender and as a "maternal practice" should force recognition of mothers as special kinds of "embodied citizens" with particular needs, rights and perspectives (Hausman 277).

Utilising theoretical frameworks offered by corporeal feminist theories, and drawing on interviews with Australian breastfeeding women, I argue that breastfeeding mothers must negotiate cultural norms and discourses which rail against their bodily experiences. Interviews with groups of new mothers suggest the embodied experience of giving breastmilk is contradictory, and may confound dominant Western models of selfhood, beauty and sexuality. From these interviews breastfeeding women can be heard as marginalised voices, with no valued model of selfhood from which to interpret their experiences thus resulting in feelings of dissonance. Furthermore, as the breastfeeding body is one at odds with contemporary ideals regarding beauty and sexuality, women in the study showed exasperation about their lactating form and revealed self-conscious tensions existing between sexuality and motherhood. For these women the lactating body became "high-maintenance" requiring careful management in both public and private domains.

METHODOLOGY

This discussion of breastfeeding is based on data drawn from group interviews involving breastfeeding mothers in Melbourne, Australia. Ethics approval was granted from La Trobe University, to recruit women through new mother's groups meetings, at suburban Maternal and Child Health Centres in Melbourne, Australia. Twenty-two women participated in four focus group interviews. The size of the focus groups depended on the number of women attending on the day; however the smallest comprised of three women and the largest had 12 women participating. Wilkinson argues that focus group interviews suit feminist analysis because they are non-hierarchical, allowing participants greater discussion opportunities. They also allow for better contextualising of information through shared dialogue (65). Topics and broad questions, introduced by the researcher, were discussed among the groups. Each interview was later transcribed, with key themes being identified. The average age of women in the study was 33 and their babies had an average age of three months. All women were born in Australia, with two identifying as Aboriginal or Torres Strait Islander. Six women had migrant backgrounds, with parents born outside Australia. One woman was a sole parent and the remaining were either married, or in a long-term heterosexual relationships. Nineteen women were tertiary educated and three had completed High School. All, except one, were employed in white-collar professional jobs prior to giving birth. Of the twenty-two women, seventeen were currently breastfeeding; one woman was both breast and bottle-feeding; and four had recently stopped breastfeeding. Pseudonyms have been used wherever names are given.

"IT'S MY BODY TOO": MAINTAINING A SENSE OF SELF

The blurred boundaries between mother and child are often experienced as a conflict, upsetting a woman's sense of autonomy and bodily integrity (Dykes; Schmied; Schmied and Barclay). Women in this study were similarly in discord about sharing their bodies and the demands of a newborn. Several women said their bodies did not feel like their own any longer. With mild ironical intent, some even made assertions to their babies that it was still their body:

> *I don't know if my body sort of feels so much mine anymore ... because it's sustaining him and it's not so much just my body anymore, you know ... I feel it you know when he's tearing at my nipple and it's like well it's my body too you know, it's not just all for you.*

> *Because it's sometimes not your body, it's theirs and I tend to fight that feeling. "No no, it's mine not yours, I'm loaning, I'm helping you out here," which is a very strange way of looking at it but it's ... how I feel.*

Interestingly, it wasn't just that sharing a body with a demanding newborn disrupted their bodily boundaries. Some also felt that they had lost any bodily privacy, because the experience of pregnancy and breastfeeding had rendered their bodies "public property" (see also Longhurst; Nash).

> *I think that starts in pregnancy and gets even more so, when you're breastfeeding ... there's no privacy about your body anymore.*

Linda Blum argues that in a medicalised model of pregnancy and breastfeeding, the mother is "treated, and pressed to treat herself as if body-less" (60). This medical model separates body from mind, objectifying the physical and placing emphasis on the product: breastmilk. It achieves this separation at the expense of the interactive process that should occur in breastfeeding (Dykes). The medical model is also child-centred, rendering the mother's subjectivity invisible to outside understandings (Wall 604). In fact, one woman said she "might as well not have been there" in her encounters with the hospital's midwives, connecting her experience to a "transition from my body to our body sort of thing." Perhaps these sentiments about women's bodies "not being their own" could be read as resistance to a hegemonic medical model in which women's subjectivities are absent, rather than read purely as a struggle between their baby's demands and their bodies.

Significantly however, the sentiments expressed are related to Western understandings of the body and subjectivity with clear boundaries between self and other. The women in this study were mostly over thirty and had professional careers before having a baby. The assumption is that they had spent the majority of their adult lives as autonomous individuals. In opposition to their pre-motherhood experience, the transition to motherhood and breastfeeding a baby on-call requires women to adopt a much less autonomous way of life governed by differing, and less individualistic, values and needs. It is this sacrifice that assaults individual understandings of self. Barbara Rothman argues that the physical embodiment and "connectedness" of motherhood contradicts and challenges aspects of liberal philosophy (59). A society committed to liberalism and the enshrinement of the autonomous self does not handle well the ideological anathema of motherhood. It is this contradiction, seen in pregnant and breastfeeding women, which confuses the dictum about individuals entering the world as autonomous, isolated beings (Rothman 59; see also Hays; DiQuinzio).

I want to challenge those cultural assumptions like Susan Maushart's (228), that conclude breastfeeding is not in women's best interests and ill-suited to contemporary lifestyles and culturally assumed notions of personal autonomy. In Western societies, such as Australia, the dominant model of selfhood conflicts with maternal embodiment and subjectivity. Women in Australia are expected to act like men within the civic sphere; that is as autonomous, liberal subjects. The problem is that there is no valid model of subjectivity to interpret their experience as breastfeeding mothers in the private sphere. The embodied state that breastfeeding magnifies is at odds with the individualised self enshrined within in our society, and breastfeeding thus becomes experienced as dissonant.

Not all women in the study, however, felt that the blurring of bodily boundaries or having sole responsibilities for sustaining a life, impacted negatively. Some women understood the sense of responsibility and shared body as empowering:

> *So it's kind of nice to feel that they are attached to you and it is that whole attachment thing just to keep them part of you for that bit longer.*

Other women described feeling "pleased" and "proud" that only *they* could comfort and feed their babies. It filled them with a sense of importance and power. Two women in the study articulated this embodied connection to their baby, describing a sense of their body as being "at one" with their babies:

> *I also find, that it's sort of like there's an attachment that no one else can have. On a couple of occasions that I've been away for more than a couple of hours, I physically can feel that there's a baby that should be here, it's that physical relationship, the attachment that you've got.*

Nerida, who was attempting to wean her baby because she planned to go back to work, said that when she bottle fed, she felt a "disconnection" with her baby and that she:

> *Can't let go of how he holds me and touches me, I can't get him this close unless he's there on my boob.*

Similarly, Dora said she was distressed when she weaned her daughter; feeling that there was a severing of a connection between baby and herself that had begun in pregnancy. Again, these experiences challenge the self/other dualism of western culture: breastfeeding blurs the boundaries between the individual and other, pointing to a need for more inclusive and fluid constructions of selfhood, which recognise the unique embodied status of maternal subjects (Van Esterik, Young).

"HIGH MAINTENANCE BODY PARTS": MAINTAINING THE IDEAL BREAST

> *Your breasts become really high maintenance body parts don't they? Because you're not used to them because before they were so benign and suddenly you go "oh my god ... this is my life."*

Iris Marion Young argues that breasts are "entwined" with women's sense of self and identity (189). She argues that in our phallocentric culture breasts predominate as inescapable signifiers of womanliness. They are fetishized, objectified pieces of flesh; constructed as solid, passive, inert; able to be handled, manipulated, measured and owned. In this construction the ideal breast is pert, firm and sits high on the chest. Most women's breasts, however, do not live up to the ideal and, as Young asserts, women do not experience their breasts in this way, especially as we age, experience pregnancy or are lactating. Young "imagines" a woman-centred view of the breasted body as "blurry, mushy, indefinite, multiple, and without clear identity."[1] It is a view directly contrasted to the "inert dead matter of the Cartesian world view" (193). Perhaps Katrina's comment above recognises this transition from the "benign" objectified breast of phallocentric culture, to a more woman-centred perspective initiated by her experience of breastfeeding. These, amongst other comments, including breasts "having a mind of their own," are distinct conceptual challenges to the object-like, solid and passive sexualised breast of Western culture's construction.

Contemporary constructions of femininity and beauty have been shown to present women's bodies as deficient, never quite reaching the standards set up by the idealised norms of beauty (Bordo). However, lactating breasts contradict the idealised, sexualised and fetishized breasts of contemporary culture. Moreover, the breastfeeding body is, as Alison Bartlett suggests, "anarchic" and "volatile," compared with the passive, pliable and controlled bodies that are culturally idealised and aspired to ("Breastfeeding, Bodies" 154). This idea became clear in the interviews when women began to talk about the way their breasts looked and felt. Some women in this study were disgruntled about their breastfeeding bodies and felt they wanted their bodies and breasts back to "normal." They disliked their bodies and breasts since having a baby and breastfeeding:

> *I can't wait until mine [breasts] dry up and shrink ... you look at them now and you can't even feel them, they're just like lumps of I don't know what.*
>
> *They're just sagging and hanging a little lower than I'd like at the moment.*
>
> *I went from an "A" cup to a double "D" and I thought these are just revolting, I want to get rid of them, they're in the way and everything doesn't fit.*

These women talked about their breasts in an objectified manner, through the phallocentric gaze that Young discusses where breasts are valued for their aesthetic appeal. Their breasts did not compare favourably to the idealised cultural breast: they sagged, were too big, or got in the way. Several other women also talked about getting their bodies "back to normal" after pregnancy and breastfeeding; normal being a body more aligned with cultural ideals of beauty. Bartlett argues that the emphasis in popular culture on restoring body shape after pregnancy and breastfeeding reflects "the social concern with maintaining and controlling the body" ("Breastfeeding, Bodies" 154; see also Nash). In fact breastfeeding promotion literature often reflects this social concern about maintenance and control, playing on women's insecurities about body image, emphasising that breastfeeding burns calories, which helps to restore the "misshapen" form back to a pre-pregnancy state (Wall 601).

"YOU'RE NOT SUPPOSED TO BE SEXY WHEN YOU'RE A MUM": MAINTAINING THE SEXUAL/MATERNAL BREAST IN PRIVATE

While Katrina said her breasts had become her "life," she also said they had become "high maintenance" referring to expressing, applying of cream to sore nipples, massaging engorged breasts and general upkeep of the lactating breast beginning from the early days of motherhood. It was a sentiment that other women in the study spoke about too. Notwithstanding these anecdotes, however, I want to argue that the breastfeeding body requires another sort of maintenance or management: that the dichotomy between motherhood and sexuality are vigilantly managed. It is the breastfeeding body in its sexual guise, as researchers have shown, that requires further erudition to explain how women manage the conflicting discourses of motherhood and sexuality (Blum; Carter; Paz Gulupo and Ayres).

Two women articulated the inherent tensions between the sexual and maternal. Jane lamented the fact that she couldn't obtain "sexy" maternity bras, as they were all practical and "daggy" and Dora commented that "people would be shocked" if breastfeeding mothers wore sexy underwear with their "breasts and cleavage hanging out" because "you're not supposed to be sexy when you're a mum." Breastfeeding, as frequently noted by other scholars, "disrupts the border between motherhood and sexuality" (Young 199) and is described as being akin to a sexual act (Giles 11). This transgression occurs not only because breastfeeding has a sexual nature about it, but also because it challenges imaginings of the sexualised breast. Young and Giles argue that in order for breasts to be sexual the maternal element must be repressed; and in order for them to be maternal they must be desexualised. Several women interviewed for this study, made clear demarcations between the maternal and sexual functions of their breasts; their breasts being sexual before breastfeeding, but being "functional" while breastfeeding:

> *Before you have a baby ... your breasts are sort of seen as sexual thing ... all of a sudden, you turn into a dairy cow ... if you thought you were sexy or attractive before, you certainly don't when you're breastfeeding, or I don't anyway.*

> Rowena: *Before breastfeeding, breasts were part of your sexual identity, your body image and you'd think about them in the clothes you wore and the bras you chose ...*
> Dora: *They were just ornaments*
> Rowena: *Now it's like well this is what they're made for*
> Dora: *They're functional*
> Rowena: *Yeah they're functional rather than sexual.*

Some women talked about sexuality in relation to the needs and desires of their partners or husbands:

> *I think for my partner ... it's hard for him to sort of reconcile both of them [the sexual and maternal images of the breast]. He doesn't like to think about it too much. For example, if I said something about breastfeeding while he was feeling sexual, he'd be like "oh no don't talk about breastfeeding now" because he just has to shut that off in his mind.*

> *Its very hard for me to make the transition of breastfeeding one hour and sexual being the next. And it feels like you're trying to keep everyone happy ... I know I need to [make the transition] for the relationship as well.*

The above comments echo advice given in breastfeeding literature, suggesting women not let breastfeeding interfere with their sexual relationships (Bartlett, "Maternal Sexuality"; Carter; Wall). Other women also discussed how to turn their partners away when their breasts were full and tender. As Pam

Carter argues, contradiction exists within the wider discourses of femininity between motherhood and heterosexuality, which require women to be good mothers and breastfeed their children whilst also ensuring their husband's needs are properly met (130). This maintains the "all give and no take" love necessary for "good" mothering, which denies women any pleasure of their own (Young 199).

Other research suggests certain liberation in women conceiving their breasts in a desexualised manner, because it signifies a perspective shift from being "sexually objectified as a woman, to serving a valued function as a mother" (Paz Gulupo and Ayres 27). There was evidence in this study suggesting that some women felt more comfortable with their bodies in the maternal role, as they felt less modesty about their breasts. The notion that a desexualization of the breasts may be liberating for women is a view that is tendered by maternalist/cultural feminism, which seeks to promote motherly and nurturing images of women, disassociating from the sexually objectified female body (Blum; Young). Conversely, others posit that it's more radical to "shatter the border between motherhood and sexuality" and reaffirm the "undecidability" of motherhood and sexuality (Young 199-200). Giles, for instance, believes that the breast is "incompletely" sexualised in Western culture (11). The idealised breast of Western culture is idealised precisely because it is *imagined* as containing none of the problematic associations with excrement, blood or childbirth, like the vagina. Giles argues for a sexual component of breastfeeding that may be celebrated, rather than feared, and that we need to affirm the real, leaking and wet breast as sexy too (11-12). Bartlett also confronts the sexuality/motherhood nexus by arguing that normal physiological responses involved in breastfeeding are part of the wider spectrum of female sexuality ("Maternal Sexuality"). It is a radical position, and as Cindy Stearns points out, "the construction of the good maternal body as being at all costs not sexual is taken very seriously by both the culture and the law" (309), highlighting the example of a young American mother investigated by Social Services after disclosing she sometimes felt aroused whilst breastfeeding. Recently, cultural antagonism toward maternal sexuality was reinforced when social networking internet sites "MySpace" and "Facebook" censored images of breastfeeding women, which were perceived as "obscene" (Ferguson; Moses).

Perhaps for this reason only three women in the study openly linked sexuality to their breastfeeding experience. Although many said they enjoyed breastfeeding once the initial period of pain and adjustment had passed, they spoke of the enjoyment in socially acceptable terms of the bonding between mother and child and about the satisfaction gained from knowing they were sustaining a life. None spoke of it purely in terms of pleasure. Jo, however, made a tenuous link between breastfeeding and sexual satisfaction:

> *It became really rewarding and really satisfying but I've also found, probably because of all the hormones, you sort of feel like you want something*

> *afterwards, something sweet or something. You feel depleted and content, like a release, almost sexual, but not really.*

After Jo spoke, the mood quickly changed with some women in the interview looking around nervously, as if disassociating themselves from her. The taboo nature of the link between sexuality and breastfeeding, at least among this particular group of mothers, was glaringly apparent. In another smaller interview, two women were quite frank about their sexuality. Sarah and Aimee acknowledged that breastfeeding had made them feel more sensual and sexy:

> *When I was in hospital … I remember feeling, wondering you know how my body would ever be sexy or attractive again but now …. my relationship with my partner is a lot closer and um, I guess you can sort of see it in two sides; you can see the biological side of your body but also the sexual side, you can have both. I actually find that breastfeeding makes me more sensual, not while, not really while I'm feeding, but in general, so um, it probably makes it easier.*

Sarah, quoted earlier, speaking about the problems her partner had separating the sexual and maternal functions of breast felt that it was easier for her to reconcile the dual roles of her breasts than for him because:

> *I've got the experience of breastfeeding and it is a sensual thing so they are separate but they're more connected for me than for him because he doesn't experience both, whereas I do.*

Sarah's comment shows an embodied subjectivity quite different from that of her partner's because, as a bystander, he doesn't experience breastfeeding as a physical, emotional and psychological presence. Here again, we find that an understanding of women's embodied experiences challenges dominant and oppressive views of breastfeeding, and of women's bodies in general. Young argues that if more women spoke about the pleasure derived from breastfeeding it would shatter the border between motherhood and sexuality, and "explode" patriarchal definitions of motherhood that require mothers to be asexual nurturers (201). Also notable in Sarah's comment is how subjectivity is sexually differentiated. The dominant Enlightenment model of subjectivity fails to acknowledge this difference, engulfing women under a male or "gender-neutral" norm. Thus the breastfeeding experience renders the sexually differentiated subjectivities of men and women more apparent.

BREASTFEEDING ETIQUETTE: MAINTAINING THE SEXUAL/MATERNAL BREAST IN PUBLIC

The issue of breastfeeding in public was a recurring theme in these interviews.

Most women expressed sentiments suggesting that breastfeeding in public intensified a negotiation between the sexual and the maternal functions of their breasts and more generally the need to manage their breastfeeding bodies. One woman experienced a negative reaction while feeding her ten-day-old daughter in the waiting room of a car dealership. Although angry at the response, she conceded that perhaps she wasn't being "discreet" enough or that maybe she should have asked someone before feeding or "turned away." For other women, too, breastfeeding in public highlighted tensions between the need to feed, and feeling they should uphold social etiquettes:

> *The thing I found was the ettiquacy (sic) you know, where can I breastfeed, like before you upset people and feeling comfortable. Because I found that as soon as he was hungry, I just wanted to feed him but ...*

> *There's (sic) people out there that do get offended when you're breastfeeding in front of them and I guess you've got to be mindful of that.*

Among one group of women, there was much talk about practices to employ and clothing to wear in order to maintain a sort of breastfeeding etiquette based on discretion. Bartlett ("Scandalous Practices" 117) highlights congruence in the fact that people who both support and oppose breastfeeding in public align often themselves with the middle class ideal of discreteness. Breastfeeding is considered acceptable in public, Bartlett argues, as long as women remain discreet. The ideology of feminine modesty or discretion, however, hides "more deeply held concerns about women's sexuality" ("Scandalous Practices" 117) and the border between motherhood and sexuality as discussed above.

Breastfeeding in public also raises issues of citizenship and the use of public space (Bartlett, "Scandalous Practices"). Until recently, the sight of women's embodied activities were relegated to the private sphere. Publicly, breastfeeding draws attention to embodied gender differences, something that has historically excluded women from the public sphere (Hausman 276). Although many public spaces and work places now have parenting rooms, "keeping the bodily flows of mothers and babies out of sight" (Bartlett, "Scandalous Practices" 112), the public world is still predominately shaped for, and by, the norms of male embodiment and autonomous selfhood, as Rachel's story highlights:

> *I was in the city, it was in a café and I walked in and there were no prams, no kids, no women, well there was one I think, but it was all business and I was like "oh god, what do I do?" and I was just panicking thinking "am I allowed to breastfeed here"? I didn't know what the rules were you know. Or do I go to toilet and then I thought that's not very healthy! But then I found a really quiet little corner and breastfed and I was lucky that the*

> *staff were really lovely and everything, but you know you just don't know what to do in those situations and this place had no baby change room, no pram access and I thought, well perhaps this is not the best place to be.*

Rachel's embodied maternal status meant she felt marginalised in a public and obviously male dominated space. Mahon-Daly and Andrews argue that breastfeeding is a "liminal" position for women, as they experience a temporary shift in subjectivity thus feeling marginalized in public places (64), an idea Bartlett takes up later in this volume. Although breastfeeding is a temporary rather than ongoing aspect of women's subjectivity, there are other times that women's embodied status reflects a distinctly gendered experience. Perhaps it would be better to challenge public citizenry, and subjectivity, rather than merely accepting women's temporary shift from "normal" subjectivity.

CONCLUSION

In this chapter I have highlighted the way in which the breastfeeding body can be experienced as "high maintenance." The embodied experience of breastfeeding requires women to both negotiate the contradictions and inadequacies of the gender-neutral Enlightenment model of selfhood because breastfeeding radically challenges self/other and mind/body dualisms. The requisites for subjectivity as they are defined and valued in contemporary society, such as autonomy and individualism, are at odds with the subjectivity of breastfeeding women thus leading some women to experience breastfeeding as a dissonance. Moreover, lactating women had to maintain the culturally created dichotomy between sexuality and motherhood in both public and private. In private women negotiated bodily experience and discourse. Health authorities and governments strenuously promote breastfeeding—yet it causes unease when performed away from the domestic realm of mothers and children because it blurs the culturally created boundaries between sexuality and maternity and draws attention to women's embodied difference.

[1]It is important to note that Young asserts she is not claiming that there is a true or authentic core of feminine identity somewhere underlying the phallocentric construction, but that it is something that needs to be made up as a political strategy to reject women" s "literal and figurative objectification" (193).

REFERENCES

Avishai, Orit. "Managing the Lactating Body: The Breast-Feeding Project and Privileged Motherhood." *Qualitative Sociology* 30.2 (2007): 135-52.

Bartlett, Alison. "Breastfeeding as Headwork: Corporeal Feminism and Meanings for Breastfeeding." *Women's Studies International Forum* 25.3 (2002):

373-82.

Bartlett, Alison. "Breastfeeding, Bodies and Choice in Late Capitalism." *Hecate* 29.12 (2003): 153-64.

Bartlett, Alison. *Breastwork: Rethinking Breastfeeding*. Sydney: University of New South Wales Press, 2005.

Bartlett, Alison. "Maternal Sexuality and Breastfeeding." *Sex Education* 5.1 (2005): 67-77.

Bartlett, Alison. "Scandalous Practices and Political Performances: Breastfeeding in the City." *Continuum: Journal of Media and Cultural Studies* 16.1 (2002): 111-21.

Blum, Linda. *At the Breast: Ideologies of Breastfeeding and Motherhood in Contemporary United States*. Boston: Beacon Press, 1999.

Bordo, Susan. *Unbearable Weight-Feminism, Western Culture and the Body.* University of California Press, 1993.

Braidotti, Rossi. *Nomadic Subjects: Embodiment and Sexual Difference in Contemporary Feminist Theory*. New York: Columbia University Press, 1994.

Britton, Cathryn. "'Feeling Letdown': An Exploration of an Embodied Sensation Associated with Breastfeeding." *The Body in Everyday Life*. Eds. Sarah Nettleton and Jonathan Watson. London: Routledge, 1998. 64-81.

Carter, Pam. *Feminism, Breasts and Breastfeeding*. London: Macmillan Press, 1995.

Dettwyler, Katherine, A. "Beauty and the Breast: The Cultural Context of Breastfeeding in the United States." *Breastfeeding: Biocultural Perspectives.* Eds. Patricia Stuart-Macadam and Katherine A. Dettwyler. New York: Aldine De Gruyler, 1995. 167-215.

DiQuinzio, Patrice. *The Impossibility of Motherhood: Feminism, Individualism and the Problem of Mothering*. New York: Routledge, 1999.

Dykes, Fiona. "'Supply and Demand': Breastfeeding as Labour." *Social Science and Medicine* 60 (2005): 2283-93.

Ferguson, Amanda. "'Lactivists' back mom in breastfeeding beef with Web site." *National Post,* September 13 2007. Acessesed 11 December 2007 <http://www.nationalpost.com/news/story.html?id=561f5869-195f-4cfc-bed4-024c3b729893&k=36166>.

Gatens, Moira. *The Imaginary Bodies: Ethics, Power and Corporeality.* New York: Routledge, 1995.

Giles, Fiona. "Fountains of Love and Loveliness: In Praise of the Dripping Wet Breast." *Journal of the Association for Research on Mothering* 4.1 (2002): 7-17.

Grosz, Elizabeth. *Volatile Bodies: Towards a Feminist Corporeality*. Sydney: Allen & Unwin, 1994.

Hausman, Bernice, L. "The Feminist Politics of Breastfeeding." *Australian Feminist Studies* 19.45 (2004): 273-83.

Hays, Sharon. *The Cultural Contradictions of Motherhood.* New Haven: Yale University Press 1996.

Kelleher, Christa M. "The Physical Challenges of Early Breastfeeding." *Social Science & Medicine* 63.10 (2006): 2727-38.

Longhurst, Robyn. *Bodies: Exploring Fluid Boundaries.* London: Routledge, 2001.

Maher, Vanessa. "Breastfeeding in Cross Cultural Perspective: Paradoxes and Proposals." *The Anthropology of Breastfeeding: Natural Law or Social Construct?* Ed. Vanessa Maher: Berg Publishers, 1992. 1-26.

Mahon-Daly, Patricia and Gavin J. Andrews. "Liminality and Breastfeeding: Women Negotiating Space and Two Bodies." *Health and Place* 8 (2002): 61-76.

Maushart, Susan. *The Mask of Motherhood.* Vintage, 1997.

Moses, Asher. "Facebook incurs lactivist wrath." *Age.* September 7 2007. Assessed 11 December 2007. <http://www.theage.com.au/news/web/facebook-bans-obscene-breastfeeding-mums/2007/09/07/1188783470779.html>.

Nash, Meredith. "Oh Baby, Baby: (Un)Veiling Britney Spears' Pregnant Body." *Michigan Feminist Studies* 19.Fall (2006): 27-50.

Palmer, Gabrielle. *The Politics of Breastfeeding.* London: Pandora, 1988.

Paz Gulupo, M. and F. Jean Ayres. "Negotiating the Maternal and Sexual Breast: Narratives of Breastfeeding Mothers." *Journal of the Association for Research on Mothering* 4.1 (2002): 20-30.

Rothman, Barbara Katz. *Recreating Motherhood: Ideology and Technology in Patriarchal Society.* New York: W. W Norton & Company, 1989.

Schmied, Virginia. *Blurring the Boundaries: Breastfeeding as Discursive Construction and Embodied Experience.* Unpublished Ph.D. Thesis, Faculty of Nursing, University of Technology Sydney, 1998.

Schmied, Virgina, and Leslie Barclay. "Connection and Pleasure, Disruption and Distress: Women's experiences of Breastfeeding." *Journal of Human Lactation* 15.4 (1999): 325-334.

Shaw, Rhonda. "Performing Breastfeeding: Embodiment, Ethics and the Maternal Subject." *Feminist Review* 78 (2004): 99-116.

Shildrick, Magrit. *Leaky Bodies and Boundaries: Feminism, Post-Modernism and (Bio)Ethics.* London: Routledge, 1997.

Stearns, Cindy. "Breastfeeding and the Good Maternal Body." *Gender and Society* 13.3 (1999): 308-25.

Van Esterik, Penny. "Thank-You, Breasts! Breastfeeding as a Feminist Issue." *Ethnographic Feminisms.* Eds. Sally Cole and Lynne Phillips. Ottawa: Carelton University Press, 1995. 75-91.

Wall, Glenda (2001). "Moral Constructions of Motherhood in Breastfeeding Discourse." *Gender and Society* 15.4: 592-610.

Wilkinson, Sue "How Useful are Focus Groups in Feminist Research?" *Developing Focus Group Research.* Ed. Rosaline Barbour and Jenny Kitzinger. London: Sage Publications, 1999: 65-78.

Young, Iris Marion. *Throwing Like a Girl and Other Essays in Feminist Philosophy and Social Theory.* Bloomington: Indiana University Press, 1990.

Receiving and Enjoying Milk

What Breastfeeding Means to Children

KARLEEN GRIBBLE

MOTHERS ARE PLACED IN an invidious position when it comes to breastfeeding in Western cultures. They are exhorted to breastfeed their babies but they face social sanctioning if they do it too frequently, too publicly, too revealingly and, above all, if they do it for too long. While breastfeeding a very young baby is considered virtuous, long-term breastfeeding is frequently viewed as perverse. Mothers who delay weaning past infancy are commonly accused of forcing their children to breastfeed because they are emotionally needy and unable to allow them to grow up (e.g. Borton 135-137; Stearns; Rowe). Even more disturbingly it has been suggested by some that mothers gain a type of sexual pleasure from breastfeeding and are therefore abusing their children by continuing to breastfeed (e.g. Stearns; Piovanetti; Wilson-Clay). These views ignore medical, historical and anthropological research supporting the normality of breastfeeding up to middle childhood (Dettwyler; Piovanetti; Sellen) and clearly flow from a cultural paradigm in which breasts have been sexualised and early weaning normalised.

The pathologising of long-term breastfeeding is problematic. It results in some women weaning before they would otherwise (Gribble, "Long Term Breastfeeding"). Many others continue to breastfeed but hide the practice (e.g. Wrigley and Hutchinson) or endure the disapproval. However, when such disapproval comes from those in authority, mothers may fear the consequences of continuing to breastfeed. The author has been contacted by women who were worried that health or education professionals were going to report them to social services for abusing their children by continuing to breastfeed. These mothers were concerned that their children might be taken from them. Whilst these fears are largely unfounded, there have been cases in the United States where children were removed from their mother's care because they were breastfeeding.[1]

However, breastfeeding is not something that mothers can do on their own; it is a cooperative activity between two individuals. In fact, strictly speaking, mothers do not breastfeed at all; it is the children who suckle at the breast and who are doing the breastfeeding. Further, research on long-term breastfeeding has identified that rather than mothers being the driver for breastfeeding continuance, it is the motivation of the children to keep breastfeeding that persuades mothers to delay weaning (Buckley, "Beliefs and Practices"; Buckley, "Comparison of Long-Term Breastfeeding"; Hills-Bonczyk et al.; Gribble, "As Good as Chocolate").

This chapter will attempt to explore breastfeeding from the child's point of view and describe what breastfeeding means to the children who breastfeed. The main source for this chapter is a study the author conducted into long-term breastfeeding involving 114 Australian breastfeeding dyads in which the child was at least two years of age. Dyads were recruited via advertisement and word of mouth. The Australian Breastfeeding Association dispersed information about the study via their network of breastfeeding support groups and the distribution of information about the study to anyone who might qualify as a participant was encouraged. As a result, descriptions of the study were posted on a number of other Internet sites and information about the study was disseminated outside the ABA network.Data for this study was generated through completion of a written questionnaire that explored mothers' opinions about their children's motivations for breastfeeding. There were also a number of questions about breastfeeding for mothers to ask their children (a detailed description of study design can be found in Gribble "As Good as Chocolate"). This chapter will include ample quotes from the mothers in this study, putting forward what they understand of their children's experience; and from children themselves; giving voice to the actual breastfeeders. It will describe how breastfeeding means pleasure, delicious food, comfort and calming, caring, security and closeness to children and how breastfeeding is normal to them. It is worth noting that while some mothers in the study articulated disatisfaction with aspects of the breastfeeding relationship, the children were unanimously positive in their expression of their experience of breastfeeding.

BREASTFEEDING MEANS PLEASURE

Mothers who have delayed weaning past infancy have indicated that the enjoyment that their child takes from breastfeeding is an important factor in their willingness to delay weaning. It is very clear to mothers that breastfeeding is pleasurable to their children. As one mother said,

> *It's his favourite thing in the whole world.*

Mothers know that their children want to breastfeed by the way in which they actively seek breastfeeding; by directly asking for it or gaining access to the breast on their own (Gribble, "As Good as Chocolate"). However, children also show their mothers that they enjoy breastfeeding in other ways. For example,

> *She strokes my breasts ... and says, "I like boobies."*[2]

He'll say things like, "I love breastfeeding mum" and after a feed, "That was wonderful."

For a while he would interrupt his feeds to tell me, "I luff dat nigh nigh boo boo mummy."

My daughter was breastfeeding when she came off, said, "milk" and then gave me the "thumbs up" sign that she used to say "good."

[He says], "I just love it."

[She says], "Mamma I like di di."

Such spontaneous expressions of enjoyment from children leave mothers with no doubt of the value their children place on breastfeeding. Further evidence that breastfeeding means pleasure to children is provided by the children's responses when they are asked why they like breastfeeding and what they feel like when they breastfeed. The most common reason that children give for breastfeeding is that they like or love breastfeeding (Gribble, "As Good as Chocolate"). Their descriptions of what they feel like when they breastfeed provides insight into why they like breastfeeding; children say that breastfeeding makes them feel happy, good, nice, warm and loved (Gribble, "As Good as Chocolate"). For example:

Nice and warm,
Nice and snuggly,
Feel good, feel happy,
I feel comfortable and I like it when you pat my hair and hold my legs.

BREASTFEEDING MEANS DELICIOUS FOOD

In the early months of life, the nutritional aspect of breastfeeding, that is the provision of breastmilk, is critically important to children. Whilst breastmilk can remain a valuable component of a child's diet well into early childhood, it is also true that its importance as a food diminishes as children grow (Buckley, "Nourishment or Nurturance"). Nonetheless, children who are old enough to be eating a wide variety and substantial amount of other food still enjoy drinking breastmilk. Mothers recognise that breastmilk is a motivator for breastfeeding and commonly indicate the taste of breastmilk as a reason for their child wanting to breastfeed (Gribble, "As Good as Chocolate"). It is common for older children to tell their mothers that they like the taste of breastmilk. For example,

He told me during the feed that the milk was "lovely."

My son says things like, "I love mummy's milk" and "you have yummy mummy's milk."

Further, when children are asked why they breastfeed the second most frequently provided reason is that they like the taste of the milk (Gribble, "As Good as Chocolate"). For example,

I love breast-milk.

I like the booby and Mummy's milk tastes yummy.

When children are asked what breastmilk tastes like they provide a range of different adjectives as descriptors, the most common of which is "*yummy*" but descriptions of the milk as "*warm,*" "*sweet*" and "*nice*" are also common. For example,

Milk is yummy,
Yummy mummy Joshy milk,
It's warm and yummy,
Yum, yum, yum, yum!
Nice, milky, like milk. I love it.

In addition to using adjectives to describe breastmilk, children also frequently compare breastmilk to the taste of a type of food. These foods include: milk, lollies, strawberries, ice cream, sugar, cordial, fruit salad, banana, mango, oranges, pear, jam, strawberry milk, chocolate milk, cows milk, rice milk, buttermilk, milkshake, peanut butter, cheese and jelly beans. It appears that the common factor in these comparisons is that children associate the flavour of breastmilk with a food they consider delicious.[3] The following exchange provided by one mother, supports this conclusion.

Mother: *What does the milk taste like?*
Child: *Warm milk.*
Mother: *Have a drink, what does it taste like?*
Child: *Cold milk. Tastes like oranges.*
Mother: *Do you like oranges?*
Child: *I love oranges!*

BREASTFEEDING MEANS COMFORT AND CALMING

Mothers note that children use breastfeeding to calm themselves (Kendall-Tackett and Sugarman) and that they find it comforting (Buckley, "Beliefs and Practices"). Breastfeeding for comfort is the reason most commonly provided by mothers for children wanting to breastfeed (Gribble, "As Good as Chocolate"). Mothers' opinion that their child finds comfort in breastfeeding comes from several different sources. Firstly, mothers have noticed that their children seek breastfeeding when they are upset or otherwise in need of calming and comforting. For example,

> *She feeds mostly when she is hurt, tired, or sick/upset, which leads me to believe that it is a source of great comfort to her.*

In addition, mothers observe that when their child breastfeeds they are calmed and comforted. For example,

> *Breastfeeding mends falls, bumps and bruises.*

> *[Breastfeeding has] amazing power ... to calm a toddler.*

> *It is an instant panacea when he is hurt, tired or upset about something.*

> *[Breastfeeding has an] instant calming influence on my daughter; she only needs two or three sucks and is "okay now."*

Toddlerhood is a developmental stage when the ability of a mother to calm her child is important. Toddlers often have much that they wish to communicate but limited ability to do so (Colson and Dworkin) and their desire for independence may outstrip their abilities. Both of these difficulties can be a source of great distress to them (Colson and Dworkin) and their distress can quickly escalate because their ability to self regulate their emotions is not yet established (Thompson and Goodwim). Many mothers view breastfeeding as a tool in their parenting repertoire that enables them to easily comfort their child when they encounter frustration or hurt. For instance,

> *Breastfeeding is such a major part of my parenting. It gives her comfort when she needs it, when we have been irritable with one another it brings us back together. It always makes her happy no matter what. If it doesn't make her happy it puts her to sleep.*

As in the previous quote, an association between breastfeeding and sleep is frequently described by mothers and the most common time for long-term breastfeeding children to breastfeed is when they are going to sleep (Gribble, "As Good as Chocolate"). The calming, comforting and sleep inducing affects of breastfeeding result from a variety of hormonal and physical mechanisms (Barr et al.; Blass and Ciaramitaro; Blass, "Consequences of Suckling"; Blass, "Mothers and Their Infants"; Blass, "Milk-Induced Hypoalgesia"; Carbajal et al.; Schore; Smotherman and Robinson; Uvnas-Moberg; Uvnas-Moberg et al.). Mothers often deliberately take advantage of the relaxant impact of breastfeeding and use it to help them to help their child to sleep. For example,

> *Getting my child to sleep with a breastfeed is much easier than any other method such as "hands on settling" or "controlled crying" as well as less traumatic for both mother and child.*

> *Such an easy way to get babies and preschoolers to sleep.*

> *She likes to feed to sleep and for both of us it is relaxing and for me an easy way to get her off to sleep.*

Breastfeeding to sleep is considered an undesirable practice in many Western cultures because it is believed that children should go to sleep without any assistance from an adult (Ferber; Hiscock et al.; Lam, Hiscock and Wake). However, the transition to sleep is stressful for many children (Green, Groves and Tegano; Sadah; Mahalski; Wolf and Lozoff) and children commonly find it difficult to go to sleep on their own (Hiscock et al.). This results in a high rate of diagnosis of "sleep disorders" in Western societies (Thunstrom; Hiscock et al.). In addition, anthropological research has concluded that cultural beliefs demanding solitary sleep are in conflict with children's psychological and biological needs (McKenna et al.). This suggests that demands that children go to sleep without adult assistance be reconsidered. It is possible that the incidence of sleep difficulties identified in Western societies would be greatly decreased if breastfeeding was considered an appropriate aid to children in going to sleep.

It is not only mothers who are consciously aware of the calming and comforting action of breastfeeding, some children are also able to verbalise their use of breastfeeds to obtain comfort and to relax. For instance,

> *If [my son] has hurt himself he has called out to me while crying that he "Needs booby to fix it better."*

> *[She has said,] "If you fall over and hurt yourself then you have non-non to make it better."*

And some children, when asked why they breastfeed, put the comforting and sleep inducing aspects forward as a reason. For example,

> *When I'm grizzly I have milk.*

> *I like it ... when I'm sad.*

> *Help John ... cry.*
> *(Mother's interpretation, "Helps John when he is crying.").*

It helps me to go to sleep.

Other children, when asked what they feel like when they breastfeed describe how breastfeeding feels calming and comforting. For instance,

Makes me feel better.

[I feel] tired, calmed down.

Some children also recognise that the calming and comforting associated with breastfeeding might assist other children. Thus, when seeing an infant or young child who is distressed, they may state that breastfeeding would help that child to calm down. For instance,

Sometimes if another child is sad he will say, "He/she sad, they want some booby."

[My son has said,] "Jack is upset mum, give him some breastmilk, that will make him better."

They both will say, "He needs some barky," if they hear a baby crying.

BREASTFEEDING MEANS "MY MOTHER IS AVAILABLE TO ME AND CARES ABOUT ME"

Mothers note that breastfeeding forces them to stop doing things and spend time with their children (Buckley, "Beliefs and Practices"; Epstein) and that sometimes their children want to breastfeed simply to have time with them.

Sometimes I think she feeds to get attention.

[She breastfeeds] to spend time with me.

In instances where a mother has a busy life, perhaps with other children to attend to, breastfeeding can provide an important link, facilitating one-on-one contact that might not otherwise occur or might occur less frequently (Epstein). For example,

[She breastfeeds for] attention and cuddles (she has to compete with two older siblings for my time!)

Mothers believe that in being available to their children and breastfeeding that they are assisting their children to feel safe and secure (Reamer and Sugarman). For example,

> *For a toddler whose world is growing and changing every day it is the constant. It helps her feel confident and secure as she approaches life from her little shoes.*

> *I think breastfeeding helps Chloe feel safe.*

> *I think she breastfeeds ... because it makes her feel secure.*

They also notice that their children breastfeed when they are feeling unsure or threatened. For instance,

> *Whenever the world seems a hostile place he asks for boobie.*

> *[Breastfeeding] helps him in situations where he feels uneasy, shy etc.*

Some children are able to express how breastfeeding helps them to feel more secure. For example, when asked why he breastfed, one child said it was *"to make me brave"* and another child said that she feels *"safe"* when she breastfeeds.

The way in which children use breastfeeding to find security when they are feeling unsure of themselves, as well as the use of breastfeeding to obtain comfort, suggests that breastfeeding is an important attachment behaviour for these children. Within attachment theory, attachment behaviours are actions that a child uses to maintain proximity to their caregiver in order to obtain reassurance and experience feelings of safety (Sutton). Attachment theory is the dominant framework within which early relationships are understood (Thompson) and the development of a secure attachment between primary caregiver and child is deemed the most beneficial type of relationship (Schore). Securely attached children use their caregiver as a base from which to explore the world and are therefore able to more effectively deal with challenges (Drury-Hudson). In addition to acting as an attachment behaviour, breastfeeding also impacts the physiology and physical circumstances of mothers in such a way as to assist them to sensitively care for their children (Gribble, "Mental Health"). Thus, breastfeeding may promote the development of a secure child-mother attachment. However, the importance of breastfeeding as an attachment behaviour also means that if breastfeeding is abruptly terminated it may have a serious adverse impact on the child-mother relationship (Ainsworth and Tracey).

BREASTFEEDING MEANS CLOSENESS AND INTIMACY

When mothers are asked what they most like about breastfeeding their most common answer is that they enjoy the closeness and intimacy associated with it. Mothers also nominate the closeness of breastfeeding as being a motivator for their children breastfeeding. For instance,

[She breastfeeds] to be close to me, the intimacy.

I think she breastfeeds because she enjoys these times of "closeness" with me.

He likes to snuggle up and be close to me.

[She breastfeeds] to be close to mummy. She has told me that the milk is warm and that she likes it so I am sure she prefers it to Milk In The Fridge but I think it is really a close cuddle at the end of the day for her.

One child when asked why he breastfed was able to express that he breastfeeds for the physical closeness, "*Like cuddling mummy, it's mine treat.*"

Children's appreciation of the closeness of breastfeeding is also evident in their descriptions of feeling cuddly or snuggly when they breastfeed. For instance,

Um, happy and cuddly.

Warm and snuggly.

Some children also say that they feel loved when they breastfeed. For example,

Close to mummy, mummy loves me.

Zoe says she feels loved when she is breastfeeding

I'm loved.

In addition to feeling love while breastfeeding, children seem to also view breastfeeding as a way of showing their love to their mother. Thus, some children when asked why they breastfeed included the giving of love in their reply saying,

Because I love you, because I love breastmilk.

I just love it, and I love you.

Observational research of the interactions between mother and child during breastfeeds provides the reasons underlying why mothers describe breastfeeding as an intimate act and why children might say that they give and receive love during breastfeeds. Such observational research has found that during breastfeeding sessions the mother and child spend time in positive mutual visual regard which is often contingent with smiling and conversation (Epstein). Tactile stimulation as mothers and children pat and caress one another has also been observed and reported by mothers (Gribble, "As Good as Chocolate"; Epstein). Thus, breastfeeding provides visual, verbal and physical intimacy.

BREASTFEEDING IS NORMAL

To long-term breastfeeding children, breastfeeding is normal: it is an ordinary activity that is integrated into their lives (Gribble, "As Good as Chocolate"). The normality with which children view breastfeeding is shown in how they talk about it. Rather than reflecting the view predominant in Western cultures of breasts as a sex organ, children view breasts as being for breastfeeding and are often quite fascinated by lactation in not just humans, but also in other mammals. For instance,

> *She loves going through my Mother and Baby magazines and seeing babies being breastfed.*

> *When friends had new babies he'd talk about the baby having the milk.*

> *She asked me if baby elephants drink mummy milk—has since asked questions about many different animals.*

> *Kangaroos have moolka memmas.*

Even where breasts are in a context not connected to breastfeeding, children may seek to understand their presentation as being related to breastfeeding.

> *John was in the shower and saw a sign about breast self-examination. After looking at the illustrations (line drawings of breast self examination in the shower, lying down and in front of the mirror) he told me that it was a sign saying how you should have a shower, get dry, put your jammies on, lie on your bed and then the baby says "milk, milk, milk" so you give it a breastfeed…a picture of bare breasts and someone handling them was understood by him to be about breastfeeding.*

> *He has commented on seeing a* Sports Illustrated *magazine that the lady had "beautiful breasts" and that she had them "all out ready for breastfeeding."*

Children may also place bottles in a context where they are used to provide breastmilk to babies. For instance,

> *Instead of making cars/planes out of Lego, Laura's favourite is a Lego breastpump… She plays with her pumps and often says that the little dolly*

> *bottles have breastmilk in them … the kids play at pumping milk and putting it in the little toy bottles before giving it to their dolls.*

The normality with which these children view breastfeeding is startling when it is compared to other research in which children considered bottle feeding the default way of feeding babies (Russell et al.). That bottle feeding might be considered normal in many Western contexts is not surprising since short durations of breastfeeding and the stigma associated with breastfeeding in public mean that breastfeeding might be only rarely seen (Cricco-Lizza "Infant Feeding Beliefs," "Student Nurses' Attidues"). In contrast, bottle feeding is familiar and visible in the public domain and television and picture books commonly present bottle feeding as the usual feeding method (Henderson, Kitzinger and Green; Henderson; Altshuler). In addition, children are socialised in the bottle feeding of babies by the routine provision of bottles with baby dolls (Gribble, "As Good as Chocolate"). What is different for long-term breastfeeding children who, rather than connecting bottles and babies connect breasts and babies and see breasts as representing breastfeeding? One can conclude that it is in the practice of breastfeeding themselves and commonly seeing other children breastfeed, including younger siblings, that they have formulated this view.

Since breastfeeding is normal to long-term breastfeeders, they see breastfeeding as an activity that they will engage in in the future. For instance,

> *[She talks] about her baby who she will breastfeed when she has milk in her "boobies."*

It is perhaps because they anticipate that they will need to know how to breastfeed when they become parents that children are interested in learning about breastfeeding. Children frequently role-play breastfeeding as a way of facilitating learning (Gribble, "As Good as Chocolate"). For example,

> *At the moment my daughter talks about "her" milk. She quite often says she needs to feed her baby and will sit down and lift her top and start breastfeeding the doll. Usually she has the doll in the right position and she checks where the doll's mouth is compared to her nipple.*

> *They … pretend to breastfeed their dolls and teddies … they will say "Dolly/teddy go to sleep now, dolly wake up, dolly have booby."*

> *She does role model me a lot and breastfeeds all her dolls and even tandem feeding two at a time.*

Learning about breastfeeding via role-play with dolls is common in cultural contexts where breastfeeding is common (e.g. Goldman and Smith; Rossie;

Thomson 38). In such contexts, dolls are considered a type of 'educational' toy (Roy; Thomson 38).

In addition to learning about breastfeeding via role play, children also discuss breastfeeding with their mothers. Their conversations reveal that this provides them with the opportunity to learn useful information about breastfeeding. This is shown in the following examples in which the demand/supply principle of milk production and the exclusivity of newborn breastfeeding are discussed:

> *She used to often talk about how the milk got there. Around 3 years she asked me "Can I help you make the milk?" I told her she just did by having a feed.*

> *Since having the baby she will say things like, "Judy only eats non-non, but I can eat other things."*

A lack of experience and knowledge of breastfeeding prior to birth has been identified as contributing to breastfeeding difficulties and early weaning (Dykes and Williams; Hill and Aldag). It is understood that breastfeeding is best learnt about over time, from childhood. These long-term breastfeeders, within an environment where breastfeeding is normal have had the opportunity to do this. As one mother described,

> *She has a real, in depth understanding of breastfeeding, how mothers nurture their young, how normal it is. What milk is, where it comes from, what it is for. We often see others breastfeeding, often see pictures, photos of breastfeeding. Already it is a part of normal life.... This is how we learn to breastfeed, by watching others.*

CONCLUSION

Mothers and long-term breastfeeding children know that there is considerably more to breastfeeding than the supply of a food. Children clearly take pleasure, find comfort and relaxation and closeness with their mother in the process of obtaining milk via breastfeeding as well as enjoying the milk itself. For mothers, hearing and seeing their child express their pleasure in this intimate and exclusive interaction remains a motivator to allow continuance of the breastfeeding relationship. These other aspects of breastfeeding should be valued and the pathologising of maternal motivations for long-term breastfeeding discontinued. We need to listen to the children.

[1]In 2001, in Illinois, a five year old boy was removed from his mother's care for six months after a baby sitter phoned an abuse hotline and reported that the child was still being breastfed (Corbett). In 2003, in Texas, four year old

and one year old boys were removed from the care of their mother for five months after staff from a photo laboratory called child protection when they saw a photograph of the one year old breastfeeding (Korosec).

[2]Quotes contain the words that children use for breastfeeding. The most common word for breastfeeding in the long-term breastfeeding study was boob/boobie followed by mummy/mumma milk, milk, breastfeed/breastmilk, feed and boo-boo. There were a total of fifty-six different names used. These names generally came into use by the child through being used by the mother or another family member for breastfeeding or being derived from a word used by the mother or other family member.

[3]There were some other interesting descriptions used by children in the long-term breastfeeding study including that breastmilk "*tastes like McDonalds*," "*beer*" and "*pink*." In regards to the child who said that breastmilk tasted like "*McDonalds*" it is worth noting that fast food corporations have spent considerable effort developing brand loyalty and desire for particular foods in very young children (Story and French). Research has found that to young Australian children McDonalds symbolises all the things that they like (Langer and Farrar). The mother of this child commented that she was not sure if the comparison of her breastmilk to McDonalds food was "*an insult or a compliment but I suppose that breastfeeding is a 'Happy Meal.'*" Given that McDonalds is a corporation that has deliberately sought to make their food attractive to toddlers it can be concluded that the child was complimenting breastmilk by comparing it to McDonalds. The mother of the boy who said that breastmilk tasted like "beer" was not aware of where this description came from. However, research has found that preschool aged children are highly attentive to the use and enjoyment of alcohol (Dalton et al.). One can speculate that this child had learnt that beer is considered an enjoyable and delicious drink in Australian culture (Pettigrew) and so thought it appropriate to compare breastmilk to "*beer*." Similarly, one could speculate that the little girl who said that breastmilk tasted "*pink*" was making a statement about her personal colour preference. Sex stereotyping of colours results in girls consistently choosing pink objects as their favourite (Picariello, Greenberg and Pillemer) and research has found that children associate the colour pink with happiness (Boyatzis and Varghese).

REFERENCES

Ainsworth, Mary D.S., and Russel L. Tracey. "Infant Feeding and Attachment." ERIC (1972).

Altshuler, Anne. "Breastfeeding in Children's Books: Reflecting and Shaping Our Values." *Journal of Human Lactation* 11.4 (1995): 293-305.

Barr, Ronald G., Simon N. Young, Rajaa Alkawaf, and Lea Wertheim. "Does Mature Hindmilk Taste Calm Crying Infants?" *Pediatric Research* 39.2 (1996): 16.

Blass, Elliot M. "Behavioral and Physiological Consequences of Suckling in Rat and Human Newborns." *Acta Paediatrica* 397.Supplement (1994): 71-76.

Blass, Elliot M. "Milk-Induced Hypoalgesia in Human Newborns." *Pediatrics* 99.6 (1997): 825-29.

Blass, Elliot M. "Mothers and Their Infants: Peptide-Mediated Physiological, Behavioral and Affective Changes During Suckling." *Regulatory Peptides* 66.1-2 (1996): 109-12.

Blass, Elliot M., and Vivian Ciaramitaro. "A New Look at Some Old Mechanisms in Human Newborns: Taste and Tactile Determinants of State, Affect, and Action." *Monographs of the Society for Research in Child Development.* 59.1 (1994): 1-81.

Borton, Leanne. "Parenting Choice or Collapse of Mutual Recognition? An Intersubjective Analysis of Extended Breastfeeding." Unpublished doctoral dissertation. California Institute of Integral Studies. 2000.

Boyatzis, Chris J., and Reenu Varghese. "Children's Emotional Associations with Colors." *Journal of Genetic Psychology* 155.1 (1994): 77.

Buckley, Kathleen M. "Beliefs and Practices Related to Extended Breastfeeding among La Leche League Mothers." *Journal of Perinatal Education* 1.2 (1992): 45-53.

Buckley, Kathleen M. "A Comparison of Long-Term Breastfeeding among Hispanics and Non-Hispanics." *Current Issues in Clinical Lactation*. Ed. Kathlen G. Auerbach. Vol. 2. Boston: Jones and Bartlett Publishers, 2002. 23-35.

Buckley, Kathleen M. "Long-Term Breastfeeding: Nourishment or Nurturance?" *Journal of Human Lactation.* 17.4 (2001): 304-12.

Carbajal, Ricardo, Soocramanien Veerapen, Sophie Couderc, Myriam Jugie, and Yves Ville. "Analgesic Effect of Breast Feeding in Term Neonates: Randomised Controlled Trial." *British Medical Journal* 326.7379 (2003): 13.

Colson, Eve R., and Paul H. Dworkin. "Toddler Development." *Pediatrics in Review* 18.8 (1997): 255-59.

Corbett, Sara. "The Breast Offense." *New York Times* 6 May 2001, sec. 6: 82.

Cricco-Lizza, Roberta. "Infant-Feeding Beliefs and Experiences of Black Women Enrolled in WIC in the New York Metropolitan Area." *Qualitative Health Research* 14.9 (2004): 1197-210.

Cricco-Lizza, Roberta. "Student Nurses' Attitudes and Beliefs About Breast-Feeding." *Journal of Professional Nursing* 22.5 (2006): 314-21.

Dalton, Madeline A., Amy M. Bernhardt, Jennifer J. Gibson, James D. Sargent, Michael L. Beach, Anna M. Adachi, Linda T. Titus-Ernstoff, and Todd F. Heatherton. "Use of Cigarettes and Alcohol by Preschoolers While Role-Playing as Adults: 'Honey, Have Some Smokes'." *Archives of Pediatrics and Adolescent Medicine* 159.9 (2005): 854-59.

Dettwyler, Katherine A. "A Time to Wean: The Hominid Blueprint for the Natural Age of Weaning in Modern Human Populations." *Breastfeeding: Biocultural Perspectives.* Eds. Patricia Stuart-Macadam and Katherine A.

Dettwyler. New York: Aldine de Gruyter, 1995. 39-73.

Drury-Hudson, Julie. "Some Effects of Attachment Disturbance on Child Behaviour." *Children Australia* 19.1 (1994): 17-22.

Dykes, Fiona, and Catherine Williams. "Falling by the Wayside: A Phenomenological Exploration of Perceived Breast-Milk Inadequacy in Lactating Women." *Midwifery* 15.4 (1999): 232-46.

Epstein, Karen. "The Interactions between Breastfeeding Mothers and Their Babies During the Breastfeeding Session." *Early Child Development and Care* 87.1 (1993): 93-104.

Ferber, Richard A. "Behavioral 'Insomnia' in the Child." *Psychiatric Clinics of North America.* 10.4 (1987): 641-53.

Goldman, Laurence, and Calvin Smith. "Imagining Identities: Mimetic Constructions in Huli Child Fantasy Play." *Journal of the Royal Anthropological Institute* 4.2 (1998): 207-34.

Green, Katherine E., Melissa M. Groves, and Deborah W. Tegano. "Parenting Practices That Limit Transitional Object Use: An Illustration." *Early Child Development and Care* 174.5 (2004): 427-36.

Gribble, Karleen D. "'As Good as Chocolate' and 'Better Than Ice Cream': How Toddler, and Older, Breastfeeders Experience Breastfeeding." *Early Child Development and Care* iFirst Article (2008): 1-16.

Gribble, Karleen D."Long-Term Breastfeeding: Changing Attitudes and Overcoming Challenges." *Breastfeeding Review* 16.1 (2008): 5-15.

Gribble, Karleen D. "Mental Health, Attachment and Breastfeeding: Implications for Adopted Children and Their Mothers." *International Breastfeeding Journal* 1 (2006): 5.

Henderson, Ann M. "Mixed Messages About the Meanings of Breast-Feeding Representations in the Australian Press and Popular Magazines." *Midwifery* 15.1 (1999): 24-31.

Henderson, Lesley, Jenny Kitzinger, and Jospehine Green. "Representing Infant Feeding: Content Analysis of British Media Portrayals of Bottle Feeding and Breast Feeding." *British Medical Journal* 321.7270 (2000): 1196-98.

Hill, Pamela D., and Jean Aldag. "Potential Indicators of Insufficient Milk Supply Syndrome." *Research in Nursing and Health* 14.1 (1991): 11-19.

Hills-Bonczyk, Sharon G., Kristine R. Tromiczak, Melissa D Avery, Susan Potter, Kay Savik, and Laura J. Duckett. "Women's Experiences with Breastfeeding Longer Than 12 Months." *Birth* 21.4 (1994): 206-12.

Hiscock, Harriet, Louise Canterford, Obioha C. Ukoumunne, and Melissa Wake. "Adverse Associations of Sleep Problems in Australian Preschoolers: National Population Study." *Pediatrics* 119.1 (2007): 86-93.

Kendall-Tackett, Kathleen A., and Muriel Sugarman. "The Social Consequences of Long-Term Breastfeeding." *Journal of Human Lactation.* 11.3 (1995): 179-83.

Korosec, Thomas. "1 Hour Arrest. When Does a Snapshot of a Mother Breast-Feeding Her Child Become Kiddie Porn? Ask the Richardson Police." *Dallas*

Observer 17 April 2003.

Lam, Peiyoong, Harriet Hiscock, and Melissa Wake. "Outcomes of Infant Sleep Problems: A Longitudinal Study of Sleep, Behavior, and Maternal Well-Being." *Pediatrics* 111.3 (2003): 203-07.

Langer, Beryl, and Estelle Farrar. "Becoming 'Australian' in the Global Cultural Economy: Children, Consumption, Citizenship." *Journal of Australian Studies* 79 (2003): 117-26.

Mahalski, Pauline A. "The Incidence of Attachment Objects and Oral Habits at Bedtime in Two Longtitudinal Samples of Children Aged 1.5 -7 Years." *Journal of Child Psychology and Psychiatry* 24.2 (1983): 283-95.

McKenna, James J., Evelyn B. Thoman, Thomas F. Anders, Abraham Sadeh, Vicki L. Schechtman, and Steven F. Glotzbach. "Infant-Parent Co-Sleeping in an Evolutionary Perspective: Implications for Understanding Infant Sleep Development and the Sudden Infant Death Syndrome." *Sleep* 16.3 (1993): 263-82.

Pettigrew, Simone. "A Grounded Theory of Beer Consumption in Australia." *Qualitative Market Research* 5.2 (2002): 112.

Picariello, Martha L., Danna N. Greenberg, and David B. Pillemer. "Children's Sex-Related Stereotyping of Colors." *Child Development* 61.5 (1990): 1453-60.

Piovanetti, Yvette. "Breastfeeding Beyond 12 Months: An Historical Perspective." *Pediatric Clinics of North America* 48.1 (2001): 199-206.

Reamer, Sue B., and Muriel Sugarman. "Breast Feeding Beyond Six Months: Mothers' Perceptions of the Positive and Negative Consequences." *Journal of Tropical Pediatrics* 33.2 (1987): 93-97.

Rossie, Jean-Pierre. "Breastfeeding of Dolls in Morocco." Email to K. Gribble. 14 Nov. 2007.

Rowe, Dorothy. "Breast Feeding: Know When to Stop…" *The Times* 5 May 2005.

Roy, Christopher D. "Mossi Dolls." *African Arts* 14.4 (1981): 47-51, 88.

Russell, Bridie, Helen Richards, Anni Jones, and Pat Hoddinott. "'Breakfast, Lunch and Dinner': Attitudes to Infant Feeding Amongst Children in a Scottish Primary School. A Qualitative Focus Group Study." *Health Education Journal* 63.1 (2004): 70-80.

Sadah, Avi. "Stress, Trauma and Sleep in Children." *Child and Adolescent Psychiatric Clinics of North America* 5.3 (1996): 685-700.

Schore, Allan. N. "Effects of a Secure Attachment Relationship on Right Brain Development, Affect Regulation, and Infant Mental Health." *Infant Mental Health Journal* 22.1-2 (2001): 7-66.

Sellen, Daniel W. "Comparison of Infant Feeding Patterns Reported for Nonindustrial Populations with Current Recommendations." *Journal of Nutrition* 131.10 (2001): 2707-15.

Smotherman, William P., and Scott R. Robinson. "Milk as the Proximal Mechanism for Behavioral Change in the Newborn." *Acta Paediatrica* 397.

Supplement (1994): 64-70.
Stearns, Cindy A. "Breastfeeding and the Good Maternal Body." *Gender and Society* 13.3 (1999): 308-25.
Story, Mary, and Simone French. "Food Advertising and Marketing Directed at Children and Adolescents in the Us." *International Journal of Behavioral Nutrition and Physical Activity* 1 (2004): 3.
Sutton, Carole. "Resurgence of Attachment (Behaviours) within a Cognitive Behavioural Intervention: Evidence from Research." *Behavioural and Cognitive Psychotherapy* 29 (2001): 357-66.
Thompson, Ross A. "The Legacy of Early Attachments." *Child Development* 71.1 (2000): 145-52.
Thompson, Ross A., and Rebecca Goodvim. "Taming the Tempest in the Teapot: Emotion Regulation in Toddlers." *Socioemotional Development in the Toddler Years: Transitions and Transformations*. Eds. Celia A. Brownell and Claire B. Kopp. New York: Guilford Publications, 2007. 320-44.
Thomson, Donald. *Children of the Wilderness*. Melbourne: Currey O'Neil Ross Pty Ltd, 1983.
Thunstrom, Malena. "Severe Sleep Problems among Infants in a Normal Population in Sweden: Prevalence, Severity and Correlates." *Acta Paediatrica* 88.12 (1999): 1356-63.
Uvnas-Moberg, Kerstin. "Oxytocin Linked Antistress Effects- the Relaxation and Growth Response." *Acta Physiologica Scandinavica* Supplementum 640 (1997): 38-42.
Uvnas-Moberg, Kerstin, Anne M. Widstrom, Giovanna Marchini, and Jan Winberg. "Release of GI Hormones in Mother and Infant by Sensory Stimulation." *Acta Paediatrica Scandinavica* 76.6 (1987): 851-60.
Wilson-Clay, Barbara. "Extended Breastfeeding as a Legal Issue: An Annotated Bibliography." *Journal of Human Lactation* 6.2 (1990): 68-71.
Wolf, Abraham W., and Betsy Lozoff. "Object Attachment, Thumbsucking, and the Passage to Sleep." *Journal of the American Academy of Child and Adolescent Psychiatry* 28.2 (1989): 287-92.
Wrigley, Elizabeth A., and Sally A. Hutchinson. "Long-Term Breastfeeding. The Secret Bond." *Journal of Nurse-Midwifery* 35.1 (1990): 35-41.

II. SHARING MILK

Perspectives on Ethics and Human Milk Banking

RHONDA SHAW

THE PHILOSOPHER ROSALYN DIPROSE has drawn attention to the invisibility of intercorporeal existence and identity in contemporary social life. For Diprose, intercorporeality is given in the lifeworld, and takes myriad forms from intangibles such as linguistic communication, gestures, movements, skills and pleasures, to more corporeally concrete substances and things. Diprose's observation is relevant to the lives of women whose identities are affected and affirmed by gift-exchange practices involving female body fluids and tissues. Breastmilk, the subject of this chapter, is one such fluid.

Although breastmilk, like tears, is often accorded deep religious significance, sitting high on the hierarchy of effluvia for its cleansing, purifying, and life-giving properties and qualities, its status as a sacred female bodily fluid cannot be universalized. The social and cultural histories of breastmilk, its relation to other body fluids such as blood and semen, as well as exchange relations involving breastmilk (i.e., wet-nursing, cross-nursing, and breastmilk donation) are complex. Contemporary understandings of breastmilk as a precious gift are bound up with new meanings of motherhood and sexuality. Although the first milk banks in the early twentieth century recompensed women for their donations and as wet nurses (Golden; Waldeck; Weaver and Williams), perceptions of human breastmilk as a gift have largely supplanted the social acceptability of payment, thus tending to morally censure its commodification.

Breastmilk has acquired public health status as liquid gold, but negative perceptions of breastmilk and of breastmilk sharing prevail. Such beliefs pertain to ideas about the sanctified institution of motherhood and how mothering care is, or should be, practiced. For many people in liberal democracies, ideal-typical mothering is conceptualized as a private and intensive relationship between a mother and her infant. Shared breastfeeding such as cross-nursing, which threatens to dissolve the boundary between presumed maternal proprietorial rights and the rights of others, upsets views of this sacred mother-child bond.

A second reason for abjecting breastmilk relates to aversion toward the exteriorization of bodily fluids generally speaking (i.e., blood, sweat, tears, vomit, phlegm, seminal and vaginal fluids, breastmilk) and fears about sharing bodily fluids. While some bodily fluids are socially acceptable, bodily secretions are more or less repugnant depending on cultural representations of the body and the gendering of bodies within specific cultures. Human breastmilk certainly ranks higher than phlegm, mucus, or excretion, but cultural perceptions of it remain ambiguous.

While Bernice Hausman (in this volume) examines fears around breastmilk as a viral fluid, fears about breastmilk are exacerbated when intimate bodily contact (like breast sharing) with unknown or non-related others is involved. Since breastmilk flows from female apertures and body parts identified as sexual, conflation of the lactating breast with the sexual or erotic breast often produces psycho-social anxiety. In order to make breastfeeding socially and culturally safe, public health campaigns and education programmes highlight the benefits of breastmilk by decontextualising it from the female body, and in so doing, sanitize the relation between women's reproductive capacities and embodiment (Bramwell 86-87). This move does little to challenge negative constructions of female bodily fluids and female sexuality, but as Ros Bramwell (86) notes, from a public health perspective the benefits of reducing morbidity and mortality rates are seen to outweigh failure to confront assumptions about gendered identities and behaviours. Donor human milk banking is a case in point. Because breastmilk donation does not involve body-to-body contact, anecdotal evidence suggests that women may support donor human milk banking where they would be rather more ambivalent about cross-nursing or wet-nursing (see Long). Notwithstanding the bodily remove breastmilk donation appears to entail, the interpersonal and institutional ethics between the parties involved are no less complex than those involving cross-nursing or wet-nursing acts and practices.

With the notable exception of Lois Arnold's work (2002, 2006a, 2006b) on human milk banking, which draws on bioethics and public health discourse to elucidate some of the salient issues, and Sarah Waldeck's essay advancing compensation for breastmilk donors, scant attention has been paid to the ethical dimensions of breastmilk donation (see also Bar-Yam, this volume). Debate on the topic is now propitious given the re-emergence of human milk banks across the globe. In this chapter I address the call for milk banking by outlining various perspectives on the gift-exchange of breastmilk through the themes of embodiment, identity, community, and generosity. This entails incorporating insights from the work of several philosophical ethicists (Macklin; Wilkinson) regarding moral principles relating to respect for persons and voluntarism, commodification and altruism, and justice and human rights. I suggest that the place of breastmilk as a body product and symbolic marker of maternal-child relations, and the cultural, ethical, and spiritual meanings and values attributed to breastmilk in ethically pluralist liberal societies warrants broader discussion than a bioethics model based on principlism[1] and public health discourse affords.

LIBERAL ETHICS

In Diprose's account of human being, as briefly sketched above, self-identity is situationally formed in relation to the identities of others. Liberal theory, by contrast, characterizes subject formation on the basis of individuation; subjects are autonomous, unitary, boundaried, and closed off from the lived bodies of other persons. The separation of individuals from other human beings is a natural state of being and a right as well as a value to be pursued (Tong). Violation of that right occurs when individuals are constrained from achieving their goals by denying them autonomy over decision-making where choices are to be made.

For liberals, breastfeeding one's infant is an antenatal or post-partum maternal choice women make on their own or in conjunction with their partners, not a decision to be dictated by breastfeeding advocates or health care professionals. In this perspective informed consent is axiomatic, and consists of a number of features: adequate disclosure of information, capacity for competence, comprehension of information, understanding of benefits and burdens, plus free and voluntary consent. Infringement of a woman's right to autonomously decide whether or not to breastfeed her infant may arise with respect to interpretations of the regulations and legislation around breastfeeding. Not surprisingly, the International Code of Marketing Breast-milk Substitutes, the United Nations Convention on the Rights of the Child (especially Article 24 (2e)), and The Baby-Friendly Hospital Initiative (BFHI) containing the Ten Steps to Successful Breastfeeding,[2] all unequivocally undertake to promote, protect and support breastfeeding, thereby highlighting its importance for the health and well-being of mothers and infants. Article 24 (2e) of the Convention, designed to protect the "best start on life" is directly related to breastfeeding; the Code expressly states that there should be "no advertising of breastmilk substitutes" and "no words or pictures idealizing artificial feeding, including pictures of infants on the labels"; and the steps in the BFHI all focus on fostering breastfeeding and ensuring its support. Needless to say, some liberals read the ratification of these documents by national governments, which are detailed in health policies, as single-mindedly elevating breastfeeding to a civic and moral responsibility for all mothers, mandating women to breastfeed. How is this so?

For Johanna Schmidt (2008), whose commentary represents this position, state sanctioned discourses such as the Code and the BFHI structure the range of possible choices for women by promoting and supporting breastfeeding above all else. While Schmidt concedes evidence for breastfeeding one's infant as the best infant feeding option health-wise, she is critical of the lack of information given to women about formula feeding, which, by omission, constructs breastfeeding mothers as good maternal citizens and others, who do not breastfeed, as morally recalcitrant. Like Jules Law (2000), who argues that scientific evidence extolling the benefits of breastfeeding is underpinned by an ideology about women's role as primary caregiver, Schmidt contends that failure to disclose all infant feeding options undermines paternal opportunity to share parenting. Not presenting the full range of infant feeding choices to women therefore limits women's right to autonomously decide whether or not to breastfeed their infants, and stigmatizes women for choosing not to breastfeed as this is seen as willful noncompliance.

In Schmidt's feminist view, it is due to the "embodied nature of breastfeeding" that the decision to breastfeed is women's "right to make alone" (71). Underpinning Schmidt's statement is the claim that body parts, products, and services such as breasts, breastmilk, and breastfeeding are personal property not community property, so decisions about how to use one's body depend on individual rights to non-interference. At the same time, Schmidt claims that the person and the body are coextensive. That is, a person's sense of self is coterminous with embodiment, but as this hermetically sealed subject is not a body-self who derives meaning vis-à-vis another or others, there is no moral obligation conferring a duty to breastfeed.

Accounts such as Schmidt's draw attention to the fact that women's general comfort and assuredness with and in their own bodies is not always a given. If the physiological dimensions of lactation are experienced as a limitation or impediment of female embodiment, then enforcing breastfeeding simply because a woman inhabits a particular kind of body curtails women's freedom. As Rebecca Kukla notes, many women experience limits to feminine bodily existence, frustrating and inhibiting their capacity to breastfeed successfully (163). Such limits include diminished milk supply due to breast augmentation; prior experiences of sexual abuse; annoyance with infants' playfulness at the breast; beliefs about breastfeeding as disgusting, unpleasant, embarrassing, or shameful; experience of body dysmorphia or negative body image; and social and existential problems related to privacy and breastfeeding. A woman's status within the family, her class positioning, her cultural and religious identification, the assertion by partners of women's conjugal duties, which can take priority over breastfeeding infants, are also factors bearing on women's ability to breastfeed.

Problems thus arise for liberals with contracts around breastfeeding that promote a child's right to be breastfed above women's right to choose. When couched paternalistically, these discourses present risks to women's self-governance.

UTILITARIANISM

Counter-intuitively, the reasons why some women do not, or cannot, breastfeed support recent calls for the provision of human breastmilk through national and global milk banking systems. In these discussions, couched in the language of public health and framed in terms of human rights, human milk banking and the less favoured option of cross-nursing are suggested as alternatives when it is not possible for a biological mother to breastfeed (see the 1980 WHO and

UNICEF joint statement [in Arnold 2002: 1] and The WHO/UNICEF Global Strategy on Infant and Young Child Feeding [2003] [in Arnold 2006a: 6]).

Although the move from breastfeeding to human milk banking endorsement is an extrapolation of international documents and health policies on breastfeeding, it should be clear that these documents do not propose the use of human milk banks for parents who "choose" not to breastfeed their children.

The utilitarian approach taken by advocates who call for the establishment and provision of human milk banking services rests on claims about the health promoting properties of breastmilk itself (See Arnold, 2006a, 2006b; Bar-Yam; Labbok). Consequently, these accounts tend to distinguish between breastmilk as a body fluid or product and breastfeeding as a process or method of breastmilk delivery. For example, in her discussion of breastfeeding and human rights, Naomi Bromberg Bar-Yam asks whether the right to be breastfed means being fed at the breast or consuming breastmilk (359). It is the mother's responsibility to breastfeed her infant, says Bar-Yam, but if this is not possible then expressing breastmilk or feeding baby human milk is not only a parental or familial obligation but also a governmental responsibility. Within such a policy framework it would not be inconceivable to offer more women the option of utilizing human milk from milk banks if they are unable or unwilling to breastfeed or express breastmilk. Naturally, policy recommendations would need to rank access to human milk according to need (premature and sick infants first), but allocation could be made along lines that take into account some of the psycho-social reasons why women cannot or choose not to breastfeed their own infants.

Critics of Bar-Yam's and Miriam Labbok's approaches might argue that splitting breastfeeding into product and process detaches the act of lactation from breastfeeding as a relationship a mother has with her infant and that this compartmentalizes the female body. For some feminists, this could mean that mothers do not need to be present to feed their infants and can return to full-time paid employment more easily, but it does not challenge the confinement of breastfeeding to the domestic realm, out of public space and away from the disapproving scrutiny of the public gaze.

COMMUNITARIAN ETHICS

Communitarianism is a broad descriptor for several approaches in contemporary political and social theory. Not all approaches grouped under this heading (e.g., ethics of care, Marxism, neo-Aristotelianism, radical feminism) would self-identify as communitarian. In common with Diprose's understanding of sociality, they do, however, share several key themes as well as objections to liberal individualism. All strands subscribe to the thesis that the social realm of human relationships is either ontologically prior to individual selves or a cherished value to which we should aspire. In health care, each would claim that the principles of liberal biomedical ethics do not always take account of lived moral life. The principles of autonomy and beneficence, for example, can be paternalistic and contradictory when they violate communitarian values about sharing child care, including breast sharing. Against a principlist approach to health care ethics, communitarians could conceivably argue that due regard be given to the rights of different cultural groups and that ticking a checklist of "informed consent," "beneficence," and so on often fails to recognize cultural specificities, especially rights to self-determination.

As stated in the introductory section to this chapter, not all body fluids and tissues are treated as equal. Cultural values and spiritual beliefs relating to conceptions of embodiment, identity, and descent affect perceptions of body fluids and tissues and this shapes views surrounding fluid and tissue donation and reception practices. Even in multi-cultural pluralist societies, where the public health emphasis is on the nutritional benefits of breastfeeding, local, social, and cultural meanings ascribed to human breastmilk may vary among different groups. Where Muslim civil law is observed, for example, links of milk kinship are important.

Milk kinship traditionally occurs by way of cross-nursing or wet-nursing arrangements, but the function of such arrangements goes beyond the provision of nutrition to the infant in establishing permissible social interaction and behaviour between kin groups (see Altorki; Cassidy and El-Tom in this volume; Khatib-Chahidi; Fortier). Jane Khatib-Chahidi, whose research focuses on Sunni Islam, explains how the establishment of milk kinship can be used to "make peace between two tribes, to consolidate clan unity, to prevent marriages, to create clients, in sum, ritually to attain objectives which lie far beyond the nursing woman's own interest" (18). Infants suckled by the same woman are obliged to support and care for her regardless of the absence of reciprocal duties and inheritance rights for the non-biologically related infant (Khatib-Chahidi 19). Once milk kinship is established, marriage between persons related by milk is barred. Although the practice of milk kinship is said to be waning in contemporary societies, the revival of interest in Islam and calls to decrease the use of infant formula globally may facilitate renewed implications of milk kinship for milk banking. Feeding a premature infant with mothers' milk pooled from a milk bank could create the problem of not knowing one's milk kinship relations and this could be socially detrimental for infants as they grow up.

Given the potential for discord with anonymous donation of human milk in these situations, a precautionary measure would be to include caveats in hospital breastfeeding policy documents to enable cross-nursing or wet-nursing arrangements. Formalizing such arrangements would require proper consent procedures in addition to donor-screening and pasteurization of milk. Implementation of cross-nursing or wet-nursing as alternatives sources of breastmilk would also cover situations where cultural protocols for infant care are deemed familial rather than individual responsibilities.

Understandably, different countries adopt slightly different milk banking policies. In the U.S., for instance, scientific reasons are given for pooling milk from several donors. Although research is presently underway, the current HMBANA practice is to pool milk from several mothers as this gives infants a mix of immunological and nutritional components (Bar-Yam, personal communication January 2009).[3] In the United Kingdom, however, where the donor milk screening guidelines are based on those of the National Blood Service, donor milk is not currently pooled between donors although several expressions of milk from a single donor may be pooled. Gillian Weaver, Chair of the United Kingdom Association of Milk Banks, points out that recipients are fed donor milk from as few donors as is practically possible but may receive milk from more than one donor. Records of donations from donors and their donations throughout the milk banking process are kept to ensure traceability from donor to recipient. Weaver explains that "these precautions came about partly as a general effort to minimize the number of donors that a recipient of any blood product or breastmilk is exposed to. It is also partly a result of the UK's experience with vCJD (variant Creutzfeldt-Jakob disease) which is thought to be transmissible via blood donations, although there is no evidence that breastmilk is a route of transmission" (personal communication February 2009).

OBJECTIFICATION, EXPLOITATION, AND COMMODIFICATION

The commercialisation of human tissue is routinely banned across the globe, although there are exceptions in some jurisdictions. A recently established California company, Prolacta Bioscience, profits from the sale of human breastmilk, but does not pay its donors. While many commentators view the sale of breastmilk as a market good to be morally reprehensible, the pivotal ethical issue, as Ruth Macklin says of body products generally, is whether commodification involves the "violation of a moral principle [e.g., respect for persons, justice] or the rights of any person or group" (106 [my insertion]). Macklin's assertion can also be applied to the gift model of altruistic fluid and tissue donation.

Although communitarians generally promote pro-social behaviours, they do not always support a feel-good view about altruistic donation of body fluids and tissues. This is not because they are in favour of commercializing breastmilk donation; some feminists, for example, would express concern that altruism can be exploitive and intrusive rather than life-affirming and world opening. They argue that valorizing women's "essential" connection to others reinforces beliefs about feminine self-sacrifice, so persuasive appeals, such as those entreating women to personally identify with recipients, may only deepen women's investments in caring protocols. Because these beliefs are affixed to perceptions of good mothering women feel compelled to engage in gift-giving practices to assuage feminine guilt about deficits to their moral character or identity as women. While these critics express reserve about women's gift-giving, they also oppose commercialization of body products and services, a position taken by human milk bank advocates.

Opposition to the commercialization of body fluids and tissues typically hinges on notions of objectification, exploitation, and commodification. There is substantial overlap between these concepts but objection to commercializing body tissues usually turns on a Kantian concept of objectification, originally formulated in Kant's second categorical imperative. Objectification is construed as morally wrong because it violates the principle of respect for persons, treating as an object that which is not an object. As Stephen Wilkinson says, this entails instrumentalisation, where people are treated as a means to an end rather than ends in themselves; and fungibility, which reduces a person's intrinsic dignity (as a person) to a price (29). Exchanging human body products and parts for a price fails to respect human beings' dignity because persons are treated as abstract resources, devoid of subjectivity, autonomy, and agency. According to this view, donors should not be financially compensated for their breastmilk because body parts and products are intimately related to persons who have intrinsic value and dignity. Once we separate bodies from persons we rob embodied human beings of something integral to their humanity. The case of breastmilk, like ovarian eggs, for example, is profound because women's identity is held to be intimately connected with sex, reproduction, and maternity. Moreover, paying a breastmilk donor as if her donation were a marketplace transaction would neutralize any meaning or motivation (aside from pecuniary recompense) the donor attaches to her act. For human milk bank advocates, this would rob it of its gift status by reducing what is currently perceived as an activity of care and concern to a fungible exchange object. To reinstitute payment for breastmilk would thus demean the donative act in the eyes of wider society, and reconnect it with a cultural history of breastmilk donation associated with a specific social class of women. For those who hold middle-class values, financial credit for breastmilk donation would be considered repugnant.

Supporters of community and hospital-based milk banks also oppose compensation for breastmilk donors and privatization of the industry. Miriam Labbok's position, for instance, is that in the "non-profit model of milk banking, milk is donated and no one makes a profit from its distribution." While this is not entirely true, since society generally profits through the improved health outcomes of its newborn, Labbok also states, "when sold, milk is turned into a commodity rather than an essential baby's food, shared freely mother to mother." Labbok is right in saying that selling breastmilk as a body product commodifies it, but it is the normative sense of Labbok's statement that is of interest here.

Many communitarians believe that health and well-being is achieved by acknowledging human existence as social and by contextualizing individuals as members of communities. For these commentators an ethical model based on altruism is morally acceptable over commercialization because when "payment is involved it debases the value of the gift" (Macklin 117). Those who hold this position argue in favour of non-commercial milk banking policies, saying that when people give donations freely they foster a culture of generosity and this nourishes and sustains human relationships. From this perspective, it might be considered parsimonious not to share or donate breastmilk especially where a woman has excess to her infant's requirements.

This view of giving is in concert with a maternalist identity politics emphasizing women's natural mothering roles, and is often articulated in breastfeeding campaign slogans such as "breastfeeding is natural and normal" and "most women breastfeed" (See Thornley et al. 4). According to maternalists women's roles correspond to specific moral codes and repertoires. They claim that "breastfeeding is associated with being a good mother" (Thornley et al. 4): the implication being that women are duty-bound to satisfy their infant's needs as a requirement flowing from the experience of pregnancy, maternity, and lactation. Since it is taken for granted that women's reproductive activities and functions are bodily and immanent, somehow presupposing reasoned self-consciousness, this line of thinking effectively precludes the possibility that women make an ethical choice to breastfeed or donate breastmilk. This is because the caring and domestic labour women undertake is deemed obligatory, issuing from the fact of being a woman and something one does passively. Giving breastmilk to milk banks, therefore, is viewed as an extension of what women are simply expected to do to fulfill their duties as mothers and moral citizens. As women's identities are intimately connected to their reproductive function, paying women to breastfeed would not only be demeaning it would also alienate women from their essential being. For critics, this position exposes some of the flaws associated with the view that only permits altruistic body tissue donation. The debate about blood donation is an instructive analogue.

Wilkinson makes the point that if "altruistic blood donation were morally obligatory, then to demand money for one's blood … would be wrong. But if, on the other hand, altruistic blood donation were supererogatory, then to demand money for one's blood wouldn't be wrong. Rather, it would be merely non-supererogatory: not good, but not wrong" (111). The same could be said of breastmilk donation. If breastfeeding one's infant is a maternal duty and breastmilk donation is seen as an extension of this duty, then we can see how payment for breastmilk donation might be considered impermissible—it would be like charging your children, and any friends they invited over for dinner, for cooking an evening meal.

For feminists the concern is that if altruistic breastmilk donation is cast as a maternal expectation and a child's right, then encouraging such donation merely reproduces asymmetric gender norms and roles rather than producing generosity as a universal trait. If this is so, then feminist economists such as Marilyn Waring have a point and the principle that is violated here is justice, since we are failing to recognize the contribution of women's labour and gift-giving to economies of exchange. On the other hand, if breastfeeding is not an essential aspect of women's being (not all women have children after all and those who do engage in many activities besides mothering), and is truly supererogatory (over and above the call of duty) then paying breastmilk donors would not demean the donative act. It may not be morally righteous, as Wilkinson says about paid blood donation, but it would still be of benefit to others and may even convey the social value of breastmilk given its remunerative recognition in the marketplace (Waldeck 1).

From the perspective of feminist economists, not paying breastmilk donors is the problem. They hold that women's non-remunerative gift of breastmilk instrumentalises women's labour in the interests of the public good (donors are used as a means to better population health outcomes), even though no money changes hands. The net result is that women's lactation work (which includes breastfeeding and breastmilk donation) remains invisible, despite the labor the breastfeeding body undertakes as a vital contribution to social well-being. As Waring says:

> Breastmilk is frequently and erroneously described as free. This is incorrect, if only from the standpoint of the energy cost to mothers and the value of their time during breastfeeding. There is also a nutritional cost. Maternal depletion is a common outcome of breastfeeding. (44)

By characterizing the lactational act as a personal sacrifice women make for their infants, Waring reveals the flip-side to the language of the gift. If "gift" is the terminology of recipients and not donors, then breastfeeding is an offering from mother to infant wrought at great expense, a form of unremunerated corporeal compensation ritualized in breastfeeding and breast-pumping regimens that continually replenish a valuable body asset. Seen in this light, there is an expectation that giving breastmilk is moral work women are expected to do as women.

Breastmilk donation, paradoxically, is assumed to be motivated altruistically. As an altruistic act or gift is one that enhances another's welfare, is voluntary, and expects no reciprocation or reward, it is this disinterest that gives the gift its noble quality. Yet motivations to donate are complex and multi-layered. In their study of the characteristics of French breastmilk donors Emilie Azema and Stacey Callahan report 60 percent of their research participants stated "too much milk" as the reason for donation, followed by 40 percent of women who indicated a "general desire to help others" (201). While this study suggests that women's motivation to donate breastmilk is pro-social to some extent, breastmilk donors are already breastfeeding their own infants so are not being induced to engage in an act they would not otherwise do (except perhaps expressing breastmilk in order to donate it). Women who have excess milk supply might then be instrumentally motivated to donate rather than "waste" their precious gift, and might otherwise experience engorgement if they did not express or donate milk. In this respect, donating excess breastmilk is not corporeally self-sacrificing like donating ovarian eggs or donating a kidney (breastmilk donation is less risky, less invasive, and breastmilk is replenishable) although admittedly, it takes more time and effort to give breastmilk than it does to give blood (since it must be hand-expressed or pumped). The point I am making is that some altruistic acts contain a reciprocity component. This does not mean that such acts are non-moral, or that getting personal satisfaction or bodily relief from giving annuls the gift, but that under a gift-exchange model there are already benefits conferred on donors.

Another objection to monetary compensation for donors, as Labbok outlines, is that it "could exploit low-income women who might be indirectly coerced into donating their milk out of economic necessity." Certainly paying for body services or products may be exploitive if money incentive induces people to become donors at risk to their own health or the health of significant others they care for, and this is one of the reasons why a gift model of donation is considered preferable to monetary compensation. The assumption is that people will give under conditions of gift-exchange, but not too much.

There is evidence to support Labbok's claim. Ana Claire Pimenteira Thomaz et al., for instance, have noted that women's motivations for breastmilk donation in Brazil in the 1940s were primarily economic; women were provided with state medical care, powdered milk and medications for themselves and their infants, as well as payment. Practices began to change when it was discovered donors' infants were suffering from the sale of their mother's milk and when milk was being diluted to increase compensation for donors (Pimenteira Thomaz et al. 74). Technically, the contemporary milk banking situation would appear to work against this risk, since, even if impoverished donors were prepared to compromise the truth about their "medical histories and lifestyles" (Waldeck 4) and jeopardize the quality of their breastmilk donations, milk banks in the U.S. have a triple screening process along the lines of blood bank protocols. This entails thorough screening by medical history, oral interview or questionnaire, serological testing of donors, pasteurization and bacteriological testing of milk (Waldeck 3), and milk pooling all of which reduce the possibility of contaminants and toxins in donor breastmilk being passed onto infants.

A further objection to paying donors is that if payment is involved then a woman may feel pressured to continue producing and donating milk even after weaning her infant. At present, milk banks only accept donations from women who have expressed milk for their own baby or who are currently breastfeeding their own children, or whose baby has died, not those who induce lactation outside of parturition. As Weaver states, "one of the assumed safeguards with donation is that the mother will have been expressing milk for or directly breastfeeding her own baby and so is at less risk of unacceptable donor behavior such as alcohol/substance misuse" (personal communication February 2009). Although the HMBANA guidelines do not specifically cover this issue, until research has been undertaken to determine the exact properties of breastmilk from relactating women such milk is not taken (Bar Yam, personal communication January 2009).

Notwithstanding guideline protocols deterring women who are not breastfeeding their own infants from donating breastmilk, a liberal rejoinder might be that the decision to continue to donate after weaning one's infant is an autonomous project voluntarily engaged in by a lactating woman, who has given her informed consent to the procedure. If this is so then a case could also be made for donating breastmilk for payment: it is not exploitive if donors are "fully informed of the purpose, procedures to be performed, the time involved, the risks, and the benefits" (Macklin 113).

CONCLUSION

This chapter has skimmed the surface of some of the ethical issues associated with human milk banking in the present. Certainly the models provided by biomedical ethics and human rights discourse provide starting points for thinking through the complexity of these issues. As Arnold argues, principlism offers checks and balances for conduct between donors, recipients, and health care professionals at an interpersonal and institutional level, and human rights protocols exhort governments to take the preventative function of dispensing human milk through milk banks into account when designing health care programmes. While these are steps in the right direction, it is worth keeping in mind Diprose's observation that our freedom to give, and this includes giving breastmilk, is limited by our "habits and capacities" in conjunction with "those of the bodies with whom we dwell" (55). This entails understanding why some women are at ease giving breastmilk to their own and to others, and how, in the process they see themselves as engaged in moral work, and how other women have difficulties doing something that seems so "natural" for some yet can feel so phenomenally alien. For this reason BFHI guidelines need to commend and incorporate protocols that are both Baby- *and* Mother-friendly so as not to alienate women who are ambivalent about breastfeeding from their babies or the health care system. Given the impact of different social and environmental factors on child and maternal health and diverse views on how to achieve health related goals, a non-paternalistic approach to breastfeeding and the use of breastmilk from human milk banks, one that recognises the values and concerns of as many cultural groups as possible at the level of policy and legislation, is also required. At the same time, non-payment for breastmilk donation should not be accepted as a fait accompli. What we need is comprehensive *localized* discussion of the complex cultural, ethical, legal, and spiritual aspects of human milk banking, and this can only be satisfactorily realised through the promotion of public dialogue and debate.

[1]Principlism is the name given to the four principles approach to normative

ethics developed by Tom Beauchamp and James Childress, based on the principles of respect for autonomy, beneficence, non-maleficence and justice. Beauchamp and Childress further specify these principles by the moral rules of veracity, privacy, confidentiality, and fidelity.
[2]Ten Steps to Successful Breastfeeding:

> Every facility providing maternity services and care for newborn infants should:
> 1. Have a written breastfeeding policy that is routinely communicated to all health care staff.
> 2. Train all health care staff in skills necessary to implement this policy.
> 3. Inform all pregnant women about the benefits and management of breastfeeding.
> 4. Help mothers initiate breastfeeding within half an hour of birth.
> 5. Show mothers how to breastfeed, and how to maintain lactation even if they should be separated from their infants.
> 6. Give newborn infants no food or drink other than breast milk, unless medically indicated.
> 7. Practice rooming-in—that is, allowing mothers and infants to remain together—24 hours a day.
> 8. Encourage breastfeeding on demand.
> 9. Give no artificial teats or pacifiers (also called dummies or soothers) to breastfeeding infants.
> 10. Foster the establishment of breastfeeding support groups and refer mothers to them on discharge from the hospital or clinic.
> (Source: WHO/UNICEF : *Protecting, Promoting and Supporting Breastfeeding: The Special Role of Maternity Services.* Geneva: WHO, 1989).

[3]Premature milk and milk of mothers on no lactose diets is sometimes processed separately.

REFERENCES

Altorki, Soraya. "Milk-Kinship in Arab Society: An Unexplored Problem in the Ethnography of Marriage." *Ethnology* 19.2 (1980): 233-244.

Arnold, Lois. "Where Does Donor Milk Banking Fit in Public Health Policy?" *Breastfeeding Abstracts* 21.3 (2002): 19-20.

Arnold, Lois. "Global Health Policies that Support the Use of Banked Donor Human Milk: A Human Rights Issue." *International Breastfeeding Journal* 1.26 (2006a): <http://www.internationalbreastfeedingjournal.com/content/1/1/>.

Arnold, Lois. "The Ethics of Donor Human Milk Banking." *Breastfeeding Medicine* 1.1 (2006b): 3-13.

Azema, Emilie and Stacey Callahan. "Breast Milk Donors in France: A Portrait of the Typical Donor and the Utility of Milk Banking in the French Breastfeeding Context." *Journal of Human Lactation* 19.2 (2003): 199-202.

Bar-Yam, Naomi Bromberg. "Breastfeeding and Human Rights: Is There a Right to Breastfeed? Is There a Right to be Breastfed?" *Journal of Human Lactation* 19.4 (2003): 357-361.

Beauchamp, Tom L. and James F. Childress. *Principles of Biomedical Ethics.* Fifth Edition. Oxford: Oxford University Press, 2001.

Bramwell, Ros. "Blood and Milk: Constructions of Female Bodily Fluids in Western Society." *Women and Health* 34.4 (2001): 85-96.

Diprose, Rosalyn. *Corporeal Generosity: On Giving with Nietzsche, Merleau-Ponty, and Levinas.* Albany: State University of New York, 2002.

Fortier, Corrine. "Blood, Sperm and the Embryo in Sunni Islam and in Mauritania: Milk Kinship, Descent and Medically Assisted Procreation." *Body and Society* 13.3 (2007): 15-36.

Golden, Janet. "From Commodity to Gift: Gender, Class, and the Meaning of Breast Milk in the Twentieth Century." *The Historian* 59.1 (1996): 75-87.

Khatib-Chahidi, Jane. "Milk Kinship in Shi'ite Islamic Iran." *The Anthropology of Breast-feeding: Natural Law or Social Construct.* Ed Vanessa Maher. Oxford: Berg Publishers, 1992. 109-132.

Kukla, Rebecca. "Ethics and Ideology in Breastfeeding Advocacy Campaigns." *Hypatia* 21.1 (2006): 157-180.

Labbok, Miriam. "Ethics, Established Breastfeeding Policy and Donor Milk Banking." Plenary Lecture presented at the HMBANA Conference November 7, 2007.

Law, Jules. "The Politics of Breastfeeding: Assessing Risk, Dividing Labor." *Signs: Journal of Women in Culture and Society* 25.2 (2000): 407-450.

Long, Debbi. "Breast Sharing: Cross-feeding Among Australian Women." *Health Sociology Review* 12.2 (2003): 103-110.

Macklin, Ruth. "What Is Wrong With Commodifiction?" *New Ways Of Making Babies: The Case of Egg Donation.* Ed. Cynthia B. Cohen. Bloomington: Indiana University Press, 1996. 106-121.

Pimenteira Thomaz, Ana Claire, Luiz Victor Maia Loureiro, Tathiane da Silva Oliveira, Norma Caroline de Mendonca Furtado Montenegro, Eglailson Dantas Almeida Junior, Claudio Fernando Rodrigues Soriano and Jairo Clado Cavalcante. "The Human Milk Donation Experience: Motive, Influencing Factors, and Regular Donation." *Journal of Human Lactation* 24.1 (2008): 69-76.

Schmidt, Johanna. "Gendering in Infant Feeding Discourses: The Good Mother and the Absent Father." *New Zealand Sociology* 23.2 (2008): 61-74.

Thornley, Louise, Anaru Waa and Judith Ball. *Comprehensive Plan to Inform the Design of a National Breastfeeding Promotion Campaign.* Wellington: Quigley and Watts Ltd, 2007.

Tong, Rosemarie. "Toward A Feminist Perspective on Gamete Donation and

Reception Policies." *New Ways of Making Babies: The Case of Egg Donation*. Ed. Cynthia B. Cohen. Bloomington: Indiana University Press, 1996. 138-155.

Waldeck, Sarah E. "Encouraging a Market in Human Milk." *Columbia Journal of Gender and Law* 11.361 (2002): 1-35.

Waring, Marilyn. "Public Forum: The Economic Value of Breastfeeding." *Proceedings 5th Biennial Conference of the Australian Lactation Consultants' Association*. Melbourne, ALCA (2000).

Weaver, Gillian and A. Susan Williams. "A Mother's Gift: The Milk of Human Kindness." *The Gift Relationship: From Human Blood to Social Policy*. Eds Ann Oakley and John Ashton. New York: The New Press, 1997. 319-332.

Wilkinson, Stephen. *Bodies for Sale: Ethics and Exploitation in the Human Body Trade*. London: Routledge, 2003.

The Story of the Mothers' Milk Bank of New England

NAOMI BROMBERG BAR-YAM

HUMAN MILK BANKING IS part of a historic and social continuum of mothers sharing the gift of themselves and their life-giving milk with other babies in need. According to Valerie Fildes (1988), this sharing is as old as time, probably beginning with mothers breastfeeding their nieces, nephews, and related children when maternal illness or death required it. As soon as there were social and economic classes, and money and goods to be exchanged, women would pay and be paid for breastfeeding. Wet-nursing, nursing the baby of another woman for pay, is a very old and respected profession. Not only have contracts for wet nurses from ancient Egypt and Babylonia been found (Fildes 6), but surviving medical texts from ancient India offer guidelines on choosing a suitable wet nurse (Fildes 9). Wet-nursing was widespread and regulated in Europe throughout the Middle Ages and onward. Many wealthy and noble European families had live-in wet nurses, whose own babies had often died. Other families sent their babies to live with wet nurses in the country. Wet nurses often had families and farms to tend, and wet-nursing provided good income and contraception. Babies lived with the wet nurse's family for about two years before returning to their own families (Fildes).

Three factors came together in the Industrial Revolution to bring about the transition from wet-nursing to human milk banking; urbanization, medicalization and industrialization. Urbanization or migration from the country to the city to work in factories, left fewer farmwives to serve as wet nurses. To fill the need, poor single urban mothers sent their own babies away to the care of relatives and friends (who fed the babies less than optimally) so that they could earn a meagre living nursing other women's babies. This brought a decline in the status of wet-nursing and was one of many factors contributing to an urban infant mortality rate of 20 percent—one in five babies died in the first five years of life (Golden 2001). Twenty percent mortality rate galvanized physicians to help, resulting in the emergence of pediatrics as a medical specialty. Pediatricians identified, screened and monitored the wet nurses for their patients, and they created special formulas for babies who did not have wet nurses (Golden 2001). Acceptance of the medicalization of infant feeding has made other changes easier to implement.

Industrialization brought fundamental changes in the way we think about work, families and machines. The invention and mass production of effective breast pumps and refrigeration led to the separation of the producer (the mother/wet nurse), the product (human milk) and the consumer (the baby) of human milk. Breastmilk, rather than breastfeeding became the commodity of exchange. Milk could be stored safely and anonymously allowing the development of milk banks.

MILK BANKING IN NORTH AMERICA TODAY

The first milk bank in the world opened in Vienna, Austria in 1909. Since the opening of the first North American milk bank at the Floating Children's Hospital in Boston in 1910, there have been numerous milk banks throughout the country. Most were hospital-based, receiving donations from local mothers and serving the hospital's premature and sick babies. As more preterm and sick babies survived, milk banking grew. Though there was some pasteurization, early milk banks generally distributed unprocessed milk (Golden).

The birth and survival of the Dionne quintuplets in Canada in the 1930s brought international attention to the Dionne family and to milk donation (see Nathoo and Ostry, this volume). Mothers from Canada and the United States donated more than 8,000 ounces of milk. In 1981, Lacie Lynnette Smith of Milburn, Oklahoma was born with a rare allergic condition and she could only ingest human milk. Because her mother was on medications, she could not nurse her. As a full term growing baby who could eat nothing else, Lacie required 200-300 ounces of milk per day. Hundreds of donors sent Lacie 24,000 ounces of milk until she began to outgrow her allergies ("Milestone"; "Okla"). In a 1999 update, Lacie was able to tolerate some foods with the help of medication, however when she is ill, even as a young adult, Lacie still relies on donated mothers' milk (Jacobs).

The 1980s brought HIV/AIDS and concerns about its spread through human milk. This led to the need for more complex and costly screening and processing procedures, which resulted in numerous milk banks closing. When Lacie Lynnette Smith was receiving milk in the early 1980s, there were about thirty milk banks. By the end of the 1980s there were only eight or nine milk banks in North America.

In 1985, the Human Milk Banking Association of North American (HMBANA) was founded. One of its primary objectives was to establish evidence-based protocols for all North American milk banks. They were published in 1990 in consultation with the United States Food and Drug Administration. HMBANA reviews and updates the Guidelines annually based on the most current research, and they serve as the basis for similar guidelines and protocols around the world (Jones).

In the 1990s evidence of the safety of pasteurized human milk and continuing research documenting the risks of formula and benefits of human milk, particularly for premature and sick babies, led to renewed interest in human milk banking. For example, research documents the risk of necrotizing enterocolitis (NEC) for premature babies who receive formula (McGuire and Anthony; Boyd, Quigley and Brocklehurst). About one third of babies with NEC do not survive. Treatment for NEC can require surgical removal of part of the intestine and can lead to lifelong gastrointestinal problems, largely preventable by feeding babies human milk.

There are two types of milk banks in North America: hospital-based and community. A hospital-based milk bank operates within a hospital facility and infrastructure, serving hospital patients first and others as milk is available. Most milk banks historically and today are hospital-based. Community milk banks are independent, charitable, non-profit institutions serving physicians, hospitals and families in their community or region. At the time of writing in 2008, there are currently ten milk banks in the United States and Canada: four of them are community milk banks and six are hospital-based.

In 2007, HMBANA banks dispensed 1,162,529 ounces of milk, more than double what they dispensed in 2000. HMBANA milk banks sent milk to hospitals in over one hundred cities located in thirty six states and five Canadian provinces (HMBANA 2008).

CASE STUDY: THE MOTHERS' MILK BANK OF NEW ENGLAND (MMBNE)

Each milk bank has its own inspiring story. The longest standing milk bank in the North America is in San Jose, California, which has been open for over thirty years. Several milk banks have opened in the last seven years. The New England region, and the Boston area in particular, are often known as a "Medical Mecca" of the world with numerous hospitals and medical schools bringing top physicians, researchers, students, trainees and patients to the area from all over the world. Yet, there was no milk bank. New England includes six small states in the Northeastern region of the United States: Connecticut, Maine, Massachusetts, New Hampshire, Rhode Island and Vermont. The most recent milk bank in this region, open between 1975 and 2001, was the hospital-based Central Massachusetts Regional Milk Bank in Worcester, Massachusetts. It was closed due to changes in administration and fiscal policies resulting from the merging of two hospitals. The newest HMBANA milk bank, the Mothers' Milk Bank of New England, is still a developing milk bank. It is a milk bank and a story in progress.

Each of us involved with MMBNE has a story that motivated our involvement. For example, two of my children were born small (2 kilos, or 4.5 pounds each) and spent time in the NICU. When Maayan was born in 1990, another baby in the NICU required human milk that her mother did not have. I was the only mother with extra milk, and I was happy to help. It was my first exposure to milk sharing. Taeer was born six years later at 32 weeks. I brought his extra milk home and, like many mothers, I could not bear to discard it, even though Taeer was breastfeeding fully. When my father became ill a few years later, we used the milk for him. While I knew that the milk was unlikely to save his life, I hope that it was able to make him more comfortable and perhaps prolong his time with us by some small amount. In looking for additional milk for my father, I discovered milk banks and learned that there was no milk bank in New England. I began researching cross-nursing, milk kinship and milk banking. After much thought, soul searching and discussions with my husband, who is president of his own non-profit institution, we decided that establishing a milk bank in New England was a valuable contribution to our community.

In late January 2006, I posted a meeting announcement on several breastfeeding listservs and the response was enthusiastic and widespread. At our first meeting, in March, we discussed whether to be a hospital or community milk bank and whether to be a local or a regional milk bank. Jane, a nurse, lactation consultant (IBCLC) and milk donor for Lacie Lynette Smith in the early 1980s, comes to each meeting from New Hampshire and serves on our education and fundraising committees. Her presence and dedication, along with emails and calls from all over New England, answered for us the question of becoming a regional milk bank.

Our Board also includes: Karen, a nurse, IBCLC, representing Boston Children's Hospital; Marcia, a retired professor of city planning; Jessica, an accountant who enjoys helping non-profit groups she cares about and keeps their books in order; David, a biochemist who researches human milk; Tanya, a writer who edits our newsletter. Our medical director, Kathie, is a neonatologist and IBCLC who lives in Connecticut two and a half hours away from Boston, and joins our meetings by phone. These are only a few of the several dozen people, primarily with older children, who give generously of their time and skills to help birth MMBNE.

The decision whether to be a hospital-based or independent milk bank involved several considerations. Hospital-based milk banks are part of the host hospital's financial and medical infrastructure, which provides salaries, equipment, supplies and space, reducing the need for fundraising. However, many North American hospitals are in financial difficulties and hospital-based milk banks are subject to fiscal cuts and elimination with no recourse, as was the case in Worcester in 2001. These financial difficulties also make it difficult for a hospital to host MMBNE. Additionally, it would be more difficult to serve the New England region. On the other hand, establishing an independent milk bank would pose several challenges: legal; financial; and educational, establishing credibility in the medical community. Though we knew it would take time, effort and funds, we decided to become an independent milk bank, and set a goal to open within two years of our first meeting, by spring, 2008.

The process of becoming a legal non-profit entity in the eyes of the Federal and Massachusetts governments took us many months, hours and the help of a (fortunately, *pro bono*) lawyer. Even our name was challenged. The term "bank" was initially turned down because of possible confusion with banks that handle money. The term "mothers' milk" was also turned down because of a defunct, but still on the record, Massachusetts business with the words "mothers' milk" in its name. At first, our legal name was MMBNE, Inc. With time, patience, good humor and the able help of our lawyer, we were able to reestablish our full name, the Mothers' Milk Bank of New England, in the eyes of the Commonwealth of Massachusetts.

As an independent institution, MMBNE must raise funds to cover all of its expenses. This is an ongoing process that has included personal appeals to our families and friends, grant proposals to regional and national foundations, fundraising events, even winning $10,000 on an online contest for our business idea (ideablob.com). Since hospitals and families pay processing fees for milk, we expect to be 70-80 percent self supporting within the first few years of operation.

Physicians in the region have little experience using banked milk. Often neonatologists first learn about banked milk when a patient's mother requests it when they cannot breastfeed fully. Lectures at conferences and hospital grand rounds have also helped educate physicians and others about milk banking and the most current research. To that end, MMBNE will sponsor a full day regional medical conference, Human Milk Banking: Preventive Medicine in Practice in the spring of 2009. We will also be hosting the 2010 conference of HMBANA, an opportunity to mark the 100th anniversary of milk banking in North America, where it began in Boston, and to bring local attention to milk banking.

In the United States, health insurance is private and diverse. Within certain legal limitations, each insurance company decides what services it will cover. In communities with milk banks, some insurance companies cover banked milk as standard care in hospitals; in others it is covered case by case. In New England, insurance companies do not routinely cover use of banked milk. Arlene, a retired attorney on our Board, is working with colleagues to develop a strategy to ensure insurance coverage for hospital use of banked milk. Educating the insurance companies is an important part of MMBNE's financial and community education agenda.

In June 2008, MMBNE opened a dispensary in a temporary space donated by the city of Newton, Massachusetts (a suburb of Boston). We receive processed milk from the Mothers' Milk Bank of Ohio and dispense it to local hospitals and families. Our clinical director, Ilene Fabisch LLLL, IBCLC refers the numerous potential donor mothers in the area to the Ohio milk bank for screening. We are seeking permanent space for our screening and processing facility. Space considerations for the permanent milk bank include appropriate electricity and plumbing for a wet lab and easy access for donor mothers, visitors and shipping personnel.

Laboratory equipment and supplies must be chosen carefully. One example is the use of glass or plastic bottles. New non toxic, BPA free plastic bottles are available, but because they are new, there is much we do not know about them. Plastic is light, unbreakable and heats the milk evenly during pasteurization. Glass is more environmentally and chemically sound, but also heavier, breakable, and because they are not of uniform quality, glass bottles do not always heat milk evenly and uniformly during pasteurization. Ilene has combined her deep passion for and knowledge of breastfeeding and her training as a medical technologist to research and evaluate every aspect of our lab. We make the best decisions we can, knowing that with new research, reevaluation may be necessary.

In addition to the milk bank facility, volunteers and professionals are working to establish milk depots throughout New England. Milk depots collect and store milk from local donors and send it to the milk bank for processing. They also raise awareness of the value and importance of breastfeeding and human milk in their communities. These will be hosted by hospitals, community centres, and mother/baby care centres.

MMBNE does not face the challenges of establishing a milk bank alone. It is part of a multinational community of milk banks who want MMBNE to succeed. Their moral and practical support has been endless and encouraging. In addition, people from all over the region and of diverse professional backgrounds give of their time, energy, resources and expertise to create and grow the Mothers' Milk Bank of New England. It is truly a community effort.

DONOR MILK SCREENING AND PROCESSING

In over 40 years of modern milk banking in North America, there has *never* been a documented case of an infant being harmed by banked donor milk (HMBANA 2008). The donation process begins with a phone call or email from a new mother interested in donating milk. Most donors are mothers of healthy full or preterm babies whose supply exceeds their babies' demand. For some bereaved mothers, the gift of milk to help another baby offers much comfort (Tully). The donor mother completes a health history, modeled after those used by blood banks, by phone and/or in writing. Her physician and her baby's pediatrician must verify the health of both mother and baby. Mothers also undergo blood tests for HIV 1 and 2, HTLV, Hepatitis B and C and Syphilis, all known to transmit through breastmilk (Updegrove). The milk bank sends donors detailed instructions and a kit for the expression and initial storage of their milk. It is delivered frozen to the milk bank or milk depot and kept frozen until pasteurization.

Milk processing also requires careful procedures and testing. In many milk banks, milk from several donor mothers is pooled to form each batch of donor milk. This allows for greater mixing of milk components. Milk banks process "preemie milk" separately from "term milk" and it is dispensed to the smallest most fragile babies. Some milk banks also separate the milk of mothers on lactose free diets. As we learn more about the changing components of milk

Table 1: Human Milk Components in Fresh Mothers' Milk, after Heating and Pasteurization, Formula and Special Preemie Formulas
Percentage of Components / Activity Present

Component	Mothers' milk from the breast	After freezing and pasteurizing	Formula	Special Formula	Function
IgA and SIgA	100	67-70	0	0	Infant's do not produce SigA until 6-9 months; active against Polio, Coxsackievirus, Herpes, CMV, RSV, Rubella, and Rotavirus
IgM	100	0	0	0	Active against CMV, RSV, and Rubella
IgG	100	66-70	0	0	Active against CMV, RSV, and Rubella
Lactoferrin	100	27-43	0	0	Protein that, binds iron required by many bacteria and thus slows bacterial growth.
Lysozyme	100	75	0	0	Enzymes that break bacterial cell walls, destroying them.
Lipases	100	0	0	0	Protect against "envelope viruses"
Mono-glycerides	100	100	0	0	Disrupts membrane coating of many viruses and protozoans destroying them.
Free fatty acids	100	100	Added to some formulas		Disrupts membrane coating of many viruses and protozoans destroying them.
Linoleic acid	100	100	Added to some formulas		Essential fatty acid; metabolic precursor for prostaglandins and leukotrienes.
Alpha linolenic acid	100	100	Added to some formulas		Essential fatty acid; metabolic precursor for docosahexaenoic acid; important for eye and brain development.
Bifidus factor	100	70-100			Promotes growth of *Lactobacillus bifidfus*, a harmless bacterium to prevent growth of harmful bacteria in the gut.
Olago saccharides	100				Bind harmful bacteria
Vitamin A	100	100			Protection against disease; gut mucosa sensitive to Vitamin A

The table is adapted from: Tully, D. B., Jones, F., & Tully, M. R. (2001). Donor milk: What's in it and what's not. *Journal of Human Lactation*, 17, 152-155.

over time, some milk banks pool milk by age of the child, thereby achieving a closer match between the milk donated and the baby receiving it. Perfect matches are not always possible since most babies receiving milk are preterm and most donors have full term babies.

To begin processing itself, each pasteurizing team member scrubs thoroughly and wears gloves, mask, hair cover and apron whenever handling milk. The thawed milk from a donor mother is transferred to glass flasks. Many milk banks culture each mother's milk for bacteria before processing. Milk from three to five mothers is then pooled, mixed thoroughly and poured into two to six ounce bottles and placed in a pasteurizer. During pasteurizing, the milk is heated to 26.5 degrees Celsius for thirty minutes. Ongoing research identifies the best way to pasteurize milk so that bacteria are eliminated but most of the beneficial components of the milk are retained. (See Table 1.) The milk is then cooled quickly and bottles sealed and marked with batch number and nutritional information. Samples from each batch of pasteurized milk are cultured and must show zero bacteria growth before it can be dispensed. Contaminated milk is discarded or used for research. Pasteurized milk is refrozen and shipped overnight to hospitals and individual recipients' homes.

According to HMBANA *Guidelines* (2007) banked milk must be dispensed by physician prescription or hospital purchase order. Most milk is used in hospitals and families at home, i.e. for adoption, surrogacy, maternal illness and low milk supply.

ETHICAL ISSUES IN DONOR HUMAN MILK BANKING

Equitable distribution of a scarce resource raises ethical issues. Lois Arnold has described the role and limits of biomedical ethical and public health ethical frames in human milk banking, and Rhonda Shaw offers an insightful analysis in this volume. Here I will briefly touch on the commodification of mothers' milk; breastfeeding and the Code; allocating donor human milk; and profit versus non-profit. Even without fully answering them, the questions raised inform how we think and how we act in our local milk banks.

COMMODIFICATION

During the Industrial Revolution human milk rather than breastfeeding became a commodity for exchange. This development is part of what makes human milk banking possible, and what informs the ethical conversation around it. Historically wet nurses have often been paid for their services. In the 1970s in the United States, human milk shifted from being a commodity for which remuneration was received to a priceless substance donated freely (Golden). More recently it has been argued that the home-based services of women, particularly a unique service such as milk donation, should be compensated monetarily (Galtry) and considered in calculation of national GDP (Smith 1998). Currently, milk banks do not pay, and do not charge for donor milk.

Table 2: Suggested Priority for Dispensing Donor Human Milk

1. *Recipient factors to consider:* Age Projected length of need Medical condition Prognosis Prevention of problems Research Ability to pay (may be a factor where medical need is not evident)	3. *Time factors to consider:* Short-term use Likely to recover Preventive treatment
2. *Maternal factors to consider:* Insufficient milk supply Medical contraindications to breastfeeding Adoption Choice	4. *Ethical values:* Community benefit (CB) Individual benefit/choice (IB)

Going from highest to lowest priority, based on these factors, from most critical (1) to least critical (3), and community benefit (CB) to individual benefit/choice (IB):

Premature infants, sick (1,2,3—CB & IB)
Premature infants, well (2,3—CB & IB)
Infants less than 12 months old with medical conditions likely to respond to donor human milk therapy (1,2,3—CB & IB)
Individuals more than 12 months old with medical conditions likely to respond to donor human milk therapy (1,2,3—CB & IB)
Research contracts for clinical use in well-designed studies (1,3—CB & IB)
Individuals more than 12 months old with chronic medical conditions and high normal functioning and low dose need for donor human milk therapy (3—CB & IB)
Individuals more than 12 months old with chronic medical conditions and high normal functioning and high dose need for donor human milk therapy (3—CB & IB)
Individuals more than 12 months old with chronic medical conditions and low normal functioning and low dose need for donor human milk therapy (IB)
Individuals more than 12 months old with chronic medical conditions and low normal functioning and high dose need for donor human milk therapy (3—CB & IB)
Infants for short term use, no specific medical condition (IB)
Laboratory research (milk that cannot be used for human consumption due to drugs used by the donor or lack of complete testing of the donor (1—CB)

From *Guidelines for the Establishment and Operation of a Donor Human Milk Bank*, Human Milk Banking Association of North America, 2007. Raleigh, NC. Reprinted with permission.

MILK BANKING AND THE CODE

How does the International Code of Marketing Breastmilk Substitutes apply to human milk banking? The Code proscribes marketing artificial milk products and bottles directly to parents. In her discussion of ethical issues in human milk banking, Miriam Labbok has argued that banked milk is not a breastmilk substitute, nor is it breastmilk, leaving donor human milk in a grey area in terms of compliance with the Code. Milk banks must educate the community about the availability of and appropriate uses for banked milk. Is this a violation of the Code? Where is the line between educating parents and marketing to them? Frequently physicians and hospitals are introduced to donor human milk when their NICU patients' parents request it. Answering such queries from parents is education. Are brochures written for parents about benefits and appropriate uses of banked milk education or marketing? Are television public service announcements and news stories seeking donors (but reading potential recipients) education or marketing? Who makes these determinations? These questions arise at MMBNE meetings and on the HMBANA milk bank directors' listserv as we all struggle to operate our milk banks in ethically responsible ways.

ALLOCATING DONOR MILK

Equitable allocation of a scarce resource involves many factors, only one of which is adequate funds. HMBANA has developed a suggested priority list for dispensing donor human milk. They considered factors related to the recipient, including age, projected length of need, medical condition and prognosis; the mother, including insufficient milk supply, medical contraindication to breastfeeding, adoption and choice; time, short term use, likeliness of recovery and preventive treatment; and ethical values, community benefit and individual benefit/choice. Going from highest to lowest priority, most critical to least critical and community benefit to individual benefit/choice, a triage of priority for dispensing milk begins with premature, sick infants as first priority, other infants less than twelve months old with varying severity of need, research contracts for well-designed studies, and individuals more than twelve months old with varying degrees of need. The list ends with infants for short term use but no specific medical conditions and laboratory research. Milk that cannot be used for human consumption for various reasons is used for laboratory research (HMBANA 2007). (See Table 2.) This triage is a helpful guideline for milk banks. Consultation with medical ethicists helps to clarify individual situations that do not fall neatly into these categories. While adequate funding is not the only issue in equitable distribution, neither can it be ignored. As MMBNE begins to distribute milk in our community we are also beginning to develop a policy regarding distribution of milk to all who need it regardless of their ability to pay the fees and shipping. While all milk banks have some funds available for needy families, there are real costs associated with operating a milk bank and we sometimes face difficult decisions in which it is important to maintain short and long term perspectives.

While there are many untapped milk donors throughout the country, currently, there is greater need for milk than there is milk available. How should milk be apportioned between non-profit milk banks producing pasteurized donor human milk and manufacturers developing and marketing human milk based pharmaceutical products for very low birth weight (VLBW) babies, sick babies, cancer patients and others? Research, development and production of these products require many ounces of human milk per ounce of medicinal product produced. Is development and sale of these pharmaceutical products justified before the number of donor mothers is increased to provide for all the babies who need the milk, and before the products have been adequately tested for safety and efficacy?

PROFIT VERSUS NONPROFIT

The use of donor human milk by for-profit pharmaceutical and other companies raises another ethical question. The primary mandate of for-profit corporations is to earn money for their stockholders. Is it ethical for these companies *not* to pay mothers for their milk? Should donor mothers' informed consent include the fact that they are providing their milk to a for-profit company at no charge? A situation in which non-profit milk banks cannot pay donors and for-profit companies must pay donors, however, is untenable. These issues are at the forefront of the milk banking ethical and policy conversation, yet to be resolved fully.

MMBNE is the newest developing milk bank in North America, though calls and emails from Oregon, Washington, Minnesota and Toronto indicate that we are, fortunately, not the last. We are part of a growing movement of professionals, volunteers and institutions dedicated to a very old and, at the same time, new and always important aspect of the health of our community.

REFERENCES

Arnold, L. D. W. "The Ethics of Donor Human Milk Banking." *Breastfeeding Medicine* 1 (2006): 3-13.

Boyd, Catherine A., Maria A. Quigley and Peter Brocklehurst. "Donor Breast Milk Versus Infant Formula for Preterm Infants: A Systematic Review and Meta-analysis." *Archives of Disease in Childhood Fetal and Neonatal Edition* 92 (2007): F169-F175.

Fildes, Valerie. *Wet Nursing: A History from Antiquity to the Present*. New York: Basil and Blackwell, 1988.

Galtry, Judith. "The Impact on Breastfeeding of Labour Market Policy and Practice in Ireland, Sweden, and the United States." *Social Science & Medicine* 57 (2003): 167-177.

Golden, Janet. *A Social History of Wet Nursing in America: From Breast to Bottle.* Ohio: Ohio State University Press, 2001.

Human Milk Banking Association of North America (HMBANA). *Guidelines for the Establishment and Operation of a Donor Human Milk Bank.* Raleigh, NC, 2007.

Human Milk Banking Association of North America (HMBANA). *Annual Report.* 2008. Raleigh, NC.

Ideablob."New England Milk Bank Voted Best Small Business Iidea in National Ideablob.com Contest." 2008. <http://www.ideablob.com/posts/157>.

Jacobs, Ruste. "Generous Mothers Save Lacie's Life." *Ardmoreite* May 16, 1999.

Jones, France. "History of North American Donor Milk Banking: One Hundred Years of Progress." *Journal of Human Lactation* 19.3 (2003): 313.

Labbok, Miriam. "Ethics, Established Breastfeeding Policy and Donor Milk Banking." Plenary Lecture presented at the conference of HMBANA, November 2007.

McGuire, W. and M. Y. Anthony. "Donor Human Milk Versus Formula for Preventing Necrotizing Enterocolitis in Preterm Infants: A Systematic Review." *Archives of Disease in Childhood Fetal and Neonatal Edition* 88 (2003): F11-F14.

"Milestone Birthday for a Three Year Old." *New York Times.* April 19, 1984.

"Okla. Couple Visit Mass. Mothers Who Are Keeping Their Baby Alive." *Boston Globe* Dec. 7, 1982.

Smith Julie P., Lindy Ingham and Mark Dunstone. "The Economic Value of Breastfeeding in Australia." *Working Papers No. 40,* National Centre for Epidemiology and Population Health, ANU Canberra, 1998.

Tully, Mary Rose. "Donating Human Milk as part of the Grieving Process." *Journal of Human Lactation* 15.2 (1999): 149-51.

Tully, Douglas B., Frances Jones and Mary Rose Tully. "Donor Milk: What's In It and What's Not." *Journal of Human Lactation* (2001)17: 152-155.

Updegrove, Kim. "Human Milk Banking in the United States." *Newborn Infant and Nursing Reviews* 5.1 (2005): 27-33.

Comparing Sharing and Banking Milk

Issues of Gift Exchange and Community in the Sudan and Ireland

TANYA M. CASSIDY AND ABDULLAHI EL-TOM

SOCIETAL BONDS HAVE BEEN forged and reinforced as a result of the sharing of breastmilk cross-culturally for countless generations. The inability (or in some cases unwillingness) of some mothers to supply their own children with milk resulted in the phenomenon of wet-nursing, a service sometimes formalised as paid employment and sometimes managed within a more cooperative framework, sometimes even religiously sanctioned. Wet-nursing has been consigned to the history books in the so-called developed world and is now being challenged, to be replaced (in an uneven and episodic manner) by "milk banking," considered a more hygienic, and controlled means to share human milk.[1] As a result of the uneven pace of this change worldwide, both wet-nursing and milk banking can form part of the life experience of two contemporary researchers. This article will focus on two examples of unpaid milk-sharing, one from Ireland and one from the Sudan, illustrating the larger implications of the "gift" of milk activating a series of expectations and obligations that anthropologists since Bronislaw Malinowski (1884-1942) have analysed in terms of structures of social cohesion. This discussion will, therefore, make use of auto-ethnography (Reed-Danahay; Ellis and Bochner 2000), the reflexive study of personal experience, in order to achieve a representative understanding of a very precise and specific experience, in a larger socio-cultural and historical context.

Tanya's experience with milk banking occurred as a result of personal tragedy. Her first son, Liam, was born prematurely in Canada and died two weeks later of necrotizing enterocolitis (NEC). While attempting to make sense of what had happened, she discovered that rates of NEC among human milk-fed premature babies were significantly lower than among formula-fed premature infants (Lucas and Cole; Lucas et al.). Unable (following birth trauma and blood loss) to express sufficient milk for Liam, formula was aggressively provided by the team in the neonatal unit in a Canadian province with no milk bank.[2] This led her to research the availability of milk banks worldwide and to begin to theorise about how and why banks flourished sporadically in different parts of the world. This research quickly took second place to the more personally urgent issue of the availability of milk banks in Ireland, where her second son was due to be born. Ireland is served by a single human milk bank in County Fermanagh which, located in Northern Ireland, and therefore under the jurisdiction of the UK department of health, functions in a cross-border context, receiving donations from north and south, and distributing across the island of Ireland on the basis of need. This bank is the only community-based bank in the UK system, rather than being a facility within an existing hospital. When making her birthing choices, Tanya and her partner chose a particular birthing hospital on the basis of its guarantee that it would apply to the milk bank if necessary.

As a result of a condition known as placenta previa, a series of dangerous bleedings led to Tanya being hospitalised. A son was born five weeks later in February, as a result of an emergency caesarean section. Like his brother, Gabriel was born ten weeks prematurely. Tanya was incapacitated, so her partner lobbied immediately for milk to be sent and for the first crucial weeks of life, he was fed on a mixture of donor milk and mother's own expressed milk. As a result, Gabriel was released early from the NICU having (unusually) suffered no infections during his stay in hospital.

The milk distribution system worked via an arrangement with Bus Eireann (the nationwide Irish bus company), involving free transportation of milk. This milk was then picked up by taxi and delivered to the hospital where it was refrigerated and used. Tanya and her partner established a telephone relationship with the staff at the milk bank placing orders through the staff in the NICU. Following Gabriel's release from hospital, the arrangement was continued at home until he was approximately one month corrected, at which time, due to supply shortages in the bank and Gabriel's thriving health, the arrangement was ended.

Fifty years earlier, on another continent, among the Berti people of northern Darfur, Sudan, another community-based milk-sharing relationship was established. In this case, it was the health of the mother which provided the main justification for the arrangement. Shortly after the uneventful birth of Abdullahi, the other author of this paper, a neighbouring mother gave birth to a son, Mohamed, under circumstances where it was lucky that both survived. As a result of this birth, Mohamed's mother was unable to breastfeed for a while, and Abdullahi's mother was enlisted to help, transforming the two infants into "milk brothers," a detailed and culturally prescribed relationship akin to blood ties in Islamic societies.

Fifty years ago, Broosh had no medical facilities and the nearest clinic was a day's journey on a donkey or a camel. Passing trucks were rare and unscheduled and most people did not rely on them for urgent journeys. A couple of traditional birth attendants helped with childbirth as a trained midwife did not appear in the town until 15 years later. Abdullahi had many friends in his early childhood but it was Mohamed who was the closest. Abdullahi's family also shared affection for Mohamed and always treated him almost as a family member. Mohamed lived only two houses away, in an identical home and both fathers had their shops attached to their respective houses. Whenever Mohamed was around during meal times, Abdullahi's late mother always kept him to share the food with the family. Mohamed's mother was among the first to show up in Abdullahi's house when extra hands were needed.

Abdullahi was around eleven or twelve when he first realized that Mohamed was more than a friend and that his special relationship with his family had its specific justification. In a casual talk that was overheard by Abdullahi as a child, a woman said to his mother: "Mohamed is a wonderful boy; it is such a shame that he cannot marry one of your daughters in the future."

Abdullahi is unable to recall whether Mohamed realized his relationship with his mother at the same time as he did but he certainly acted as a second child to Abdullahi's mother. Mohamed and Abdullahi attended the same educational establishments right up to university level. Later, both went to work for different organisations away from Broosh. Every two or three years, they visited Broosh, sometimes together but often separately. In his visits home, Mohamed always went to Abdullahi's mother with gifts and was treated as a returning child. Abdullahi responded to Mohamed's kindness to his mother by treating his in a similar fashion even though she is not Abdullahi's milk mother.

Separated by space and time, both Gabriel and Mohamed were provided with life-sustaining milk from women other than their own mother, a need which their respective communities helped to provide. Thinking about the changes over time and across cultures with regards to breastfeeding is important for understanding responses in circumstances where this most natural form of nutrition is not directly available. Rather than choosing (for whatever reasons) artificial feeding, the historically more prevalent and religiously defined relationship of wet-nursing versus the modern sterile medicalized aspects of milk banking is key to our tale.

BREASTFEEDING

The WHO Global Data Bank on Breastfeeding and Complementary Feeding shows that in the Sudan breastfeeding rates as of the turn of the millennium were between 95 to 98 percent for initial feeding rates. After Sudanese children reach one year of age, these rates drop substantially, and urban rates are much lower than rural rates, with Darfur having the highest percentage of breastfeeding. On the other hand, Ireland has one of the lowest rates of breastfeeding in not only Europe, but the world generally (WHO Data Bank), with not even forty percent reporting any breastfeeding. Historical data is provided for the UK and Northern Ireland which also has a very low rate of breastfeeding initiation. These data suggest that the breastfeeding rates around the United Kingdom in the 1940s and 1950s were over ninety percent, but began to drop in the 1960s, and were to reach a particularly low point in the 1970s.

In October of 2006 Irishhealth.com online published the results of a survey asking why there were such low rates of breastfeeding in Ireland. They reported that although almost a quarter of the respondents felt there was a lack of support from the hospital staff; over forty percent felt that the main reason was a sense of "fear or embarrassment." A year earlier, Irishhealth.com also reported Maureen Fallon, the National Breastfeeding Coordinator, as saying that "a number of mothers have been asked to move or leave hotels, public houses and other social events," despite research indicating that Irish people were "very accepting" of a mother's need to breast feed outside of the home. Fallon went on to say, "Our aim is to make breastfeeding a normal and unremarkable part of child rearing. We want to have a society that values breastfeeding and doesn't bat an eyelid when a woman chooses this option" (Condon). Clearly the sexualisation of women's mammary glands at the expense of their reproductive nutritional qualities, are key to the establishment of this ideal. Research published in the *Irish Medical Journal* by Connolly and colleagues also found "embarrassment" to be a major detriment to breastfeeding over bottle feeding choices.

For a number of reasons, in most parts of Africa artificial feeding has never been as widespread. The expense, the lack of facilities to properly prepare the formula, and the high rates of illiteracy, has all contributed to the disastrous consequences associated with the use of formula on the African continent. Bottle-feeding is much more common in the urban centre of Kartoum (WHO). Family law among the Berti is an approximation of Islamic law. This fact has its history in pre-British colonialism whereby family relations are derived from Islam, with only minor local variations. Family law runs parallel to other laws that are either of national or local bases and are often at odd with Islamic principles.

Traditionally, mother's milk for two complete years is regarded as ideal for a baby. Obviously, this ideal cannot always be adhered to. Breastfeeding for two years requires collaboration of senior female relatives as well as the husband. Following practice reminiscent of the WHO doula system, the Berti commission a senior female relative to advise young mothers on how to breastfeed while other relatives take over routine housework. If the mother experiences some difficulty at first, the breast is massaged with sesame oil and the young mother is encouraged to continue trying until milk flow is secured. Early milk (colostrum) is regarded as especially crucial for healthy progress of the baby and is often fortified by butter made of goat or cow milk. This butter is the only external feeding given to the baby in the first five to six months. Modern medical personnel in the area now advise against the use of butter but are rarely listened to. The use of butter at this early stage is similar to the practice of giving dates to a newborn reported in central Sudan but unknown to the Berti. As it is reported in central Sudan, as soon as the baby is born, the Traditional Birth Attendant (TBA) chews a small piece of date and then deposits it in the mouth of the baby. Dates were regarded as the Prophet's favorite fruit and are hence intended to be the first food the baby tastes in their life (El-Tom 1996).

The father's commitment is important for maintaining the ideal of breastfeeding for the duration of two years. Parents of the breastfed baby are expected to abstain from having sex for the entire duration of breastfeeding. This is to ensure avoidance of pregnancy believed to spoil the milk of the lactating mother. The local view asserts that as soon as the mother gets pregnant, her milk is no longer suitable for breastfeeding. In their words, the milk then belongs to "the baby inside the womb rather than the one outside." It is understood that the breastfed baby will be harmed either by being weaned prematurely or being fed on defective milk. Such milk is seen to be a common cause of a particular type of diarrhoea which is tested by pressing a thumb on the forehead of the sickly child and observing how the skin bounces back into position. If the skin is too slow when bouncing back, the diarrhoea is certainly caused by defective milk due to pregnancy. Modern medics take this as a likely sign of malnutrition. The Berti agree but see the cause differently, giving it a moral twist. In their culture, this is indicative of callous parents who are irresponsible enough to sacrifice their baby for their own pleasure. High significance attached to breastfeeding for two years among the Berti is unmistakably of Islamic origin.[3]

Global efforts have been in place for a number of years to try to combat the cross-cultural differences in breastfeeding rates, including a WHO recognition that all children should be exclusively breastfed for the first six months of their lives (WHO), and the WHO UNICEF hospital friendly initiative which is designed to encourage increased breastfeeding rates particularly in countries where these rates have dropped tremendously. Despite these efforts inequity continues to exist around the world, therefore making it even more difficult when breastfeeding difficulties occur. Mothers who are unable to breastfeed, but recognize the need and importance of such nutrition for their infants, and wish to provide human milk from another woman, are once again cross-culturally specific in their possible choices.

WET-NURSING

The Berti in the Sudan make little fuss about wet-nursing. Chances are wet-nursing is much more prevalent than is talked about. As Abdullahi's biography illustrates, people recognize the relationship but they do not boast about it. This reticence perhaps resides in the fact that wet-nursing is a gift that one gives without expecting any direct gratification and that its very essence is undermined by boasting. The value of children in the society, and the centrality of that to motherhood and hence femininity, colludes in its disguise. Few women would want to admit to their inability to breastfeed their babies and their surrogate mothers may prefer not to expose them as unfortunate mothers. Moreover, surrogate mothers may find it denigrating to reduce their service simply to a commercialized transaction. Indeed the altruistic value embedded in wet-nursing defies boasting about it as it reduces it to an individual enterprise. Yet, long term as it may be, personal gain accruing out of wet-nursing cannot be underestimated. In a society where children and grandchildren constitute the only old age insurance, it makes little sense to forgo a milk-adopted child for short-term commercial gain. Although Abdullahi's mother did not need to rely on Mohamed for her old age support, it would have been difficult for him not to help her, should she need his support.

Given the relative marginality of the Berti within Arab-Islamic culture, it would perhaps be safe to say that adoption of wet-nursing is either inspired and/or augmented by Islam. It is common knowledge among the Berti that Prophet Mohammed himself was wet-nursed. School children across Muslim Sudan can even name Halima Alssadiya as his wet-nurse. However, details of Islamic theological debate on wet-nursing have not filtered into Berti's collective memory of Islam. Such knowledge is, nonetheless, available to local religious leaders. What is striking is the right of the mother to abstain from breastfeeding and her entitlement to support in case of divorce at the time of breastfeeding. Moreover, Islamic edicts oblige the "father" and not the mother to shoulder cost of breastfeeding. At the same time, Islam instructs that the mother should be allowed to breastfeed her child even if the father of the baby is divorced.

The Quran is also quite explicit on its edict that a wet-nurse should be paid for her service. That also applies to the mother who is divorced at the time of breastfeeding. It is here that the Berti offer a different interpretation. Among the Berti, wet-nursing belongs to the so-called "gift economy" domain. In anthropological terms this is an exchange based on reciprocity, which involves a give and take interaction. Often these types of exchanges do not involve money, and generally occur between social equals, often related by kinship or marriage, or in this case creating kinship and marriage ties. The value of the gift is not specified and neither is the time of repayment. So important is this gift that it is as close as familial gifts. It is done for altruistic reasons and for enhancing community relations. That of course does not preclude the wet-nurse receiving personal gifts in return. It might be strange to contemplate how the early Arabs had commercialised wet-nursing in the seventh century while the Berti have not done so in the twenty-first century. The Berti are certainly not new to commodity economics. Nonetheless, they opted not to apply commodity economy to wet-nursing. We must caution that this fact can only be laboured up to a point. After all, most societies including modern ones combine both commodity and gift economy in their cultures. For example, blood banks as well as milk banks in the United Kingdom currently operate under gift rather than commodity economies (Oakley and Ashton).

At a different level, the Berti are careful regarding selection of a wet-nurse: certain women do not make good wet-nurses, being likely to transmit diseases to the breastfed baby and or convey undesirable characters. Some diseases like TB, epilepsy, mental illness and leprosy are believed to run in certain families and might be transmitted through wet-nursing. Peculiarly, the Berti also think certain ethnic groups have a tendency to turn into haunting ghosts after death. That feature too is likely to be transmitted through breastfeeding. As far as possible, women of bad moral character are equally to be avoided as possible wet nurses. Little differentiation is made between learnt character and attributes that are of biological nature. Some of these perceptions can be found in early Islamic exegeses. (It is to be noted that Bani Saad were regarded as the best Arabic speakers at the time and it was they who provided Halima Assaidya [of Bani Saad ethnic group] who wet-nursed the Prophet himself.)

Wet-nursing is also restricted by consanguinial relationship of the baby to the potential nurse. The Berti are aware of future marriage restrictions imposed by wet-nursing. As their culture lays preference for marriage within the group, wet-nursing within the group is only reluctantly pursued. Furthermore, the Berti do not have to worry about unknowingly breaching the marriage code related to wet-nursing. Wet-nurses come from the community and they and their children are known to all.

It is interesting that within the heritage of Old Testament narratives shared by Jews, Christians and Muslims alike, wet-nursing receives special attention. There is a long, but currently often forgotten tradition in Catholicism associated with the wet-nursing of foundlings in particular following the tradition of Moses, recorded in the Book of Genesis (Exodus, II, 7-9). The reputed founder of monotheistic religion is therefore associated with a milk-sharing arrangement, albeit one which paradoxically reinstated his real mother as milk mother in place of an adoptive mother. It is reasonable to suppose that this story asserts the importance of Hebrew milk as an antidote or at least corrective to an Egyptian upbringing: not so much "blood will out" as "milk will out."

The historian Janet Golden has pointed out that the majority of wet nurses in late nineteenth-early twentieth-century America were foreign born, particularly Irish born women. Given widespread prejudice against Irish immigrants to the United States, this preference deserves careful consideration. Paradoxically, the pseudo-Darwinist taxonomies that created categories of animality and promoted Anglo-Saxons as a more highly evolved order of being may well have helped advertise Irish women as productive bovines, closer to being functioning mammals than their more refined employers and therefore worth paying for their milk services. At the same time there were moves to improve the milk available to children generally through the establishment of cow's milk depots (first in France, and then later in both Britain and North America). Attitudes towards beneficial features of these non-human milk depots varied between establishing contact with mothers to advocate breastfeeding to offering cleaner safer "artificial" milk products. In Ireland, on February 22, 1908, a lecture discussing infantile mortality given to the Women's National Health Association, calls for a milk depot in Ireland, stating that there has been a reduction in breastfeeding which is leading to an increase in death among infants ("Women's National Health Association: Infantile Mortality"). Even in the infancy of their profession, paediatricians fully recognized the immeasurable value of human milk over what they labelled purposefully "artificial" choices, but how to provide alternatives to growing number of women having supply problems, not to mention medical difficulties associated with premature birth, became the focus of the modern medicalized version of milk banking.

MILK BANKING

Historically milk banking is understood to have begun in Vienna (1909) and in Boston (1911), and were both linked to increasing survival rates of the prematurely born, and to infants who are without their original mothers, specifically in "foundling hospitals" (Jones). In the 1930s, the development of milk banks was accelerated in part due to the impact of high profile multiple births, such as the Dionne Quintuplets in Ontario and the St Neots Quads in England. Such cases generated both media fascination and consequent milk drives. In the latter part of the twentieth century, milk banking has had to engage two major setbacks. The strength of formula companies in the post-World War Two environment led to a dramatic decline in all forms of human milk feeding in the 1950s and 1960s. Although breastfeeding and milk banking resurfaced in the 1970s, milk banks would close in large numbers in the 1980s in response to the HIV/AIDS epidemic. Given the slightest prospect of spreading the virus through milk, the banks were regarded as too dangerous to continue. It is instructive to reconsider again a comparison between donated blood and donated milk at this point. Nobody argued for the closure of blood banks in the 1980s, only for the strict testing of their stocks. This is presumably because there is no multi-billion formula blood industries that can claim to replace donor blood. Eventually the case began to be made that milk can and should be tested and guaranteed on the same basis as blood, and banks began to reopen, though in a very uneven fashion across the world. Immensely popular in Brazil, and growing in popularity in some parts of Europe and the United States, milk banks were recently re-established in Australia, and there are plans to re-establish other banks in Canada.

Milk banking has been expanding since the mid-1990s, and its various health benefits have been increasingly recognised. In Africa, the two main places where milk banking has grown most are in Cameroon and South Africa. The latter is unique in that it provides milk to orphans of HIV/AIDS mothers. The former is run on a very low budget and also has links to the combating of HIV/AIDS.

In Ireland, milk donations are accepted from mothers who complete a telephone questionnaire thereby fulfilling a series of minimum health criteria. The milk is collected and sent to the bank in Fermanagh to be tested and pasteurised. The bank carefully catalogues all donations, which are traceable to source at every stage of preparation and distribution. A key feature of this arrangement is anonymity. The parents of children who receive donor milk are unaware of its source, although Tanya was informed (unofficially) of the fact that a particular individual had been responsible for a disproportionate amount of her son's intake. Although this arrangement precludes the possibility of personal contact with donors, it establishes a very strong psychological sense of an imagined community, a community of gratitude that extends towards anyone who has ever given milk. This was particularly noted during a trip to Canada where Tanya's partner encountered a woman who had given milk in Vancouver (milk which her son could not possibly have received). The experience of being the parent of a donor milk recipient also encouraged reflection on the success of an arrangement which largely avoids the cash nexus altogether. The most vulnerable people in Ireland are fed and nurtured through the most perilous portion of their lives without any need for money to change hands.

The urgency inherent in the situation of being the parent of a premature infant fast-tracks a familiarity with all aspects of milk banking, which leads in turn to a sense of estrangement from the majority of the population, for whom milk donation remains (in Ireland and elsewhere) a strange and even disturbing development. For example, during an interview on Radio Telefís Éireann (the Irish national radio and television network) given by Tanya and her family, the interviewer asked how either parent might react to the instinctive distaste associated with this form of giving. While travelling by train with a container of donor milk, Tanya's partner was challenged by other passengers as to the contents of the bulky container, to whom he was inclined to confidently offer at least one hundred guesses. This very estrangement from the general population is derived from a peculiar experience and only reinforces a sense of community identity associated with everybody associated with giving, receiving, and administering donor milk.

Feeding by donor milk remains a rare and short-term alternative to direct breastfeeding or formula feeding. Choosing donor milk is not however a choice defined as "between" breast and formula, since it is based on a firm moral choice that affirms breastmilk as preferable to formula milk. Donor milk is not chosen in preference to direct breastfeeding (which may continue to be attempted) but as the second best available option if direct breastfeeding is impossible. Morally and politically, as a breastmilk recipient, Tanya and her partner became eager supporters of boycotts of formula companies, and increasingly angry about attempts by such companies to advertise within hospitals and other medical environments.

The community milk bank represents therefore a kind of invisible community based on a unique and invaluable form of giving. This community represents a body that is derived from neither the public nor the private sector, traditionally understood. It is not directly founded on structures of reciprocity, long familiar via anthropological models, since it is based not on exchange but on giving without expectation of any reward. It is however derived from a deep-rooted societal obligation to feed children on the part of mothers whose own supply enables them to expand their own maternal role beyond their immediate offspring. Milk banking therefore celebrates an ideal of motherhood that transcends narrow or constraining definitions of "the domestic sphere."

CONCLUSION

There can be no doubt that Berti culture is fully in support of breastfeeding and that it is equally accommodating for wet-nursing. While the influence of Arab-Islamic culture is evident, survival of strong breastfeeding culture among the Berti is due to their poor exposure to modernity. Invariably, breastfeeding has declined in all Muslim societies which have given way to the modern way of life. Sadly, this may also be the future of Berti society, and the time is ripe to counter such influence. In this regard, efforts must be made to preserve the current preference for extended breastfeeding in the area. As far as wet-nursing is concerned, we can be assured that it is well grounded in Berti culture. Nonetheless, wet-nursing in Berti culture is community-based, a situation which cannot necessarily be sustained in the future. As the society becomes more individualistic and urban-oriented, wet-nursing will face a formidable challenge. In the current wet-nursing arrangement, the possibility of a person unknowingly marrying a milk sibling is beyond contemplation. This situation will not remain the same if milk of unknown donors is used.

In a rural Berti setting a modern milk-banking system may be both unnecessary and unpractical. This is due to poor infrastructure as the entire area lacks transport, communication networks, electricity and reliable health amenities. Additionally, population is sparse in the area. Luckily, there is ample scope for the current community-based wet-nursing to be enhanced. Restrictions based on traditional health beliefs can be exploited here, while the exclusion of potential wet-nurses based on a belief in ghosts must be negotiated. Prospects for the introduction of milk banking are far better in the urban areas where modern facilities are already in place. Moreover, community-based wet-nursing is unlikely to be sustained in urban zones. Hence, milk banking could serve as a back-up if not an alternative to community-based wet-nursing, but not one that startles the mass media with any urgency.

Human milk banking operates on very different scales, as the various chapters in this volume attest. Human milk may be pooled, pasteurised and distributed in a very anonymous fashion, or it may be donated by a comparatively small number of regular donors who may or may not be known to one another, creating a knowable community of donor-recipients. In Ireland there is a continuing need to encourage healthy mothers to provide human milk to their infants. A society that desexualizes the breast, and does not impose a sense of impropriety on the lactating mother, is therefore crucial.

The two stories offered by the two authors of this chapter illustrate the transhistorical and cross-cultural persistence of the idea of mothers' milk being shared at times of need. The strategic and ideological variety and versatility of milk-sharing only adds to its power and its promise as a central component of an ongoing global struggle against Infant Mortality, a struggle that will not be defined by the "First World" conferring scientific benefits on the "Third" but rather by the sharing and adaptation of examples of good practice wherever they can be found.

Neither Tanya nor her partner are under the delusion that a milk bank would have definitely saved their son Liam's life, but they are convinced that their son Gabriel benefited immensely from the donor milk he received, as are both Abdullahi, and the now professional adult Mohamed regarding his milk ties. It is their hope, and a goal of this paper, that other babies will, like Gabriel and Mohamed, have statistical and medical evidence in their favour, and have access to human milk.

[1]Recent discussions have argued for the use of the terms "cross-nursing" or "cross breastfeeding," suggesting that ultimately "both wet-nursing and cross-nursing" can be classified along a continuum of reciprocities from symmetric to asymmetric relations" (Shaw 2007:443). This more generous definition of wet-nursing fits better with the Muslim translation of this concept.

[2]Since the late 1980s with the medical scare associated with HIV/AIDS, all but one of the Canadian milk banks was closed (Jones).

[3]Due to limitations of space, details regarding the Islamic verses associated with breastfeeding have been omitted from this discussion.

REFERENCES

Condon, Deborah. "Breastfeeding Discrimination Remains." *Irish Health* website. 2005. <http://www.irishhealth.com/index.html?level=4&id=7958&ss=maureen%20fallon>. Last visited April 2, 2008.

Connolly, Claire, Cecily C. Kelleher, Genevieve Becker, Sharon Friel and Saoirse Ni Gabhann. "Attitudes of Young Men and Women to Breastfeeding." *The Irish Medical Journal* 91.3 (1998): 88-89.

Ellis, Clair and Arthur Bochner. "Bringing Emotion and Personal Narrative into Medical Social Science." *Health* 3 (1999): 229-237.

Ellis, Clair and Arthur Bochner. "Autoethnography, Personal Narrative, Reflexivity: Researcher as Subject." *Handbook of Qualitative Research*. Second edition. Eds N. K. Denzin and Y. S. Lincoln. Thousand Oaks, CA: Sage, 2000. 733-768.

El-Tom, Abdullahi Osman. "Traditional Practices and Perinatal Health in a Sudanese Village." *CURARE: Special Issue* on *Early Childhood* 9 (1996): 1-20.

El-Tom, Abdullahi Osman. "Female Circumcision and Ethnic Identification in Sudan with Reference to the Berti of Darfur." *GeoJournal*. 46 (1998): 163-170.

Golden, Janet. *A Social History of Wet Nursing in America: From Breast to Bottle*. Cambridge: Cambridge University Press, 1996.

Jones, Francis. "History of North American Donor Milk Banking: One Hundred Years of Progress." *Journal Human Lactation*. 19.3 (2003): 313-318.

Lucas, Alan and Timothy J. Cole. "Breast Milk and Neonatal Necrotising Enterocolitis." *Lancet* 336 (1990): 1519-1523.

Lucas, Alan, Ruth Morley, Timothy J. Cole and Sheila M. Gore. "A Randomized Multicentre Study of Human Milk Versus Formula and Later Development in Preterm Infants." *Archives of Disease in Childhood* 70 (1994): 141-146.

Malinowski, Bronislaw. *Argonauts of the Western Pacific: An Account of Native Enterprise and Adventure in the Archipelagoes of Melanesian New Guinea.* London: Routledge and Kegan Paul. [1922] 1964.

Oakley, Ann and John Ashton, eds. *The Gift Relationship: From Human Blood To Social Policy.* New York: The New Press, 1997.

Reed-Danahay, Deborah. *Auto/Ethnography*. New York: Berg, 1997.

Shaw, Rhonda. "Cross-Nursing, Ethics, and Giving Breast Milk in the Contemporary Context." *Women's Studies International Forum* 30 (2007): 439–450.

World Health Organization (WHO). *Global Strategy for Infant and Young Child Feeding*. Geneva: World Health Organization, 2003.

"Women's National Health Association: Infantile Mortality." *Irish Times* 22 February 1908: 9.

Going With the Flow

Contemporary Discourses of Donor Breastmilk Use and Breastmilk in a Neonatal Intensive Care Setting

CAROL BARTLE

THE COMPETING DISCOURSES POSITIONING breastmilk as both life-saving for low birth weight babies in neonatal intensive care units (NICUs) and as a potentially contaminated bodily fluid in the same settings, creates tensions between the interested actors within this techno-scientific setting. Not 'having enough' breastmilk and having to use infant formula also represents a source of stress for mothers with babies admitted to NICUs. Availability of donor breastmilk banking facilities in NICU settings could ameliorate these stressful situations and protect babies from infant formula interventions. Currently in New Zealand there are no formal and/or regulated donor human milk banks. This situates concerned midwives, nurses, mothers and families, who wish to avoid infant formula and give babies breastmilk exclusively, in the difficult position of either accepting infant formula for hospitalised neonatal unit babies, when a mother's own milk is not fully available, or attempting to access donor-milk from informal sources.

To establish the feeding trajectories and types of milk feeds in a cohort of neonatal babies in one New Zealand NICU, an audit of 303 babies was undertaken in 2002 (Bartle). This group represented all babies admitted within a six-month period. In this audit it was found that some babies received breastmilk, either expressed or directly from the breast as their first feed. Other babies received a combination of expressed breastmilk and infant formula and others formula alone. Although the nineteen babies in the twenty-four to twenty-seven weeks gestation group all received breastmilk as their first tube feed, eleven babies out of the thirty-six in the twenty-eight to thirty-one week gestation group received infant formula as a first feed. The NICU had a high initiation rate of expressing/breastfeeding with 94 percent of mothers commencing breastmilk provision and the majority of babies receiving some breastmilk during their NICU stay. There was a high level of infant formula use however. Exclusive breastfeeding rates were low at ten percent despite 46.2 percent of babies in the cohort being thirty-seven weeks gestation or above. A recommendation from this audit was that access to screened pasteurised donor breastmilk via a regulated breastmilk bank would be a valuable development for this NICU. After this audit was finished a qualitative research project to investigate supports and barriers to breastfeeding in NICUs was carried out and completed in 2005 (Bartle 2005). This research project involved thirteen women participating in semi-informal interviews during the time their babies were in the NICU and up to six months after the babies went home.

Breastmilk is constructed as desirable, life saving, sometimes hard to produce, and an essential product at the same time as it causes a degree of uneasiness in some contemporary neonatal intensive care environments. Research and evidence indicate that using donor breastmilk is life-saving and life-enhancing for preterm babies in NICU (Arnold 2002; Fewtrell; Lucas and Cole). Breastmilk, however, may continue to be regarded as insufficient in amount, inadequate in content or easily replaceable with novel milk formulas in these high-tech, cultural oases as evidenced by the widespread use of these products as either partial substitutes or as additions to 'fortify' breastmilk (Bartle 2002; Schanler 1998, 2001). Freely available infant formula products, which appear to be considered safe, postpone the urgent consideration of formal human milk banking facilities in New Zealand. Using donor breastmilk, gifted from other human mothers, is not actively or openly encouraged in New Zealand neonatal units, necessitating some degree of breastmilk-baby-mother advocacy 'work'. This has the potential to create a climate of unease amongst mainstream unit staff and position donor-milk advocates and mothers who request donor-milk as difficult or risk-taking.

PRECIOUS BODY FLUID BREASTMILK

For the majority of mothers with babies admitted to neonatal intensive care units breastmilk quickly becomes a precious liquid which they work very hard to obtain by regular breast expression (Albright; Kavanaugh, Mead, Meier, and Mangurten; Kavanaugh, Meier, Zimmermann and Mead; Lucas; Shearer; Sherman; Sykes; Thoms). Establishing lactation, under stressful conditions, without a baby suckling, can become an overwhelming undertaking at times (Killersreiter, Grimmer, Buhrer, Dudenhausen and Obladen). Some professional literature suggests that mothers may feel like breastmilk providers rather than mothers (Bradfield; Hill, Aldag and Chatterton) and maternal stress related to milk volumes obtained is prevalent (Flacking, Nyqvist, Ewald and Wallin; Hill, Hanson and Mefford; Kavanagh, Mead, Meier and Mangurten; Lefebvre and Ducharme).

During semi-informal interviews for the qualitative research project I undertook, mothers described their distress when unable to establish an 'adequate' breastmilk supply, the pressure felt when breastmilk supplies were 'low' or 'dwindling' and the ever present 'threat' of their babies being given infant formula (Bartle 2005). Olivia[1] described her experiences with trying to provide 'enough' breastmilk (Bartle 2005: 61).

> Olivia: *Well, every time your milk drops you look at it and go [pause] 'Oh my God I'm failing', because you can't really be a mum up here. It sort of compounds it, I suppose, and you do feel like you're just* hopeless *really ... everything I tried just [pause] wasn't working 'cause I'd just stress more and more and more.*

Another participant in the same study, Tara, was also feeling distressed because a flatmate had accidentally defrosted the home freezer and her stores of breastmilk had to be discarded. Following this, Tara then received an added setback when her NICU breastmilk was discarded due to it being left in the fridge for over 48 hours. Protocol in this particular unit indicated that breastmilk has to be frozen, if unused, at 48 hours after expression. Tara described concerns about her baby being given infant formula (Bartle 2005: 69).

> Tara: *Like last night I was getting a bit worried. I don't want her going on formula. I thought that if I had all that [breast] milk supply at home I would have been alright but I knew I didn't have that to back me up and to keep her going for a while.*

Mother participants quickly became engaged with the concept of breastmilk as precious and essential and then later obsessed with the NICU 'safety in numbers' culture, which sees all amounts expressed from the breast observed, assessed and measured by mothers and nurses and calculated in measured syringes by staff members. Breastfeeding as a meaningful and significant mother-baby process in its own right is lost and breastmilk becomes just another product. Annemarie Mol and Jessica Mesman suggest that food in the NICU becomes a fluid and a series of numbers (430). Mol and Mesman describe a difference between an infusion and a breastfeed, "a dripping infusion is a meagre substitute for the warmth of a breast flowing with milk" (431). Whether the dripping infusion is intravenous fluids, or the barely noticeable flow of breastmilk from a syringe down a feeding tube, the amounts are measured carefully and this is generally out of the control of mothers. One mother (Bartle 2005) found comfort in the safety in numbers approach.

> Jan: *It's a very nice, safe feeling, environment up there ... I really like knowing amounts and knowing that they were always full and never hungry.*

Jan later discontinued breastfeeding in the NICU, in favour of the security of measured amounts of breastmilk in bottles. Shortly after Jan's baby went home, infant formula feeds were commenced as this enabled Jan to more effectively continue the routine schedule she had become accustomed to in the NICU.

Glenda Wall suggests that when the medical model dominates breastfeeding thinking, mothers become "disembodied providers of breastmilk who must be educated and scrutinised" (594). Hilde Lindemann Nelson describes how women may be seen as "maternal background" or as "means to other's ends" with mothers viewed as "objects to be managed and monitored" (3). In an environment as baby-focussed, weight-focussed, nutrient-focussed and number-focused as NICU, women's breastmilk insecurities may increase and breastmilk and breastfeeding experiences become managed products rather than embodied mother-baby processes. Breastmilk also becomes easily replaced or altered with infant formula products which are always on hand and commercially marketed as scientific, reliable, nutritionally complete and safe.

INADEQUATE BODY FLUID BREASTMILK

Breastmilk, mother's own and donor, is viewed by many health professionals as being a crucial part of infant health and neonatal intensive care treatment (Arnold 2002, 2006a, 2006b; Balmer and Wharton; Human Milk Banking Association of North America; Lucas and Cole; Tully, Jones and Tully; Wight). In some NICU settings, however, breastmilk may be viewed as inadequate in amount in the first few days, when colostrum is produced in physiologically small amounts[2] and then inadequate in content necessitating the addition of a cow's milk-based fortifier to increase the protein and calorie intake of very preterm babies (American Academy of Pediatrics; Atkinson; Kuschel and Harding; Moro and Minoli; Schanler 1998, 2001; Schanler and Hurst). M. M. Ziemer and C. George suggest that supplementation of human milk with formula may be necessary for most low birth weight infants due to the difficulties mothers have in providing enough breastmilk. The reasons given are difficulties in establishing lactation or maintaining lactation using a breast pump, unavailability of breastmilk due to travelling distances and personal stress of NICU mothers (37). Unavailability of donor breastmilk in such situations is a signifier of the absence of baby 'feeding care' and a lack of attention to the baby's 'internal embodied integrity' and this results in the risky practice of infant formula supplementation when mother's own milk is not available.

Making sense of conflicting messages about breastmilk may be problematic for women establishing lactation in the NICU. Breastmilk appears to be simultaneously constructed as important and also inadequate or easily replaceable. Although breastmilk is treated as an essential component of a baby's care and often recognised as being a "medicine rather than food" (Meier 318), practices that undermine breastmilk may begin almost simultaneously to affect its 'status'. If 'breastmilk is best' in NICU and promoted as such, then mothers can be forgiven for thinking that the naturally small amounts of colostrum after birth should be enough for their babies in most cases. If 'breastmilk is best' and associated with such improved outcomes in NICU babies, then mothers may be confused about why a cow's milk fortifier is added to their breastmilk. If breastfeeding is valued as a process with benefits of its own rather than a 'breastmilk product in a bottle', why are some nurses quick to suggest using bottles and teats? These issues dominate breastmilk and breastfeeding discourses within NICU settings and as a medical consensus on infant formula additives and other feeding practices has not been achieved, parental and staff confusion is understandable.

Practices differ within New Zealand units and between different NICU settings. For example some practitioners do not routinely add cow's milk fortifier to breastmilk unless a baby is not gaining weight whereas others add fortifier routinely. Certain NICU protocols give instructions to add fortifier to breastmilk at the cot-side just before giving the feed and other protocols dictate that fortified feeds may be pre-made for a twelve hour period and stored in a designated fridge. Some NICUs avoid bottle-feeds completely for breastfeeding babies to protect breastfeeding and others commence bottle-feeds alongside breastfeeds when babies are barely transitioned to full oral feeding.

DANGEROUS BODY FLUID BREASTMILK

A paradoxical situation appears to exist in some neonatal intensive care environments. The evidence-based, extensively researched literature about the life-saving properties of breastmilk sits uncomfortably alongside the concerns about a potentially infected female body fluid. This creates an uneasy alliance between breastmilk and its users. Staff members 'working' with breastmilk participate in a range of practices from wearing gloves and protective eye goggles when decanting breastmilk, to wearing gloves when assisting a mother to breastfeed (Bartle 2005). One of the participants in my NICU research project spoke of being perplexed when a nurse put gloves on to assist with latching her baby on the breast, saying that it made her feel "dirty" (Bartle 2005). Risk discourses about exposure to the body fluids of 'others' for health workers are expanded to include breastmilk, despite no documented evidence of any infection of workers exposed to breastmilk. Infection of a baby receiving the 'wrong' breastmilk is reported once only due to staff error (Human Milk Banking Association of North America 2005). Information from La Trobe University Department of Microbiology suggests that it would take at least three weeks of feeding breastmilk infected with a virus or bacteria to a baby before that baby potentially became infected.[3]

Prior to commencing the research project interviewing mothers about their NICU lactation and breastfeeding experiences I facilitated a focus group with a self-selected 'naturally occurring' (Kitzinger 300) group of NICU staff who talked about donor breastmilk. Some insights into the attitudes of neonatal staff regarding the use of donor breastmilk may be useful, as 'in-house' culture may have a positive or negative effect on women who may be considering using donor-milk for their babies, with or without the provision of milk banking facilities. The six nurse participants in the focus group were all women and generally supported donor-milk use in the NICU, but this acceptance was framed within a legitimate medical discourse. One participant spoke about a particular incident in the NICU and of why she thought nurses had difficulty in this situation, supporting a mother who had donor breastmilk available for her baby from a screened donor and who had also signed an indemnity form:

> Focus group member 4: *I think they [nurses] felt that if they actually ... because they were wondering in that case that if further down the track there was legal issue taken then they would be held accountable, even though there was an indemnity form signed. I think that was where people [nurses] were coming from. They would be responsible for administering it [donor breastmilk].*

The focus group member indicated that the fear of medico-legal aspects appeared to prevent some nurses from being donor-milk advocates for mothers and babies. Even with mother consent, donor screening and an indemnity form signed by the mother receiving the donor milk for her baby, it appeared that some nurses may have remained vulnerable to the concept of possible future legal repercussions if they actively became involved in this uncommon activity. Another situation discussed during the focus group was related to mothers making their own decisions and using donor breastmilk for their NICU babies. If the decision was taken completely out of nursing hands, as in the case of a mother with a NICU baby who used her sister's breastmilk for her baby, without asking 'permission', that seemed to ease the problem for some nurses, according to the focus group discourse . A nurse could then avoid a potential conflict situation with a mother who wished to use donor milk and passive nurse support of donor milk usage could be quietly undertaken without fear of negative backlash from colleagues.

Invisibility of practice, enables 'different' behaviours to take place without attracting increased surveillance and results in avoidance of the label 'difficult' or 'non-compliant' or having the behaviour closed down by medical authority. However, the success (or failure) of an 'alternative' practice remains invisible to all but those few co-conspirators. Participation in the usual acceptable practices of the NICU—babies having infant formula when breastmilk supplies are limited—is constructed as 'normal' and 'what most mothers are doing' so visibly opting out of 'normal' and deciding to use donor breastmilk can result in some degree of stigmatisation and the questions, 'is there something wrong with you?' (Greenhough 1146), and 'why are you being difficult or why are you taking this risk?'

There was a general agreement and recognition amongst focus group members about the negative effects of infant formula on babies.

> Focus group member 3: *I just get so mad when they start putting formula down [down a baby's feeding tube]. I get so angry because there's just no way that it's any better. They've got to have breastmilk....*

Given the awareness of the negative health effects of infant formula on babies generally, it is interesting that medico-legal issues related to giving babies these imitation products was not reported as a nursing consideration, but instead fears about potentially dangerous donor-milk were reported. The authority of a medicalised nutritionist[4] voice about infant formula products and their suitability, tolerance and safety seems to overwhelm nursing and parental concerns and decision-making attempts and the infection risk discourse surrounding breastmilk is prevalent. Medically authoritative voices questioning infant formula products in NICU settings appear to be uncommon in New Zealand as are medical voices in support of human milk banking and donor milk use.

AUTHORITATIVE KNOWLEDGE AND 'BEING TAKEN SERIOUSLY'

When Brigitte Jordan discusses the notion of authoritative knowledge, her central observation is, "that for any particular domain several knowledge systems exist" (56). Some knowledge systems are privileged above others because of a structural superiority and this knowledge comes to be seen as "natural, legitimate and in the best interests of all parties" (57).

Susan Wendell uses the term 'cognitive authority'[5] to describe how authority is necessary to succeed in having "one's description of the world taken seriously, believed or accepted generally as the truth" (5). The different actors participating in decisions about breastmilk, donor breastmilk and using infant formula construct and make meaning of the discourses in this environment. What is said and what is written and how these relate, contradict, justify or reinforce certain practices but not others, is of interest. Diverse positions on feeding issues, and diversity of meanings, identify power relationships which give certain discourses legitimacy whilst disqualifying other knowledges. Making sense of what is going on in relation to others involves processes of dialogue and critical reflection which draw on concrete human experience (Dahlberg, Moss and Pence 107) and which also allow consideration of a diversity of information. When a medicalised discourse is dominant and results in 'different', even robustly researched information being de-legitimised, making sense of this 'other' information and utilising this for practice is problematic.

When Opie (cited in Henwood and Pidgeon 22) argues that a "valorising of quantity serves to conceal the significance of events that are either fleeting, infrequent, or about which little is said," it highlights the importance of hearing voices that have remained silent, or been silenced in this neonatal culture. The 'fleeting, infrequent, easily dismissed accounts' which are subjugated, by authoritative universal recommendations, are essential contextual pieces of the neonatal feeding 'jigsaw' which are missing. Given that these missing pieces cover a range of solid research including the dangers of infant formula, benefits associated with breastmilk and donor breastmilk, successful models of human milk banks and the rights of parental decision making, which include informed consent and informed refusal, this silencing of voices is significant. How staff support, make sense of, or resist dominant practices and how mothers negotiate, resist and make sense/meaning of feeding information within this powerful system warrants further attention.

BREASTMILK WITHOUT THE MOTHER

Jaimie Smith-Windsor (2) discusses situations where technology displaces motherhood and infancy 'without motherhood' becomes possible. Mothers are discharged from the post-natal ward leaving their babies in the NICU. This situation potentially causes not only feelings of loss but may result in mothers feeling as if providing breastmilk is the 'best' or the 'only thing' they can do. Mol and Mesman point out that, "many forms of social control rely on the erasure or silencing of various workers, on deleting their work from representations of their work" (425). Visible breastmilk represents the 'work' of the mother and supplying breastmilk situates a mother in the role of disembodied, often absent, nomadic[6] breastmilk provider. The stresses, complexities, influences on and realities of this expressing 'work' done by the mother are effectively deleted. Even discussions about this 'work' are limited and seemed to be confined to a token inquiry by nurses to mothers. Lactation, breastmilk and breastfeeding rarely made an appearance as a topic of importance in the clinical notes of the babies in my feeding audit and research project.

In situations where mothers are struggling to provide breastmilk for their babies, milk from a human milk bank, donated by "donor mothers [who] are 'fed by' stories of the recipients" (Arnold 2006: 9) is valuable. "Fed by" is a term used by Lois Arnold, who has written extensively about human milk banking, to indicate the sense of reciprocity involved in the donor experience—the gift of breastmilk and the received satisfaction for the donor who is emotionally 'fed' by positive stories about the baby recipients. Donor breastmilk is gifted to mothers by other mothers and when this practice is visible, valued, able to be discussed and part of a recognised and legitimate system, it is rendered more meaningful.

SUBTERRANEAN DONOR BREASTMILK

NICU authoritative breastmilk and feeding discourses may create a narrow range of conformist behavioural parameters or acceptable practices for mothers, with minimal possibilities of negotiation. Subsequent increases in stress may occur as mothers try to reconcile the contradictory statements and practices. Accepting infant formula causes stress for many mothers and using screened donor breastmilk against perceived or real medical and nursing opposition may equally cause stress, guilt and fear of personal repercussions. Some women, empowered by supportive networks, are making informed decisions to give their babies donor breastmilk from screened mothers and making informed refusals of infant formula. The informal mothers' milk bank is alive and well, thriving but fragile. When informal, out of the mainstream practice becomes visible, it is open to censure from medical authority and has the potential to create increased hostility towards and surveillance of the participants and supporters.

Human milk banks are thriving in many parts of the world and now opening again in Australia with the Perron Rotary Express Milk (PREM) Bank operating in Perth at the King Edward Memorial Hospital, a community milk bank at the John Flynn Hospital in Tugon on the Gold Coast, and another in Melbourne at the Mercy Hospital for Women. It is hoped that this represents just the beginning of an Australian and New Zealand shift in thinking which will lead to informal donor human milk banks transforming into visible, approved, supported, acceptable, treasured facilities and being counted as providers of a valuable mother-to-mother-to-baby gift of breastmilk when needed.

[1]Participant pseudonyms were either chosen by the women involved in this study or by the researcher with participant consent.

[2]NICU fluid requirements in the study NICU (Bartle 2002) are generally 65mls/kg/day on Day 1, 90mls/kg/day on Day 2, 120mls/kg/day on Day 3 and 150mls/kg on Day 4. Volume of colostrum varies between 0-5mls at the first breastfeed. Average amount taken by a well baby in the first 24hrs has been calculated to be between 7-123mls (Kent).

[3]See Table 4 at http://www.latrobe.edu.au/microbiology/milk.html

[4]Michael Pollan uses the term nutritionism, attributed possibly to Gyorgy Scrinis, a sociologist, who described margarine as the ultimate nutritionist product—"able to shift its identity depending on the prevailing winds of dietary opinion" (27). This can be likened to infant formula identity—constantly changing with new and novel non-food ingredients being added, to provide whatever seems important at the time to 'imitate' breastmilk, make health claims and increase the product cost, medical and consumer attraction and profits.

[5]A term 'borrowed' from Kathryn Pyne Addelson and by Ssuan Wendell.

[6]Kyro Landzelius describes "navigation between home and hospital" as "circumstantial nomadism" and suggests that the "enforced migrations" between home and the NICU causes psychological issues for mothers similar to those experienced by refugees. NICU mothers are described as being, "exiled from traditional maternal identities and role expectations" (331).

REFERENCES

Addelson, Kathryn Pyne. "The Man of Professional Wisdom." *Discovering Reality: Feminist Perspectives on Epistemology, Metaphysics, Methodology and Philospphy of Science.* Eds. Sandra Harding and Merrill B. Hintikka. New York: Kluwer, 1983. 165-186.

Albright, Lisa. "Persevering with a Premie." *New Beginnings* 11 (1994): 76-77.

<http://www.lalecheleague.org/NB/NBMayJun94p76.html>.

American Academy of Pediatrics. "A Policy Statement: Breastfeeding and the Use of Human Milk." *Pediatrics* 115.2 (2005): 496-506.

Arnold, Lois D. W. "The Cost-Effectiveness of Using Banked Donor Milk in the Neonatal Intensive Care Unit: Prevention of Necrotising Enterocolitis." *Journal of Human Lactation* 18.2 (2002): 172-177.

Arnold, Lois D. W. "The Ethics of Donor Milk Banking." *Breastfeeding Medicine* 1 (2006a): 3-13.

Arnold, Lois D. W. "Global Health Policies that Support the Use of Banked Donor Human Milk: A Human Rights Issue." *International Breastfeeding Journal* (2006b): 1-26.

Atkinson, Stephanie A. "Human Milk Feeding of the Micropremie." *Clinics in Perinatology* 27.1 (2000): 235-247.

Balmer, Susan E. and Brian A. Wharton "Human Milk Banking at Sorrento Maternity Hospital, Birmingham." *Archives of Disease in Childhood* 67.4 (1992): 556-559.

Bartle Carol. *A Feeding Audit in Neonatal Intensive Care*. Unpublished Audit. 2002.

Bartle Carol. *Mothers' Experiences of Initiating Lactation and Establishing Breastfeeding in a Neonatal Intensive Care Environment*. Unpublished Master's thesis. University of Otago. 2005.

Bradfield, Orma M. *Issues of Power and Control Within Women's Experiences of Breastfeeding Following Childbirth.* Unpublished Masters Thesis. Deakin University. 1995.

Dahlberg, Gunilla, Peter Moss and Alan Pence. *Beyond Quality in Early Childhood Education and Care: Postmodern Perspectives*. London, Philadelphia, Routledge Falmer 1999.

Fewtrell, Mary S. "The Long-Term Benefits of Having Been Breastfed." *Current Pediatrics* 14 (2004): 97-103.

Flacking, Renee, Kerstin H. Nyqvist, Uwe Ewald, and Lars Wallin. "Long-Term Duration of Breastfeeding in Swedish Low Birth Weight Infants." *Journal of Human Lactation* 19.2 (2003): 157-165.

Greenhough, Beth. "Situated Knowledges and the Spaces of Consent." *Geoforum* 38 (2007): 1140-1151.

Henwood, Karen and Nick Pidgeon. "Remaking the Link: Qualitative Research and Feminist Standpoint Theory." *Feminism and Psychology* 5.1 (1995): 7-30.

Hill, Pamela D, Jean C. Aldag and Robert. T. Chatterton Jr. "Breastfeeding Experience and Milk Weight in Lactating Mothers Pumping for Preterm Infants." *Birth*, 26.4 (1999): 233-238.

Hill, P. D, K. S. Hanson and A. L. Mefford. "Mothers of Low Birthweight Infants: Breastfeeding Patterns and Problems." *Journal of Human Lactation* 10.3 (1994): 169-176.

Human Milk Banking Association of North America. *The Value of Human milk: A Position Paper on Donor Milk Banking.* (2003): 1-4. <http://www.hmbana.org/position.htm>.

Human Milk Banking Association of North America (HMBANA). *Best Practice for Expressing, Storing and Handling Human Milk in Hospitals, Homes and Child Care Settings.* 2005.

Jordan, Brigitte. "Authoritative Knowledge and its Construction." *Childbirth and Authoritative Knowledge: Cross Cultural Perspectives.* Eds. Robbie E. Davis-Floyd and Carolyn. F. Sargent. Berkeley: University of California Press. 1997. 55-79.

Kavanaugh, Karen, Linnea Mead, Paula Meier and Henry H. Mangurten. "Getting Enough: Mother's Concerns About Breastfeeding a Preterm Infant After Discharge." *Journal of Obstetric, Gynecologic and Neonatal Nursing* 24.1 (1995): 23-32.

Kavanaugh, Karen, Paula Meier, Beth Zimmermann and Linnea Mead. "The Rewards Outweigh the Efforts: Breastfeeding Outcomes for Mothers of Preterm Infants." *Journal of Human Lactation* 13.1 (1997): 15-21.

Kent, Jacqueline C. "How Breastfeeding Works." *Journal of Midwifery & Women's Health* 52.6 (2007): 564-570.

Killersreiter, Birgit., Ingrid Grimmer, Christoph Buhrer, Joaquin W. Dudenhausen, and Michael Obladen. "Early Cessation of Breast Milk Feeding in Very Low Birth Weight Infants." *Early Human Development* 60 (2001): 193-205.

Kitzinger, Jenny. "Introducing Focus Groups." *British Medical Journal* 311 (1995): 299-311.

Kuschel, Carl. A. and Jane. E. Harding. "Multicomponent Fortified Human Milk for Promoting Growth in Preterm Infants." *Cochrane Review*: (2004). <http:www.cochraneconsumer.com/Content.ASP?ID=CO0000000564>.

Landzelius, Kyra. M. "Charged Artifacts and the Detonation of Liminality: Teddy-Bear Diplomacy in the Newborn Incubator Machine." *Journal of Material Culture*, 6.3 (2001): 323-344.

Lefebvre, Francine and M. Ducharme. "Incidence and Duration of Lactation and Lactational Performance Among Mothers of Low-Birth-Weight and Term Infants." *Canadian Medical Association Journal* 140 (1989): 1159-1164.

Lindemann Nelson, Hilde. "Feminist Therapies for Low-Birthweight Babies." *Medical Humanities Report* 22.1 (2000). <http://www.bioethics.msu.edu/mhr/oof/feministtherapies.htm>.

Lucas, Jodie. G. "Ryan Can Nurse Today." *New Beginnings* 14.1 (1997): 24-25. <http://www.lalacheleague.org/NB/NBJanFeb97p24.html>.

Lucas, Alan and Tim. J. Cole. "Breast Milk and Neonatal Necrotising Enterocolitis." *The Lancet* 336 [8730] (1990): 1519-1523.

Meier, Paula. P. "Supporting Lactation in Mothers with Very Low Birth Weight Babies." *Pediatric Annals* 32.5 (2003): 317-325.

Mol, Annemarie and Jessica Mesman. "Neonatal Food and the Politics of Theory." *Social Studies of Science* 26 (1996): 419-444.

Moro, Guido. E. and Iolanda Minoli. "Fortification of Human Milk." Paper presented at the *Nestle Nutrition Workshop Series: Nutrition of the Very Low Birth Weight Infant*, Warsaw, Poland, 1998. 18-19.

Pollan, Michael. *In Defence of Food*. New York: Penguin Books, 2008.

Schanler, Richard. J. *Fortified Human Milk: Nature's Way to Feed Premature Infants. Journal of Human Lactation*, 14.1 (1998): 5-11.

Schanler, Richard. J. "The Use of Human Milk for Premature Infants." *Paediatric Clinics of North America* 48.1 (2001): 207-219.

Schanler, Richard. J. and Nancy. M. Hurst. "Human Milk for the Hospitalised Preterm Infant." *Seminars in Perinatology* 18.6 (1994): 476-484.

Shearer, J. "Malachi's Breastfeeding Story." *Aroha* 4.2 (2002): 11-12.

Sherman, Yehudit. "Premature Arrival." *New Beginnings* 20.3 (2003): 98-101. <http://www.lalecheleague.org/NBMayJun03p98.html>.

Sykes, Melissa. "Breastfeeding Multiples: Breastfeeding Premie Twins." *New Beginnings* 12.2 (1995): 58-59. <http://www.lalecheleague.org/NB/NBMarApr95p58prem.html>.

Smith-Windsor, Jaimie. "*The Cyborg Mother: A Breached Boundary*." *Theory, Technology and Culture* 27 (2004): 1-2, Article 137. <http://www.ctheory.net>.

Thoms, Marlene. "*Breastfeeding Our Miracle Baby*." *New Beginnings* 11.1 (1994): 11-12. <http://www.lalecheleague.org/NB/NBJanFeb94p11.html>.

Tully, Douglas. B., Frances Jones, and Mary Rose Tully. "Donor milk: What's In It and What's Not." *Journal of Human Lactation* 17.2 (2001): 152-155.

Uuay, Ricardo and Patricio Peirano. "Breast is Best: Human Milk is the Optimal Food for Brain Development." *American Journal of Clinical Nutrition* 70.4 (1999): 433-444.

Wall, Glenda. "Moral Constructions of Motherhood in Breastfeeding Discourse." *Gender and Society* 15.4 (2001): 592-610.

Wendell, Susan. *The Rejected Body: Feminist Philosophical Reflections on Disability*. Routledge. 1996.

Wight, Nancy. E. "Donor Human Milk for Preterm Infants." *Journal of Perinatology* 21 (2001): 249-254.

Ziemer, M. M. and C. George. "Breast Feeding the Low-Birthweight Infant." *Neonatal Network* 9.4 (1990): 33-38

Wet-nursing, Milk Banks and Black Markets

The Political Economy of Giving Breastmilk in Canada in the 20th and 21st Century

TASNIM NATHOO AND ALECK OSTRY

PRACTICES FOR GIVING BREASTMILK have varied enormously throughout Canadian history. In colonial Canada, formal and informal networks of women sharing and selling breastmilk were shaped by the cultures that women brought with them from the Old World. For example, in New France, wealthier families followed the wet-nursing practices of the upper classes of France. One of the earliest documentations of wet-nursing in Canada describes how Pierre Guy, an eighteenth century Montreal merchant, hired a wet-nurse for each of his fourteen children. They were "put out to nurse" in neighboring parishes days after they were born where, if they survived, they remained until the age of two (Clio Collective 78). While little data remains on early Canadian breastfeeding practices, given the historical absence of feasible alternatives, breastmilk through maternal breastfeeding and wet-nursing were likely the primary means for nourishing infants until the late nineteenth century. By the beginning of the twentieth century, practices of giving milk were altered by new technologies, government interest in breastfeeding promotion, the rise of scientific medicine, and changes in the societal value placed on breastfeeding and breastmilk. In this paper, we explore the interconnections between broader social change and the ways in which women have provided breastmilk to their own and other women's infants through wet-nursing, donating to milk banks, and sharing breastmilk through informal networks.

MILK FOR THE NATION, 1900-1930

The economic and social transformations that occurred in Canada between 1850 and 1920 contributed to the development of an environment in which extended periods of breastfeeding were neither possible nor always desirable. Industrialization, immigration, and urbanization resulted in smaller families, increased isolation, and a growing dependence on professional rather than informal support (Prentice et al.). These socio-demographic changes likely resulted in fewer opportunities for milk sharing between women. Another consequence of these dramatic structural transformations was an increasing awareness of a variety of social problems by activists and government, including the high rates of infant mortality.

Most industrializing nations at the end of the nineteenth century initiated a "fight against infant mortality" (Rollet 38). In Canada, interest in infant mortality at the municipal and provincial levels began around 1910. The political emphasis on saving the lives of infants were intertwined with discussions on the need for workers in an industrializing society; the new science of eugenics with its emphasis on "race" degeneration; and nationalistic discussions in both English and French Canada which were concerned with the survival of the "white" nation and "the survival of the race," respectively. In 1910, 1911, and 1912, the Ontario government published three reports on infant mortality (MacMurchy, *Infant Mortality: Special Report*; MacMurchy, *Infant Mortality: Second Special Report*; MacMurchy, *Infant Mortality: Third Report*). They described the extent and causes of infant mortality and were filled with strategies for solving the high rates of infant mortality, including establishing infant welfare clinics in poor neighborhoods, campaigns for clean milk legislation, the provision of state pensions and nursing allowances for breastfeeding mothers, increased supervision and care for mothers by physicians and nurses, and enforcing legislation for patent food advertisements which described their products as the "perfect substitute for mother's milk." Central to all of these discussions was the role of breastfeeding:

> The Most Important Thing: One thing we know about Infant Mortality. If the baby is nursed by its mother the chances are that it will live. If the baby is fed in any other way the chances are great that it will die. (MacMurchy, *Infant Mortality: Special Report* 5)

Following the First World War and the worldwide flu pandemic, rebuilding the population and the strength of the nation became a priority for the federal government. The development of the first national department of health led to efforts to address infant mortality. The first edition of federally-sponsored *The Canadian Mother's Book* was published in 1921 and over 150,000 copies were distributed by the end of the year. Nearly 1 in 4 Canadian mothers received a copy between 1921 and 1932 (Lewis and Watson 11). Through the widespread dissemination of advice literature, mothers were informed that they were responsible for the well-being of the nation and were encouraged to make "Maternal Nursing the Canadian Way" (MacMurchy, *Canadian Mother's Book* 74).

The introduction to *The Canadian Mother's Book* informed women that only dedicated mothers could make up for the losses suffered during the First World War.

> The Government of Canada, knowing that the nation is made of homes, and that the homes are made by the Father and Mother, rec-

> ognizes you as one of the Makers of Canada. No National Service is greater or better than the work of the Mother in her own home. The Mother is 'The First Servant of the State'. (MacMurchy, *Canadian Mother's Book* 5)

The manuals commented on how bottle-fed babies were nine times more likely to die during infancy than were breastfed babies. Mothers were advised to exclusively breastfeed their babies for nine months as it was "safer, easier, cheaper, wiser, and more successful" (MacMurchy, *Canadian Mothers' Book* 30) than bottle-feeding.

The breastfeeding messages contained in the federal advice literature were echoed in the public health and professional literature and in public and intellectual discussions about the importance and role of mothers in society. These messages also contrasted with a growing awareness that rates of breastfeeding had been steadily declining throughout the first two decades of the twentieth century. While the exact reasons for the decline were difficult to pinpoint, rates appeared to be decreasing most rapidly among women of higher social class, women who were born in Canada, and women in urban areas. These trends suggested that breastfeeding was beginning to take on new meanings and value amongst various social groups and that women's choices about infant feeding were more strongly influenced by other contextual and individual factors (Brown, *The Ability of Mothers*; Brown, *Problems of the Rural Mother*).

FROM COMMODITY TO CHARITY: DONATING MILK IN THE 1930S

Although government and other individuals and organizations concerned with infant mortality continued to promote breastfeeding into the 1930s, rates continued to decline, mirroring trends in other industrializing nations including the United States (Apple; Nathoo & Ostry; Wolf). Breastmilk alternatives, primarily based on cow's milk, became increasingly popular and technological innovations began to offer women other mechanisms for obtaining breastmilk.

In the 1930s, another alternative to cow's milk formulas became available to mothers with the opening of the first breastmilk bank in Canada. Milk banks had been growing in popularity outside Canada during the 1910s and 1920s. By 1929, over twenty cities in the United States were providing bottled breastmilk to sick and premature infants (Golden 193). The first "human milk depot" in Canada opened in the mid-1930s at the Royal Victoria Hospital in Montreal. According to a report in Toronto's *Globe and Mail*, breastmilk was frozen and distributed free. In their first year, the hospital distributed over sixty-seven gallons. In its 1936 annual report, the hospital described a 50 percent decrease in infant mortality ("Death Rate Cut by Human Milk").

The emergence of milk banks symbolically represented the decline of the traditional wet-nurse. Milk banks paid lactating mothers per ounce for their

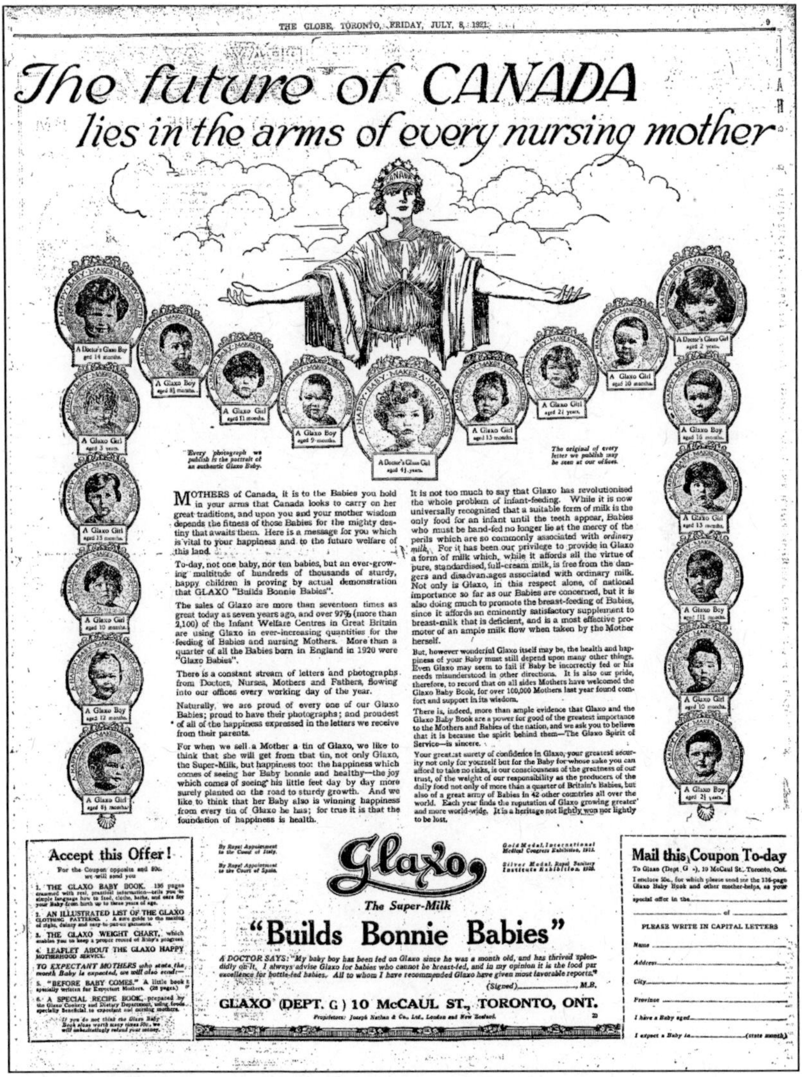

Figure 1: The message that mothers were responsible for the health of the nation was also reflected in advertising (including for breastmilk alternatives) and other domestic advice literature. (The Globe *8 July 1921*)

milk and generally distributed the pooled and pasteurized milk to mothers of needy infants. Physician Frederick Tisdall in the 1942 edition of his child advice manual *The Home Care of the Infant and Child*, commented that,

> Due to the progress made in the artificial feeding of infants and the fact that breastmilk can now be obtained in most cities, it is very

> seldom necessary to procure the services of a wet nurse. Today in the children's hospitals of most cities, breastmilk is available for use when necessary. It is obtained from mothers throughout the city, who, for one reason or another, are willing to sell it. (Tisdall 87)

Formal networks for obtaining breastmilk through health services appear to have replaced more informal (for example, milk sharing between family members and neighbors) and sometimes unregulated commercial or "black market" arrangements.

Although breastmilk continued to be viewed as a commodity, a new perception of breastmilk donation as a charitable act also emerged in the 1930s. This is particularly well demonstrated in the case of the birth of Dionne quintuplets. On May 28, 1934, Yvonne, Annette, Cécile, Émilie, and Marie were the first known set of identical quintuplets to survive and consequently made world headlines. Following their birth, mothers from both Canada and the United States were eager to donate breastmilk to the quintuplets to aid in their survival. One mother commented: "I suppose my part in the lives of the quints was minimal but it was a small satisfaction for me—and a fun thing for our family" (quoted in Arnup 69). In the months following their birth, the quintuplets received over 8,000 ounces of breastmilk that had been boiled, bottled, and shipped by rail and air to their home in northern Ontario (Berton 63). Breastmilk had now become a product valued separately from the practice of breastfeeding.

SCIENTIFIC MEDICINE AND THE "DESKILLING" OF MOTHERS, 1930-1970

In the early part of the century, infant feeding was the focus of the specialty of paediatrics. Motivated by a desire to find alternatives to breastmilk for orphaned infants and the infants of mothers who were unable or chose not to breastfeed, paediatricians exerted much time and energy in the development of infant formulas. Gradually, the training of physicians in infant feeding began to focus exclusively on the development and proper use of breastmilk alternatives and the myriad circumstances in which breastfeeding could go awry. While many leading pediatricians would agree that breastfeeding was superior to the alternatives, this commitment was not universal among these specialists and, among general practitioners, there was a tendency to switch to bottle-feeding at the first sign of difficulty (Nathoo and Ostry; Comacchio; Brown, "The Ability of Mothers").

In the past, many mothers turned to their extended families or women in their communities for assistance with childbirth and for advice on childrearing (Benoit 359). In Canada, these traditional female support systems began to change dramatically in the mid-twentieth century. By the 1930s, urbanization, immigration, rural isolation, and declining fertility meant many women did not have an extensive network of female advice and experience to draw upon. These traditional support systems were gradually replaced with institutional systems. Throughout the 1930s, the medical supervision of mothers and infants through both public and private services became increasingly routine, and members of the scientific and medical fields became central figures in dispensing advice on the care and feeding of children (Comacchio; Prentice et al.). One of the consequences of socio-demographic change in conjunction with scientific and medical involvement in infant feeding was the "deskilling" of mothers so that many women did not have the practical knowledge or social supports to successfully breastfeed.

The most important newly emerging institutional system, in terms of its impact on breast feeding, was mediated by the shift of birthing from home to hospital and the increased control over infant feeding advice this gave to nurses and physicians. For example, while, in 1940, approximately 35 percent of Canadian women gave birth in hospitals by 1960, almost every women birthed in hospital (Ostry, 2006). Birth was transformed from a social event, often attended by informal caregivers to a medical event supervised by medically trained professionals many of whom were unable and uninterested in coaching women to breastfeed.

Fears about infant mortality had greatly diminished from earlier decades and breastfeeding was not as valued for its life-saving properties. Sterilized cans of evaporated milk were now widely available either to be directly fed to infants or used as the main dilutant for infant formulas. As well, pasteurized milk and clean water were increasingly available. Under these new conditions, alternatives to breast feeding were safer and physicians had one less reason to advocate breastfeeding than they may have had in the past.

Meanwhile, in the community, breastfeeding seemed to have fallen out of favor. In 1950, Hilary Bourne, a physician in the Department of Obstetrics and Gynecology at the Royal Victoria Hospital in Montreal commented that,

> It is a well-known fact that the worst place in the world as regards breast feeding is the United States; Canada runs a close second. It is also well known that the European, and in particular the Scandinavian, countries are best in this regard. The difference, however, is not due to geographical location, or anatomical development, or even physiological insufficiency. The great difference is one of temperament, education, and so-called modern living. (Bourne 969).

National data on breastfeeding practices between 1965 and 1971 reveal that breastfeeding initiation rates across Canada were 26 percent with approximately two percent of mothers breastfeeding exclusively (that is, no supplements of formula). At three months, 75 percent of infants were no longer being breastfed (Myeres 200-11). Breastfeeding practices seemed to have reached an all-time low.

SOCIAL MOVEMENTS, A NATIONAL CAMPAIGN, AND "GIFTS" OF FORMULA, 1970-2000

The 1970s marked another changing tide in breastfeeding practices. New social movements revived women's networks of breastfeeding knowledge and increasing international attention to the marketing practices of infant formula companies and their deleterious effects abroad and in Aboriginal communities highlighted the value of breastfeeding. Throughout the 1970s and early 1980s, breastfeeding initiation rates grew from approximately 25 percent to 65 percent (McNally, Hendricks and Horowitz 102). The federal government, with the support of the Canadian Paediatric Society and La Leche League Canada, launched a promotion campaign designed to increase knowledge about the value of breastfeeding amongst health professionals and mothers. A key part of this campaign was to highlight the detrimental effects of free "gifts" of infant formula in hospitals. Throughout the 1980s and 1990s, numerous professional associations, groups of mothers, and activists advocated for hospital practices that were "Baby Friendly" and supported successful breastfeeding initiation. Even though support for breastfeeding increased significantly during this period, resources to support milk banks dwindled and the distribution of breastmilk through this avenue declined.

In the 1970s, breastfeeding became a part of several political and social movements. Interest in breastfeeding was rekindled by the emergence of the natural childbirth movement and the "second wave" of feminism. Although neither of these movements directly addressed breastfeeding, this period of social activism resulted in small groups of women questioning and challenging the dominance of scientific medicine. Women "reclaimed" their bodies and infants from professional experts and began to recreate and share their knowledge gathered from personal experience.

In terms of breastfeeding, one of the most important developments was the emergence of La Leche League in Canada. The first groups started in Quebec in the early 1960s and were followed by groups in Ontario and Alberta. By 1965, there were five groups in Canada (some of which are still in existence). A description of the mother-to-mother approach used by the League and its early formation in Canada can be found in a letter in a women's advice column in *The Globe and Mail*, dated 18 July 1968.

> I am one of those women who always wanted to nurse her babies. I got off to a terrible start in the hospital with our first baby, but one of my friends put me in touch with the then president of the Childbirth Education Association in Toronto. She had nursed four children and had taken it upon herself the task of helping mothers who need another mother to give moral support and knowledge about the womanly art of breastfeeding. Within a week or so my sore nipples were healed and our baby plainly preferred my milk to formula. I was

> so grateful to this mother that I asked her what I could do in return. She suggested that I form a La Leche League in Toronto. This I did a couple of years later (1965). (Thompson W4)

In part, the organization was a response to the dearth of information available on breastfeeding. According to one newspaper commentator, "There is no folklore in our society about breastfeeding so women who try it may feel isolated" ("Doctors, Fashion, Status Vary Attitudes of Breast-Feeding in Canada." W03). By 1970, there were over twenty groups and fifty leaders (Audy 82-83). In the early 1980s, the League worked in conjunction with the federal government to develop materials for mothers and played an important role in reviving the sharing of knowledge about breastfeeding between mothers. The League continued to grow throughout the 1980s and peaked in the early 1990s with nearly 300 groups and about 640 Leaders. In 2004, the league had 188 groups and 466 leaders (Audy 83).

Another social movement abroad contributed to growing discussions among new mothers, health professionals, and government regarding the value of breastfeeding. Beginning in the 1960s, infant formula companies began aggressive marketing strategies in the developing world. Activists and advocates reported on how the marketing and increased use of infant formula was resulting in innumerable cases of often fatal diarrhea, dehydration, and malnutrition (Baumslag and Michels 150). But these conditions were not limited to the developing world. Throughout the 1970s, reports on the detrimental effects of increasing use of infant formula in Aboriginal communities across Canada also emerged (Kome T2; Hogan P15).

The work of activists across the world eventually culminated in the well-known Nestle Boycott. In 1977, the Infant Feeding Action Coalition (INFACT) launched a boycott of Nestle on 4 July 1977. In early 1978, the campaign spread to Canada, New Zealand, and Australia. By 1980, it had spread to the United Kingdom; by 1981, to Sweden and West Germany; by 1982, to France. In Canada, organizations involved in the boycott included the Anglican Church of Canada, the United Church of Canada, the Canadian Religious Conference, the Canadian Nurses Association, the Toronto City Council, the Toronto Board of Health, and the Toronto Board of Education (Van Esterik, *Beyond the Breast-Bottle Controversy* 8). The scale of the boycott was unparalleled. In 1981, one survey estimated that three in ten Toronto residents were aware of the boycott and one in ten were actively boycotting the company's products ("Canada: 10% Toronto Residents Actively Boycott Nestle").

One of the outcomes of the boycott was the development of the WHO Code to regulate the promotion of baby foods. The Canadian government committed to implementing the Code's provisions across the country. A national survey in 1982 provided more conclusive evidence on the impact of infant formula marketing on Canadian women's infant feeding decisions (Health and Welfare Canada, *Canadian Infant Feeding Patterns* 8). The survey revealed that 71 percent of all mothers received a free sample of commercial infant formula in hospital. The survey examined the age at which breastfeeding stopped in relation to whether or not mothers received a formula sample. Within the first month, almost three times as many mothers gave up breastfeeding in the "sample" group as in the "no sample" group. Mothers who received a sample were much more likely to introduce formula sooner than were mothers who did not receive a sample. Further, the sample that mothers received in hospital had a clear influence on the brand choice of the first formula used. The donation of a particular brand of infant formula by a hospital resulted in the choice of that brand by 80 percent to 90 percent of mothers.

Efforts to increase awareness about the WHO Code amongst health professionals were one aspect of the broader breastfeeding campaign launched by the federal government in the early 1980s. Other activities included the development of educational materials for both health professionals and mothers. Throughout the 1980s and 1990s, the Canadian Institute of Child Health took a leadership role in promoting family-centred maternity care in Canadian hospitals which also included support for breastfeeding (Health and Welfare Canada, *Family-Centred Maternity and Newborn Care*; Post). Unfortunately, infant formula manufacturers were only required to comply with the WHO Code on a voluntary basis and hospital practices, particularly with respect to free "gifts" of formula, remained far from ideal. A 1993 survey revealed that 23.8 percent of hospitals reported routinely giving sample packs containing formula to breastfeeding mothers and 82 percent of hospitals had an exclusive contract with a formula company (Levitt et al. 183). In 1996 the Breastfeeding Committee of Canada launched the WHO/UNICEF Baby-Friendly Hospital Initiative to "protection, promote and support breastfeeding" in Canada. By 1999, there was only one hospital in Canada which qualified for Baby Friendly status (Breastfeeding Committee for Canada 1).

While formula remained readily available to mothers, breastmilk through milk banks did not. An absence of historical records on milk banks from the 1930s through to the early 1980s makes it difficult to track changes in the decline of milk banks. However, it appears that, in tandem with the declining breastfeeding rates between the 1930s and early 1960s, milk banks decreased in popularity and accessibility. In the early 1980s, twenty-three milk banks remained in Canada. Fears about viral transmission, especially HIV/AIDS, gradually led to each of these closing until only one remained at British Columbia's Children's and Women's Hospital. While preferable to infant formula, breastmilk through milk banks was clearly difficult to obtain (Jones, "The History of Milkbanking").

Regardless of the many barriers to breastfeeding success, rates continued to increase throughout the 1980s. After the dramatic spurt of the late 1970s, initiation rates in 1982 were 69.2 percent (Health and Welfare Canada, *Canadian Infant Feeding Patterns* 3). Two national surveys in 1994 showed that breastfeeding initiation stood at 73 percent with 40 percent of mothers breastfeeding for less than three months (Health Canada, *Canadian Perinatal Surveillance System* 9).

THE RE-COMMODIFICATION OF BREASTMILK, 2000 AND BEYOND

Since the 1970s, public awareness of the value of breastfeeding has continued to grow; in 2003, 85 percent of mothers in Canada initiated breastfeeding. However, in the 2000s, the value that many individuals and groups place on breastmilk appears to be contributing to an increasing trend towards the commodification of breastmilk (Van Esterik, *Contemporary Trends in Infant Feeding Research* 276). At the turn of the twenty-first century, informal networks of women sharing breastmilk appear to be re-emerging alongside the growth of milk banks. While the idea of breastmilk as a commodity is not new, it is to the highly capitalized and complex market environment of the 2000s.

In the 2000s, the demand for donated human breastmilk has been increasing in response to the increasing value placed on breastmilk (Tully, Lockhart-Borman and Updegrove). In Canada, while there are efforts to set up milk banks in Quebec, Alberta, Saskatchewan, Nunavut, and Ontario, there is only one milk bank operating at B.C. Children's and Women's Hospital in Vancouver, British Columbia (Kopun). While the demand for milk is increasing, the bank is not accessible to most mothers with its focus on hospital patients as well as premature infants, formula intolerant infants, and infants of HIV-positive mothers. In 2004, 255 babies received milk from the bank (Nicholson 1-2). Also, while the milk is technically donated and distributed for free, milk bank recipients have to pay a processing fee of approximately three dollars for 2.5 ounces. In 2006, an article in the *Toronto Star* reported on a family that found the Vancouver milk bank on the internet (Kopun). The family spent $160 per week on breastmilk plus $100 to have it delivered (packed in ice) by courier.

Using US figures, enough breastmilk from a milk bank for one infant for six months could cost as much as $18,000 (even though the price of breastmilk from milk banks is intended only to cover processing fees). As formal means for obtaining breastmilk can be difficult to access and costly to obtain, women are developing unofficial "milk sharing" networks as a response. Reports from across Canada and the U.S. describe the development of a breastmilk "black market." Women on the internet and in classified ads are developing their own networks for sharing, swapping, and selling breastmilk. An article in the *Globe and Mail* in 2007 on "the return of the wet nurse" described one woman's experience:

> When Toronto mother Janet Belray was diagnosed with breast cancer in her right breast, a mastectomy and chemotherapy ended her six-month old son's breastfeeding at least a year earlier than she'd intended. A close friend organized six "milk mamas," including one woman Mrs.

> Belray had never met, to pump for baby Julian until he was 11 months old. "It was the single most amazing thing these women could have done for me," says Ms. Belray, who celebrated her milk donors at a "weaning" brunch at a Toronto restaurant. (Pearce L1)

The view of breastmilk as a commodity seems to have re-emerged after a hiatus of approximately 70 years. However, unlike earlier periods, the re-commodification of breastmilk in a highly globalized and neo-liberal environment presents numerous ethical questions and raises public health concerns. Unlike historical wet-nursing, where infants received milk from one woman, the sale of breastmilk results in one infant receiving milk from multiple women. In 2006, Health Canada released a warning about the sale and distribution of human milk obtained from the internet or sold directly by individuals (Health Canada, *Information Update* 1; Jones, "From the Chair": 3). The advisory highlighted concerns about disease transmission through breastmilk, especially where medical information is lacking (e.g., HIV, staphylococcus aureus), as well as risks from improper handling and storage. Thus far, there has been minimal discussion of the need for regulation or whether informal mothers' networks should be allowed to thrive as they have done historically. These networks are also challenging the view of milk donation as a philanthropic endeavor that emerged in the 1930s. While many women are happy to donate their milk to needy infants, other women believe their work should be compensated, like sperm or eggs in the United States (Austin).

An initiative in the United States has also generated discussion and concern in Canada and other jurisdictions about potentially coercive practices. The California-based company Prolacta Bioscience has recently started selling its own brand of breastmilk at ten times the price of milk available from milk banks. Some worry that their donation and collection system pressures women to donate. Others question the ethics of having women donate for free and then having the hospital and Prolacta profit from it (Ensor B1; Bernhard 1).

As the value of breastmilk continues to grow in the twenty-first century, concern about potentially exploitive practices in both formal and informal settings will be likely to continue (see Shaw, this volume). Current trends in giving milk have been shaped by class, politics, science, technology, and socio-demographic forces. Consequently, resolving these new ethical tensions and public health concerns will require both an understanding of history and the collective action of networks of women, government, and industry.

REFERENCES

Apple, Rima D. *Mothers and Medicine: A Social History of Infant Feeding, 1890–1950. Wisconsin Publications in the History of Science and Medicine.* Madison: University of Wisconsin Press, 1987.

Apple, Rima. *Perfect Motherhood: Science and Childrearing in America.* New Brunswick, NJ: Rutgers University Press, 2006.

Arnup, Katherine. "Raising the Dionne Quintuplets: Lessons for Modern Mothers." *Journal of Canadian Studies* 29.4: 65-81.

Audy, Fiona. "The Year of the Group: History of LLL Canada." *Leaven: La Leche League's International Journal for Leaders* 40.4 (2004): 82-83.

Austin, Marsha. "Sides Clash over Putting Price on Mothers' Milk." *Denver Post* 26 March 2006, Final Edition: A-01.

Baumslag, Naomi, and Dia L. Michels. *Milk, Money, and Madness: The Culture and Politics of Breastfeeding.* Westport, Conneticut: Bergin & Garvey, 1995.

Benoit, Cecilia. "Rediscovering Appropriate Care: Maternity Traditions and Contemporary Issues in Canada." *Health and Canadian Society: Sociological Perspectives.* Eds. David Coburn, Carl D'Arcy and George Torrance. 3rd ed. Toronto: University of Toronto Press, 1998. 359-78.

Bernhard, Blythe. "Breast-Milk Clinic Confronts Criticisms." *Knight Ridder/Tribune News Services Orange County Register*, 2005.

Berton, Pierre. *The Dionne Years: A Thirties Melodrama.* Toronto: McClelland and Stewart, 1977.

Bourne, Hilary B. "Breast Feeding." *The Canadian Nurse* 46.12 (1950): 969-71.

Breastfeeding Committee for Canada. *The Implementation and Evaluation of the Baby-Friendly Initiative in Canada: Final Project Report 1999-2002.* Toronto: The Breastfeeding Committee for Canada, 2002.

Brown, Alan. "The Ability of Mothers to Nurse Their Infants." *Canadian Medical Association Journal* 7 (1917): 241-49.

Brown, Alan. "Problems of the Rural Mother in the Feeding of Her Children." *The Public Health Journal* 9.7 (1918): 297-301.

"Canada: 10% Toronto Residents Actively Boycott Nestle." *INFACT Update* (1982): 54. Cited in Chetley, Andrew. *The Politics of Baby Foods: Successful Challenges to an International Marketing Strategy*. New York: St. Martin's Press, 1986.

Clio Collective, The. *Quebec Women: A History*. Trans. Roger Gannon and Rosalind Gill. Toronto: The Women's Press, 1987.

Comacchio, Cynthia R. *Nations Are Built of Babies: Saving Ontario's Mothers and Children 1900-1940.* Montreal: McGill-Queen's University Press, 1993.

"Death Rate Cut by Human Milk." *Globe and Mail* 22 April 1937: 10.

"Doctors, Fashion, Status Vary Attitudes of Breast-Feeding in Canada." *Globe and Mail* 27 August 1964, sec. Family: W03.

Ensor, Deborah. "Land of Milk and Money; Breast-Milk Enterprise Raises Concerns among Those Who View Collection and Distribution as a Philanthropic Endeavor." *San Diego Union-Tribune* 12 February 2006, sec. Local: B-1.

"Glaxo the Super-Milk: The Future of Canada Lies in the Arms of Every

Nursing Mother." Advertisement. *Globe and Mail*, 8 July 1921: 5.
Golden, Janet L. *A Social History of Wet Nursing in America: From Breast to Bottle*. Cambridge: Cambridge University Press, 1996.
Health and Welfare Canada. *Canadian Infant Feeding Patterns: Results of a National Survey, 1982*. Ottawa: Minister of Supply and Services Canada, 1984.
Health and Welfare Canada. *Family-Centred Maternity and Newborn Care: National Guidelines*. Ottawa, 1987.
Health Canada. *Canadian Perinatal Surveillance System - Breastfeeding*. Ottawa: Health Canada, 1998.
Health Canada. *Information Update: Health Canada Raises Concerns About the Sale and Distribution of Human Milk*. 2006. Health Canada. Available: <http://www.hc-sc.gc.ca/ahc-asc/media/advisories-avis/2006/2006_56_e.html>. Sept. 11 2006.
Hogan, Denys. "Churches Fight Formula Promotion Nestle Smarting from Boycott." *Globe and Mail* 15 December 1979: P15.
Jones, Frances. "The History of Milk Banking." 2003. Human Milk Banking Association of North America. Available: <http://www.hmbana.org/index.php?mode=history>. July 31 2006.
Jones, Frances. "From the Chair." *HMBANA Matter* 3 (2006): 3.
Kome, Penney. "Formula-Feeding Is Hurting Native Infants' Health: MD." *Globe and Mail* 16 July 1981: T2.
Kopun, Francine. "Investing in Motherhood." *Toronto Star* 19 February 2006: D03.
Levitt, Cheryl A., Janusz Kaczorowski, Louise Hanvey, Denise Avard and Graham W. Chance. "Breast-Feeding Policies and Practices in Canadian Hospitals Providing Maternity Care." *Canadian Medical Association Journal* 155.2 (1996): 181-8.
Lewis, Norah, and Judy Watson. "The Canadian Mother and Child: A Time-Honoured Tradition." *Health Promotion* Winter 91/92 (1991/92): 10-13.
MacMurchy, Helen. *Infant Mortality: Second Special Report*. Toronto: The Legislative Assembly of Ontario, 1911.
MacMurchy, Helen. *Infant Mortality: Special Report*. Toronto: The Legislative Assembly of Ontario, 1910.
MacMurchy, Helen. *Infant Mortality: Third Report*. Toronto: Legislative Assembly of Ontario, 1912.
MacMurchy, Helen. *The Canadian Mother's Book*. The Little Blue Books, Mothers' Series No. 1. Ottawa: Department of Health, 1923.
McNally, Ellen, Suzanne Hendricks, and Isadore Horowitz. "A Look at Breast-Feeding Trends in Canada (1963-1982)." *Canadian Journal of Public Health* 76.March/April (1985): 101-07.
Myeres, Allan W. "A Retrospective Look at Infant Feeding Practice in Canada: 1965-1978." *Journal of the Canadian Dietetic Association* 40.3 (1979): 200-11.

Nathoo, Tasnim and Ostry, Aleck. *The One Best Way? Breastfeeding History, Politics, and Policy in Canada*. Waterloo: Wilfrid Laurier University Press, 2009.

Nicholson, Patricia. "Inside Canada's Breast Milk Bank." *Medical Post* August (2005): 1-2.

Ostry, Aleck. *Change and Continuity in Canada's Healthcare System*. Vancouver: University of British Columbia Press, 2006.

Pearce, Tralee. "Breast friends." *The Globe and Mail* 1 May 2007: L1.

Post, Shirley. "Family-Centered Maternity Care: The Canadian Picture." *Dimensions in Health Service* June (1981): 26-31.

Prentice, Alison, et al. *Canadian Women: A History*. Toronto: Harcourt Brace Jovanovich, 1988.

Rollet, Catherine. "The Fight against Infant Mortality in the Past: An International Comparison." *Infant and Child Mortality in the Past.* Eds. Alain Bideau, Bertrand Desjardins and Hector Perez Brignoli. Oxford: Clarendon Press, 1997. 38-60.

Thompson, Elizabeth, "Group aims to teach the art of breastfeeding." *The Globe and Mail* 18 July 1968: W4.

Tisdall, Frederick F. *The Home Care of the Infant and Child.* New York: New Home Library, 1942.

Tully, Mary Rose, Laraine Lockhart-Borman, and Kim Updegrove. "Stories of Success: The Use of Donor Milk Is Increasing in North America." *Journal of Human Lactation* 20.1 (2004): 75-77.

Van Esterik, Penny. *Beyond the Breast-Bottle Controversy.* New Brunswick, N.J.: Rutgers University Press, 1989.

Van Esterik, Penny. "Contemporary Trends in Infant Feeding Research." *Annual Review of Anthropology* 31 (2002): 257-78.

Wolf, Jacqueline H. *Don't Kill Your Baby: Public Health and the Decline of Breastfeeding in the Nineteenth and Twentieth Century.* Women and Health: Cultural and Social Perspectives. Columbus: Ohio State University Press, 2001.

III. MILK POLITICS

Breastfeeding and HIV/AIDS

Critical Gaps and Dangerous Intersections

PENNY VAN ESTERIK

THIS CHAPTER[1] EXPLORES THE role of breastfeeding and breastfeeding advocacy in the context of HIV/AIDS. The transmission of HIV through breastfeeding creates an excruciating dilemma for many mothers who are HIV positive. Often they are told to make a choice between breastfeeding and replacement feeding with infant formula without receiving sufficient information on the least risky way to feed their infants. In other places, they are not given a choice. In contrast, transmission of HIV through breastmilk is a relatively minor concern for AIDS researchers considering the importance of other modes of transmission, the overall demands for more effective prevention, and better access to treatment worldwide. However, the subject is of central importance to child feeding advocates who seek interventions to prevent HIV transmission that do not also undermine child feeding programmes.

Many health professionals, social scientists and breastfeeding advocates have made direct contributions to research directed towards preventing and treating HIV/AIDS. I have made no such contribution. I write from the edges of HIV/AIDS research, having been drawn to this work indirectly in the context of other work, first in Thailand dealing with gender issues, and second in relation to international advocacy work on breastfeeding. I have worked at the edges, in the spaces between, in a few of the gaps. But perhaps by focusing on the gaps, the spaces between and the pieces that don't fit the HIV/AIDS paradigm, we can bring new questions into focus. This chapter provides a personal response to attempts to understand HIV as a gendered public health issue by examining discourses surrounding breastfeeding and HIV/AIDS at two conferences: the first, at York University, May, 2006 on *Gender, Child Survival and HIV: from evidence to policy;* and the second, the *International AIDS Conference* (IAC) in Toronto, Canada, August, 2006. The chapter concludes with an assessment of the challenges of bridging the many divergent frames of reference exposed at these conferences, in order to create the possibility for an effective advocacy and policy response to breastfeeding and HIV/AIDS.

WHAT WE KNOW (OR THINK WE KNOW)

While epidemiological and biomedical research on the transmission of HIV through breastmilk and prevention-of-mother-to-child-transmission (PMTCT) is progressing, corresponding research on gender inequalities, embodiment, stigma and contagion is less well developed, and less integrated into broader discussions of maternal health and child survival. Since it was discovered that breastmilk could transmit HIV (Ziegler, Cooper, Johnson & Gold, 1985), there has been a concerted effort to discover the best infant feeding regime to keep the babies of HIV-positive mothers healthy and free of the virus. Although we recognize the fact of HIV transmission through breastfeeding, the exact mechanisms are still unclear.

To simplify the complex and ever-changing scientific evidence, it is often difficult to identify the timing and source of transmission of HIV. Even if we could be sure whether the transmission was intrauterine, perinatal or postnatal through breastfeeding, it is difficult to know if an infant is infected until they are about six weeks old.

Many women and infants have received single dose nevirapine to prevent transmission during labour and delivery. HAART reduces transmission through pregnancy, delivery and exclusive breastfeeding to around two percent. A child breastfeeding from a woman who is HIV positive has about a 14 percent risk of infection when neither receives any antiretroviral therapy (ART). Consider a community with a 20 percent HIV infection rate; only three infants out of 100 are likely to be infected through breastfeeding, leaving 97 who would benefit from breastfeeding. The 2006 updated WHO policy on HIV and infant feeding states:

> Exclusive breastfeeding is recommended for HIV-infected women for the first six months of life unless replacement feeding is acceptable, feasible, affordable, sustainable, and safe for them and their infants before that time. When replacement feeding is acceptable, feasible, affordable, sustainable, and safe, avoidance of all breastfeeding by HIV infected women is recommended. At six months, if replacement feeding is still not acceptable, feasible, affordable, sustainable, and safe, continuation of breastfeeding with additional complementary foods is recommended, while the mother and baby continue to be assessed. All breastfeeding should stop once a nutritionally adequate and safe diet without breastmilk can be provided. (WHO)

But because of difficulties surrounding both exclusive breastfeeding and exclusive replacement feeding, infants often receive mixed feeds, the option most likely to kill babies, particularly in the global south. However, replacement feeding is assumed to be easier in the global north where facilities for the safe use of replacement feeds are widespread. When the risk of an infant dying from not being breastfed is greater than the risk presented by a HIV-positive mother's breastfeeding, then mothers are advised to exclusively breastfeed their infants.

Recent evidence has produced the surprising results that exclusive breastfeeding for three months led to the same transmission rates as exclusive replacement feeding (Coutsoudis, Pillay, Spooner, Kuhn, and Coovadia). In addition, programs that inform women of the dangers of mixed feeding, prevent and treat potential breast problems such as cracked nipples, and advise the use of condoms to prevent further infection during the period of lactation have been effective at reducing the transmission rate (cf. LINKAGES).

The dilemma for breastfeeding policy is that while we know that exclusive breastfeeding is the single most effective intervention to prevent infant death (cf. Jones et al.) when there are no effective vaccines to prevent transmission of HIV or cure AIDS, what boosts immunity and provides food security for infants—breastmilk—can also transmit HIV. While researchers are actively assessing the risk of transmission of HIV through breastfeeding, mothers and child feeding advocates are equally concerned about the long term survival and health of infants. These widely shared discourses around breastfeeding and HIV/AIDS permeated both conferences and should have provided a common basis for discussion.

THE YORK CONFERENCE

My experience of organizing and hosting a conference on *Gender, Child Survival and HIV/AIDS: From Evidence to Policy*, at York University (May 2006) revealed mammoth disconnections between how the infant feeing issue is framed in the global north and the global south. Sponsored by a number of academic programs at York University, local NGOs, and the World Alliance for Breastfeeding Action (WABA), an international NGO based in Malaysia, the conference aimed to bring together academics, women's health activists, HIV/AIDS workers and breastfeeding advocates. I was the conference organizer, ably assisted by Francoise Guigne (who is currently completing Master's research on breastfeeding and HIV).

Our conference at York focussed not on all those affected by AIDS, but on women; and not all women, but on mothers bearing children. And we drew attention to a particular route of transmission: through breastfeeding, rather than transmission during pregnancy or childbirth. We knew that the topic would not be easy to talk about. There were conceptual difficulties, scientific difficulties, political difficulties and advocacy difficulties, to name a few. Delegates had ample opportunity for participation, but we came from many different worlds and brought many diverse perspectives to the discussion, from local Canadian mother-to-mother support groups, to Christian NGOs working on AIDS education in African cities. Even Canadian and Ugandan doctors participating in the conference worked in very different worlds. We viewed the conference as an opportunity to bring these diverse perspectives together for a critical examination of breastfeeding and the role of gender in health research, and how evidence is used (or not used) to direct policy relevant to women's health, infant health, and HIV/AIDS. We also wanted to address "the gender gap" in HIV research and prevention.

The transmission of HIV through breastmilk is only one small part of the problem facing women who are HIV positive. Nearly half the people living with HIV/AIDS are female. Women have higher viral loads, are often diagnosed later, and have poor access to care and medications. They are most often the caregivers for HIV positive family members, and most likely to be exposed to abuse and violence. Thus, gender inequity underlies the marginalization of women living with HIV, and discussions of child survival and feeding must be considered within the context of poverty, poor access to treatment, drugs and medical care. When ART is available, it is often given only long enough to reduce the risk of transmission during birth; the emphasis is often on preventing HIV transmission to infants rather than improving the health of mothers and infants.

Gender biases have had a profoundly negative impact on women through gender insensitive language that blames women for infecting their partners and infants; through inappropriate, authoritative counselling style; and through treatment that focuses only on reducing the transmission of the virus to the newborn, ignoring women's health needs in the process. Women are more vulnerable to HIV infections biologically because they are twice as likely as men to be infected from one act of unprotected sex, and culturally, because of pervasive gender inequalities.

The conference asked how women were moved aside and ignored for so long in HIV/AIDS policy and treatment. When attention was on women, we noted that it was often on sex workers, ignoring the fact that sex workers are also mothers. When attention was on mothers, treatment was often directed to them only to prevent transmission to their infants. In the early eighties, women, mothers and children were ignored when policy makers looked at risk categories—"the 4H's"—homosexuals, hemophiliacs, heroin addicts and Haitians, and when we shifted to talking about risk behaviours in the late eighties, breastfeeding mothers still didn't fit in.[2] When analysts focused attention on carrier fluids, most attention was on blood and semen rather than breastmilk.

When attention focused on semen as the carrier fluid, we learned a great deal about prevention and treatment from gay men's groups. When the circulating medium was blood, we also learned from hemophiliac support groups. We wanted the York conference to explore what gets revealed when we examine breastmilk as the carrier fluid. What new processes can be understood when we look at mothers who breastfeed and at breastfeeding support groups? How do the questions change? And how can groups working to support breastfeeding mothers further support the research and policy work of AIDS advocacy groups? To make this commitment visible, we handed out the red ribbons of AIDS advocacy pinned together with the gold bow of the breastfeeding mother and child.[3] We took these arguments to the male dominated HIV support groups to attract them to the conference, and many were persuaded.

In preparation for the conference, we reviewed available literature on the subject. But when we reviewed HIV/AIDS materials, breastfeeding was mentioned only as part of PMTCT strategies, usually drug-based clinical trials; when we reviewed gender and HIV/AIDS materials, we found another gap; there was no reference to breastfeeding or the infant feeding problems faced by HIV-positive mothers. In fact, in the global north, many people expressed the belief that HIV positive women should not even have children.

A closer examination of the York conference illuminates the difficulties of meeting the lofty objectives to "fill the gender gap" and "fill the breastfeeding gap." The gaps didn't line up. What was a gap, an absence, for some, was a gaping wound for others. What is the significance of the fact that gaps exist, but that they do not line up? Never have I experienced such a disconnect between the way the problem of breastfeeding and HIV/AIDS was framed in industrial and resource poor countries, in the global north and the global south.

Among North American service providers, academics and NGOs, I was repeatedly told that breastfeeding for HIV-positive mothers was not an issue for research, treatment or prevention, and there was nothing to discuss. In fact most refused to enter into discussion. They thanked us for the invitation, but declined to participate in the conference, preferring to concentrate on other issues relevant for women—microbicides, female condoms, and sexual rights. They "solve the problem" for HIV positive pregnant women by providing ART in late pregnancy, and requiring exclusive replacement feeding from birth. No breastfeeding is permitted, and women who breastfeed a child knowing they are HIV positive could be accused of child neglect. For North American women, there is no choice, thus no problem, and no issue to debate. No consideration was given to the possibility that North American women might have difficulty accessing infant formula, or that some North American women wanted to breastfeed exclusively. Nevertheless some individuals and groups agreed to participate out of solidarity; others out of an interest in gender and HIV; and some came to the conference out of a desire to have a platform to complain about the fact that when treatment for women was discussed in North America, it was framed as necessary to prevent the transmission of HIV to their newborns, not "for them" as HIV positive women. Some came with a heavy chip on their shoulders ready to confront activists who were doing exactly what we were doing, drawing attention to mothers and newborns, rather than to women per se. From them, there was not just disinterest but active resentment.

In contrast, when the call for conference abstracts went out, the response from South Asia and African countries in particular was overwhelming. Finally, they said, a forum to help "fill the gap" with discussion of research and interventions on the important subject of infant feeding among HIV positive and negative women, and women who do not know their status. We received abstract after abstract on how to handle the difficult choices HIV positive women must make. These included problems about lack of adequate counselling about infant feeding options, problems of maintaining exclusive breastfeeding as a viable option to reduce transmission of HIV, and the challenges of encouraging exclusive breastfeeding considering the fact that breastfeeding support had almost disappeared in those same countries and communities because of HIV/AIDS.

Many complained of the lack of follow up on the survival of infants of HIV-positive mothers given replacement feeds. And others, totally committed to replacement feeding in industrialized and developing countries, raised the problem of the fact that replacement feeding was not available when needed or it was too expensive for mothers to purchase.

In many resource poor communities, use of replacement feeds raises familiar problems—need for clean reliable water source, adequate conditions for sterilization or hygienic preparation, cash for purchase. Contaminated feeding bottles and over-dilution of infant formula do not disappear in the context of HIV/AIDS. But the discourse has changed from the early days of the Nestle boycott. The old rhetoric of the breast-bottle controversy becomes a tragic, ironic double bind, advocacy turned inside out, where companies supplying the replacement feeds of infant formula were heralded as "the good guys," and the breastfeeding advocates, "the bad guys" with their heads in the sand, ignoring, as one participant said, "the fact that breastmilk causes AIDS."

Many conference participants, particularly health activists, addressed the fact that the reduction in facilities to support maternal and child health generally was a direct result of American policies to remove support for services that could be construed as linked in any way to women's reproductive rights. The "ABC" (abstinence, be faithful, use condoms) criteria for PEPFAR (U.S. President's Emergency Plan for AIDS) funding was ridiculed by participants from the global north and global south, as insulting, ineffectual and unrealistic for women, offering nothing relevant to solving HIV positive women's problems, particularly infant feeding.

The extent to which the gaps did not line up was brought home to me in exchanges with a Ugandan doctor at the York conference. As we began to educate each other about the way we approached breastfeeding, one Ugandan doctor exploded with anger about what she called "a vicious double standard." She viewed PMTCT and AFASS, as global strategies that said a Ugandan baby's death didn't matter as much as an American baby's death and that was why Ugandan babies were allowed to be breastfed. But the death of a white American baby matters; therefore American mothers were told not to breastfeed. Marion Tompson, a founding mother of La Leche League, was devastated to learn how her work and the work of others to maintain breastfeeding support in the face of HIV/AIDS was interpreted. She wrote to her colleagues: "And then it all poured out, her perception that women in Africa were being encouraged to breastfeed because African babies were expendable and no one cared if they got AIDS and died. But in industrialized countries, breastfeeding was strictly forbidden to prevent any of those babies from getting AIDS!"[4] The Ugandan doctor was surprised that some North American women who were HIV positive wanted to breastfeed their babies, even against "doctor's orders," risking having their children taken away from them. The heated exchange cleared the air somewhat, and increased understanding, as the American, Asian and African participants learned how their words and actions had been mutually misinterpreted.

The conference task of producing a consensus statement on transmission through breastmilk was particularly challenging. The conference exposed how the transmission of HIV through breastmilk evoked personal, emotional, political and cultural struggles over the value and meaning of maternal and infant bodies in the context of economic and gender inequalities. Nevertheless, we accomplished the task between May and July in time to bring the statement to the IAC.[5] (The struggle over language and the politics of track changes is another paper.)

THE INTERNATIONAL AIDS CONFERENCE (IAC), TORONTO

Breastfeeding and HIV/AIDS did not figure prominently at the *International AIDS Conference* (IAC) in Toronto, August, 2006; breastfeeding did not fit in well with the discourse on sexual and reproductive health, nor men having sex with men. The major scientific panel on PMTCT was rejected from the scientific programme, and was presented as a satellite panel at 7:00 am, at the cost of several thousand dollars (paid for by a health NGO who could have used the funds more effectively elsewhere).

While lining up to register for the IAC, I struck up a conversation with a representative from People Living With AIDS from Uganda. I wanted her to distribute the joint statement from the York conference. Her concern—no, anger—when I mentioned I represented a breastfeeding advocacy group was striking and painful. She repeated over and over, "if you are HIV positive, you must do everything you can to prevent the transmission of HIV to your child. Isn't it worth suffering for three or four months to save your child?" She discussed the clash between building up of immunity in the infant by breastfeeding and the breaking down of immunity by HIV. This was the heart of the anger-making tragedy for her. She took out this anger on breastfeeding advocacy groups, who, she said, should not be promoting breastfeeding, but should instead help break down the stigma in her country of not breastfeeding.

She spoke of her friend who didn't want to tell her partner she was HIV positive, so she breastfed her first baby who is now HIV positive. For the second baby she refused to breastfeed and the baby is free of HIV. Now the first child blames her mother, asking why her sibling is healthy and she is sick. The woman in line didn't know she herself was HIV positive and breastfed her daughter for four months. When they both got sick, they were both tested and found to be HIV positive. Her daughter is a teenager now, and getting treatment. The woman tried traditional medicine and herbs first, but lost her appetite, and if she ate before she took the herbs, she vomited her food and wasted it. Now both she and her daughter give talks about preventing HIV infection. Not breastfeeding is included as a prevention strategy for avoiding HIV transmission. When I mumbled something about wanting to help, she asked me to help raise money to subsidize infant formula in the villages of Uganda. Needless to say, I kept the joint statement, pins and other advocacy materials from the York conference in my bag.

At the IAC, I also learned how upsetting it was to health workers in Maternal and Child Health who have been trained to support breastfeeding to be told now to advise women not to breastfeed. As one explained, we went from "breast is best" to "breastmilk is a poison that kills babies." South African researchers deplored the rate of burnout among HIV counsellors advising women on infant feeding options. They quit in large numbers. This lack of job satisfaction is a much bigger problem in the global south than in North America where support for breastfeeding is stronger at the level of rhetoric than practice, where breastfeeding is considered a lifestyle choice, and conditions for the safe use of replacement feeds are assumed to be universally available.[6]

Stephen Lewis's keynote address at the closing plenary summarized eighteen key points from the IAC conference. The gender activists anticipated a strong attack on gender inequality, and were not disappointed. Ending domestic and sexual violence against women is an unambiguous good. Increasing treatment and care for children and orphans is another unambiguous good. Everyone agrees in principle and in practice. There are no longer two sides to the question of violence against women. The breastfeeding activists hoped he would call for more research on mother to child transmission and support for exclusive breastfeeding, perhaps with a link to gender inequality. We were disappointed. Between violence against women and care for children was a brief point about childhood sexual abuse, a subject covered by children and violence. We were left to wonder why Lewis failed to address the complexity of the infant feeding dilemma, since he was key in initiating the subject at a breastfeeding and HIV/AIDS conference in Tanzania a few years before.[7] Perhaps it has something to do with the lack of interdisciplinary integration in research and policy development. While many researchers call for race, class and gender to be considered in HIV/AIDS research, medical science rarely trains health professionals to do class or gender analysis. It is the social sciences that specialize in this kind of analysis. Something very powerful happens when you take the best of the social sciences and combine it with clinical expertise, but health professionals should be cautioned against practising social science without a license.

The seventeenth IAC was held in Mexico City in August, 2008. As part of the committee organizing the social science track, I had the opportunity to review abstracts and meet other committee members, all with their own agendas for the meetings. Once again, breastfeeding was of minor interest except for the PMTCT reports on drug trials considered relevant to clinical and scientific tracks. With a strong representation from gender networks, sexual and reproductive rights were prominent in the Mexican IAC program. But sexual and reproductive rights advocates pressed for discussion of rights to abortion, family planning and sexual pleasure, and did not consider breastfeeding as a reproductive rights issue. Breastfeeding advocates at the meeting reported that the WHO recommendations on breastfeeding were not discussed or questioned during the conference. NGO participants requested more information to disseminate in Latin America where HIV-positive mothers were forbidden to breastfeed, denying them the right to make to an informed choice.

Those working in international health or HIV/AIDS work know that present conferences are understood by reference to past conferences. HIV/AIDS research and policy is shaped by non-binding documents produced at earlier conferences and at United Nations' agencies:

> As 'language' is quoted and repeated from one conference document to the next and as states begin to conform their practices, or at least their discourse, to the norms expressed therein, some of what is agreed upon at global conferences gradually will become rules of 'customary international law'. (Riles 2008: 9)

IN SEARCH OF BRIDGES

These conferences revealed—at times painfully—some unstated corollaries about breastfeeding and HIV/AIDS. In the global south, breastfeeding matters and was hard to give up, both personally and socially. Giving up breastfeeding was a necessary sacrifice, "a sacrifice for the baby." Mixed feeding was often the result. Mixed feeding was not recognized as dangerous because it was accepted as the normal way to feed a baby before the HIV/AIDS crisis. There was no discursive space for recognizing that replacement feeding was killing babies. Instead, the message was that breastfeeding kills babies, and replacement feeding will save them.

In the global north, breastfeeding as a mothering practice is less valued, and was perceived as easy to give up, since medical professionals already viewed replacement feeding as equivalent or even better than breastfeeding. The distrust of breastfeeding and breastfeeding advocacy groups in Canada was re-enforced recently when *Chatelaine*, a leading Canadian women's magazine, published an article headlined, "Breastfeeding Sucks" (60). The article refers to the "pro-breastfeeding tyrants," the "evangelism" of the "boob squad" who use "scare tactics" to stifle women's choices, and concludes, "We might have to suck up the pain of breastfeeding, but we can spit out the piety of the breastfeeding bullies." This attitude explains in part why many North American women's groups concerned about HIV/AIDS were not willing to participate in the York conference, and what makes international collaboration between global north and global south on gender and HIV issues so challenging.

How can we address the problems of infant feeding and HIV/AIDS policy when there are so many gaps in our knowledge and when the gaps do not line up? How can we build bridges when the issues in the global south/global north are conceptual inverses of each other, or to paraphrase Annelise Riles (2001), "the policy inside out"? I conclude with a few questions that need to be answered before we can "bridge the gaps":

1. What happens when the global north advises the global south on this issue? Many large international bilateral and multilateral projects send foreign experts to advise on gender and HIV issues in southern Africa and elsewhere. Infant feeding is often not included in the workplan. When breastfeeding doesn't matter in the global north, it may not be addressed appropriately in international projects.

2. Why is informed choice configured so differently in the global north and the global south? There is no choice of infant feeding for HIV positive women in the global north, and only the rhetoric of informed choice in the global south. While the numbers of women making these decisions, and their access to treatment differ by country, the concept of informed choice should be examined more seriously, and should not differ so dramatically in the global north and south.

3. How can breastfeeding advocates avoid being placed in the "dissenter box" when they call for surveillance of survivor rates for different feeding modes or more research on the mechanisms of transmission through breastmilk? Calling for more research on exclusive breastfeeding still feels like suggesting lemon and garlic as treatment for the disease. Can we avoid the dissenter/scientist split altogether, so that calling for more research on exclusive breastfeeding or monitoring HIV positive women who "break the rules" and breastfeed, is not interpreted as anti-science?[8]

4. How can we reconceptualize risk to find a compromise between the idea that any risk is unacceptable, and the everyday lived reality that we all live with a range of risks as a part of life? AFASS is part of a discourse of mastery that says any risk is unacceptable. Breastfeeding has risks; not breastfeeding has more risks. But actions to control risk often create other unnamed risks. Policies such as AFASS rarely deal with the complexities around different perceptions of risk, including emotional or psychological risk, and the potential for racial bias, as revealed by these conference stories.

5. What concepts and policies address the mother-infant dyad, rather than treating mothers and infants as separate competing individuals? The latter individualistic approach meets western feminist standards for treating women as individuals, but it does not address the synergetic interdependence of mothers and infants so crucial for all discussions of intersubjective experiences like breastfeeding. In the context of HIV/AIDS, keeping mothers healthy is the best way to keep infants and children healthy.

6. Why were alternatives such as pasteurising breastmilk not explored as rigorously as replacement feeds? Why was exclusive breastfeeding not originally supported as the best policy option for all mothers? Support for EBF does not pit HIV/AIDS objectives against other primary health care objectives, HIV negative women against HIV positive women, nor the global north against the global south; the most cost-effective intervention—EBF—also happens to be the best solution to a number of related problems.

7. How can universal health policies such as AFASS, other WHO documents and human rights issues be translated into local vernaculars that civil society NGOs can use or modify to meet local conditions? And how can they be wiped from those same vernaculars when they are found to be inadequate or need to be replaced, as with the various iterations of WHO guidelines on this subject?

8. How can we create solidarity and support among women and women's health advocacy groups, and other single-issue advocacy groups working on HIV/AIDS? Can we build on commonalities, try to meet regularly at international events to develop shared objectives, and maximize synergies by not working too narrowly on our "own issues"?

The 1990 *Innocenti Declaration* on the protection, promotion and support of breastfeeding was the first United Nations policy document related to infant feeding that did not target industrial and developing countries separately. This policy initiative had the potential to add new and powerful unifying language to breastfeeding protection and support. Similarly, the Code for the Marketing of Breast Milk Substitutes applies equally in the global north and global south, although consequences are greater in the global south.

Contexts differ, but the documents have universal relevance. International health policy such as AFASS carries many underlying assumptions, however: that all women in the global north can replacement feed safely, and do not value breastfeeding; that all women in the global south cannot replacement feed safely, and that breastmilk and milk or soy based replacement feeds are equivalent. As these conferences revealed, all these assumptions are false. Acting on such assumptions reveals the cracks in the myth of international solidarity.

Bridges appear when least expected, when we remain open to the opinions and experiences of others. On this subject, we need to avoid premature closure, with both biological and cultural explanations. Breastmilk may indeed be a dangerous fluid carrying virus into the bodies of uninfected newborns, but it is simultaneously food security for infants, and may, in future research, provide the key to understanding immune processes, suggested by the survival of infants exclusively breastfed; this makes gender-sensitive research and policy around exclusive breastfeeding a critical gap to fill.

[1]This title of this chapter is part of the title for the 2006 American Anthropology Annual meetings, where I presented an earlier version of this paper.

[2]A black, fuzzy stuffed animal made by Giant Microbes, for sale at a science

museum in Toronto, comes with a note that says HIV is transmitted through unprotected sexual contact, sharing needles, during pregnancy and childbirth, or through breastfeeding.

[3]WABA made these ribbon/pin combinations into pins and distributed them at the IAC conference in Toronto.

[4]I thank Marion Tompson for sharing these very personal email communications with me.

[5]The consensus statement can be accessed through the WABA website <http://www.waba.org.my/pdf/JointStatement_hiv.pdf>.

[6]More research is needed about how poor HIV positive women in the global north are expected to obtain and use replacement feeds.

[7]HIV and Infant Feeding: A Report of a WABA-UNICEF Colloquium, September, 2002.

[8]One of the most rewarding moments following the York conference was when members of two different groups who were considered dissenters said that this was the first time they had been given the opportunity to speak at a conference. Their positions were listened to respectfully, critiqued effectively and they were not shut down.

REFERENCES

"Breastfeeding Sucks." *Chatelaine* November 2006: 60.

Coutsoudis, A., K. Pillay, E. Spooner, L. Kuhn and H. M. Coovadia,. "Influence of Infant Feeding Patterns on Early Mother-to-Child Transmission of HIV-1 in Durban, South Africa: A Prospective Cohort Study. South African Vitamin A Study Group." *Lancet* 354.9177 (1999): 471-6.

Jones, G., R. Steketee, R. Black, Z. Bhutto and S. Morris. (2003) "How many child deaths can we prevent this year?" *Lancet* 362.9377 (2003): 65-71.

LINKAGES. "Reducing Mother-to-Child Transmission of HIV Among Women Who Breastfeed." *Spotlight* April 2004.

Riles, Annelise. *The Network Inside Out*. Ann Arbor: University of Michigan Press. 2001.

World Health Organization (WHO). *HIV and Infant Feeding. Report of a Technical Consultation*, October 25, Geneva, Switzerland. 2006.

Ziegler, J. B., D. A. Cooper, R. O. Johnson and J. Gold. "Postnatal Transmission of AIDS-associated Retrovirus from Mother to Infant." *Lancet* 1.8434 (1985): 896-8.

From Maternal Love to Toxic Exposure

State Interpretations of Breastfeeding Mothers in the Child Welfare System

JENNIFER A. REICH

BREASTFEEDING HAS BECOME A symbolic marker of maternal commitment and has been endorsed in public health campaigns as unequivocally good. Simultaneously, the content and quality of breastmilk has been called into question as mothers' imperfect diets, alcohol or drug use, or disease status allow breastmilk to be seen as toxic to their infants. Nowhere are these complicated and contradictory meanings of breastfeeding more evident than in the child welfare system. This chapter uses qualitative ethnographic data collected in the child protective services system (CPS) to show how nursing mothers and breastfeeding as a practice are read in different ways.

Parents come to the attention of the CPS system because of a report that a child's safety is in jeopardy. The parents that enter the system are seen as inadequate care providers but are usually provided rehabilitative services. Judges and social workers then examine and reexamine parental progress toward state-defined rehabilitation and assess whether a child may safely return home. Many cases that enter the system involve infants and young children, in part because of state policy that defines prenatal and parental drug use as incompatible with parenting. As a result, mothers who wish to breastfeed are read in varying ways. In some cases, a mother's desire to breastfeed communicates a commitment to her baby and a symbolic desire to parent effectively. In other cases, judges view mothers' milk as dangerous—most commonly because of suspicions of maternal drug or alcohol use—and will legally bar a mother from continuing to breastfeed. In this chapter, I examine two cases of breastfeeding mothers to show the complicated ways state actors interpret the lactating mother. I then juxtapose these cases with my own treatment as a breastfeeding (and frequently pumping) researcher to illustrate the complex and contradictory meanings applied by state actors and examine how those interpretations differentially make breastfeeding practice visible.

BACKGROUND

Data come from a larger study of one unnamed Northern California county

(Reich, *Fixing Families*). Families most often enter the system when someone calls the agency to report concern, and after some vetting, they are investigated by a social worker. Additionally, newborns who test positive at birth for illicit drugs or who are born to a mother who has been identified as posing a risk to her baby (this includes prior CPS involvement) are frequently reported to CPS. After a child is placed in state custody, parents are expected to appear in court within a few days. A judge will usually offer them a case plan that most often includes requirements for drug testing, parenting classes, and counseling, and rules for visitation with their children. Should they comply with these orders and demonstrate themselves as reformed, their visits with their children will increase until they regain custody.

This system is a civil one, which means that the burden of proof to find a parent responsible for the accusations levied against them is based on a preponderance of the evidence, or as attorneys describe it, "50%+1." This is a much lower standard than that used in a criminal court, which requires proof beyond a reasonable doubt. This is designed to allow protecting children to take precedent over efforts to prove guilt. It also allows decisions to be made about families based on a belief in the likelihood that particular acts that endangered children occurred, rather than the certainty that they did.

Of the hundreds of cases I observed, few involved breastfeeding mothers. However, the cases discussed in the following sections provide an example of what Michael Messner suggests "presents the researchers with an opportunity to excavate gendered meanings and processes through an analysis of institutional and cultural contexts" (766). Thus, these cases are not representative of the majority of the kinds and courses of cases that wend through this system. Nonetheless, they illustrate the complex interpretations of the lactating body in the eyes of the state and its actors.

THE PROBLEM OF THE DRUG-USING MOTHER

The last twenty years has marked a heightened increase in public concern about drug use during pregnancy. Beginning in the 1980s in the United States, reports of crack cocaine use were reported in gendered ways. Crack reportedly increased women's sexual libido, the likelihood that they would prostitute themselves for drugs, and exterminated their maternal instinct, resulting in the neglect of children (Gomez).

The newborn baby whose mother had used crack during her pregnancy—known as the "crack baby"—became a potent symbol of the crack epidemic and accompanying war on drugs. Crack babies reportedly were more likely to be born prematurely, to be smaller in length (Chasnoff et al., "Temporal Patterns of Cocaine Use") to be "irritable, inconsolable, developmentally delayed, and incapable of love," and were expected to be learning-disabled (Siegel 255). Although most of the reported damage of drugs was overstated (Vidaeff and Mastrobattista), it nonetheless served as a rallying cry for greater state intervention. Illustrating its success, by 2000, at least 200 women from more than 30 states had been arrested and criminally charged for alleged drug use or other behavior during their pregnancies (Center for Reproductive Law and Policy). Outside of criminal prosecution, this increased awareness heightened child welfare agencies' concern about drugs and defined maternal failings as possessing a particular kind of immorality—allowing Americans to wonder what kind of selfish or evil woman would subject an innocent baby to such toxins.

CHILD WELFARE AND MATERNAL FAILINGS

The charge of the CPS system is to protect children who face imminent danger in their homes or from their parents or care providers. In general, CPS concern over parental drug use presumes that drug use is intrinsically incompatible with parenting for two reasons. First, there is a widespread belief that women who use drugs during pregnancy cannot parent. The logic goes that a woman who has jeopardized her baby's health in utero has proven herself unfit to mother ex-utero. And if she wouldn't abandon drugs while pregnant, it seems unlikely she will do so after birth.

The second rationale reflects a presumption that children of drug addicts do not receive adequate care. In reality, research on this issue is mixed, in large part, because it is difficult to untangle maternal substance use from neglect, and thus, compromised physical safety. Because many substance-involved mothers are poor, many of the problems attributed to maternal drug use may in actuality be the effects of poverty. Additionally, many existing studies examine families who were reported to child protection agencies, and thus may not include families where maternal substance use has not affected child well-being (Noble et al.). Nonetheless, concern over parental drug use has informed CPS policy and has led to an increase in cases. More subtle but also informing CPS practice is concern about breastfeeding. Once newborns are outside what is seen as their mothers' potentially poisonous bodies, babies are believed to be easier to protect. However, breastmilk represents a new risk.

TOXIC BREASTMILK AND RISKS TO INFANTS

Information about toxins in breastmilk has been assembled piecemeal. Much of the literature is comprised of case studies, trickling into news reports. For example, in 2007, warnings were issued about codeine use while breastfeeding (FDA), while others reported toxins in breastmilk (Williams; Cohen; Dorea; Washam), including from herbs and herbal supplements (Chien et al.; Washam). Some point to theoretical risks of medication use, but few identify actual risks (Stowe; Stultz et al.; Schirm et al.; Begg et al.). Addressing this, the American Academy of Pediatrics has attempted to clarify that not all prescription drugs require cessation of breastfeeding, as is often advised (AAP Committee on Drugs). There is little rigorous medical research of illicit drug exposure via breastmilk. One 1987 article described a case of a two week old infant exposed to cocaine through breastmilk (Chasnoff, Lewis and Squires), while others discuss potential risks of drug exposure (Young, Vosper and Phillips; Golding; Das).

Even lacking a strong scientific basis, tainted milk remains an issue. In 1992, a mother was sentenced to six years in prison for causing the death of her infant daughter by delivering methamphetamines to her through breastmilk (Associated Press). This case remains exceptional but suggests the culpability mothers face in providing tainted breastmilk. Because the CPS system is a civil one with a lower burden of proof, judges need only decide that there is some likelihood that breastfeeding could harm a child to address it specifically. System actors look for signs of risk to children by interpreting parents' behaviors, personality, and willingness to be rehabilitated. The following sections examine two cases of lactating mothers and shows how early impressions of them as mothers and breastfeeders shaped their cases.

BREASTFEEDING AND THE BENEFIT OF THE DOUBT

Lisa Flynn, a white woman in her early twenties, first entered CPS when a friend molested her five-year-old daughter, whom, in the view of the system, she had failed to protect. Sixteen months later, Lisa's newborn baby James was automatically made a dependent of the court since Lisa had an on-going case relating to her daughter who remained in foster care. Social workers and attorneys agreed to allow Lisa to keep physical custody of James. In this unusual situation, Lisa was both the parent attempting to reunify with her son and the equivalent of a foster parent who cares for a child whose custody belongs to the state.

As Lisa entered court for the first hearing about James, she walked with the newborn lying in her arms breastfeeding. During the short hearing, the social worker recommended keeping James with her. The other attorneys agreed. Lisa's attorney noted that she and the baby had been tested for drugs at the hospital at birth and had both tested negative. The judge agreed to allow Lisa to keep James with her and ordered her to continue her case plan on James's sister, which included parenting classes, individual counseling, and drug testing, and to allow for paternity testing (since a different man than the one Lisa identified claimed to be the biological father). She politely agreed.

In thinking about the social workers', attorneys', and judge's unusually generous interpretation of Lisa as a parent, it is likely that Lisa's blonde hair, fair skin, and appropriate dress may have allowed state actors to identify with her more than they usually do. However, many other white clients are treated with far more suspicion. What marks Lisa as unlike virtually all parents entering the courtroom is that she did so while breastfeeding. Her desire to breastfeed James silently communicated her concern for her son's well-being, as the "breast is best" campaign has suggested. Symbolically, Lisa invoked powerful middle-class images of competent mothering, even as she was a mother who failed to protect her daughter. In presenting herself this way, she allowed court officials and state actors to feel uncharacteristically optimistic about her ability to regain legal custody of her son; having him in her care meant that she was on her way.

Lisa's case slowly disintegrated. Although she had been ordered to participate in services more than sixteen months prior, she had not done so. She also had not regained custody of her daughter. In a later hearing about her case, a social worker submitted a report to the court detailing her concerns:

> *Mother failed to complete court ordered reunification services designed to help her overcome the problems which led to the initial removal and continued custody of the child's half-sibling. The child's mother has a substance abuse problem from which there is no evidence she has rehabilitated from, which renders her incapable of providing adequate care and supervision for the child in that she failed to comply with court ordered drug testing.*

In detailing her non-compliance with services, the social worker defines her as a failed mother. Because she hasn't proven to the contrary, she should be understood as a woman with a drug problem. Between her daughter's removal and her son's birth, Lisa tested positive for marijuana on eight occasions and for methamphetamines twice. Although this suggests that she had in fact used drugs, there was no concern that she was a habitual user. If there had been, she would have been legally barred from breastfeeding, as many mothers are. Instead, she failed to defer to the court and provide evidence of her abstinence, ignored a policy by which each missed drug test is administratively considered a positive result, and allowed herself to be recast as a failure, uncommitted to her children.

In the coming months, views of Lisa worsened. The attorney for the county called her "flaky and hard to get a hold of." The child's attorney voiced frustration that she was uncooperative in letting her check on the baby, as she is required to do. (She did note that when she finally saw the baby, he looked well.) Though attorneys and social workers voiced their concerns, the judge left James with Lisa but forcefully warned her that if she did not cooperate with her social worker, he would remove James. She said she understood. Few thought Lisa was incapable of providing care, impressions shaped at that first hearing. However, Lisa continued to ignore her case plan and refused to present herself as willing to improve. Her case continued to worsen until James was removed from her care.

THE PRESUMED TOXIC MOTHER

Audrey Simpson, a nineteen year-old white woman, entered the CPS system when police seized large quantities of drugs and cash belonging to Miguel, her twenty-seven year-old live-in boyfriend. As police searched the apartment,

Miguel assured her, "[he] kept telling me, they're bluffing, Audrey. They're not going to take you to jail; you had nothing to do with this." After several hours, the police found illicit drugs and money. They arrested both Audrey and Miguel and called CPS to place their four-month-old daughter Cara in protective custody.

Initially, Audrey expected to be released, but when her sister came to post her bail, she discovered that the amount had been raised significantly and she was unable to help. After mandatory home evaluations and background checks, Cara was placed with Audrey's sister. However, for the first two weeks of Audrey's incarceration, Cara was in a foster care placement. As an exclusively breastfed baby, the separation was difficult for them both. Audrey explained, "It was hard because I was breastfeeding her. She was four months, four and a half months old, and I was breastfeeding her. The foster mother said that she didn't eat for two days."

Audrey recognized that the police and social workers were concerned that she was exposing Cara to drugs through breastmilk. She remembers,

> *They took Cara straight from me and took her straight to the hospital and did toxicology on her because I was breastfeeding her and they wanted to make sure she didn't have withdrawal symptoms. She came out negative.*

From there, Cara was placed in a foster home. After refusing to eat for two days, Audrey says Cara "took to the bottle and she's been on the bottle ever since." According to Audrey, the social worker explained that she was forbidden to breastfeed the baby, "even though I wasn't on drugs when I got arrested." While the separation was difficult for Cara, it was also difficult physically for Audrey. Recalling the experience in jail, she explained,

> *My chest was leaking. And I kept wanting to go to the medical floor but they wouldn't let me so after that they started making me take anti-inflammatory pills. And when I got out my chest was so small all the milk was dried up anyhow. And when I got out I tried to pump my breasts because they don't have a pump at the [jail] hospital; I was having to do it every night before I went to bed -- I was trying to do it. Because they said if it builds up over 24 hours you can get an infection or something like that. So I would sit there at night and try to do it manual into a cup because I thought I was going to get out sooner … Then once I got out I tried to use a breast pump but then I went to court and they said I couldn't breastfeed her anyhow so I just quit altogether.*

By the time her CPS case came to court roughly thirty days after her arrest, criminal charges against her had been dropped. Nonetheless, in this civil system, was she was treated as potentially dangerous to her child. For the following two months, she was required to complete three drug tests each week and parenting classes, and was allowed to visit her daughter who remained with her sister. Audrey explained that, "after the six clean drug tests they said I could start trying to breastfeed but Cara has nothing to do with me now." After adjusting to the bottle, Cara was uninterested in resuming breastfeeding.

Although drug testing presented challenges to her efforts to keep a full-time job, most difficult for her was her lack of parental autonomy. She explained,

> *It's been hard. Really hard. I mean I've never left my daughter alone except for maybe a half an hour.... And for them to grab her from me and then to walk straight out the door and then I knew; in a matter of seconds I lost my life, my love, my daughter and I was just crazy. It all happened so fast. And now I'm just trying to deal with it.*

One particularly challenging aspect of her separation from her daughter was being asked to a use a vocabulary that suggested that someone else was like her daughter's mother. As the court referenced the foster mother, Audrey became upset. "I said she's the caretaker, not the foster mother, ya know. It was hurting me inside to call someone else her mother." Both the vocabulary of an alternative mother and the view of her as irrelevant to her daughter's nutrition and wellbeing speak to her demoralizing experience in the system.

READING THE LACTATING BODY

In taking Lisa and Audrey's cases side by side, we see the complex and contradictory ways that breastfeeding signals maternal commitment and danger. Lisa, a mother who had already failed to protect one child and had in fact tested positive for drugs, was allowed to continue breastfeeding. In contrast, Audrey, a young mother with no history of drug use but one who was arrested for a drug-related offense, was legally barred from breastfeeding until she could prove that she was drug-free. By the time she was able to do so, her ability to breastfeed had been irreparably damaged. Criminal charges against her were dropped within two weeks of her arrest and after 60 days of drug testing three times each week, Audrey never once tested positive.

In evaluating these two cases, we have an opportunity to explore how state actors interpret the lactating body. It is not my intent to argue whether these women should or should not have been allowed to breastfeed. Rather, in evaluating their different treatment by the same court (and judge), we can unpack the cultural assumptions of the maternal body and the differences context makes. In both, we see the subjective nature of assessments of child risk and how first impressions—or initial stories—of clients shape court orders.

First, the first impression the court forms—whether a woman is a mother or a hazard—shapes much of case outcome. One could imagine that had Audrey entered the courtroom for the first time breastfeeding, she may have been seen as a committed mother. Instead, she was first perceived as the girlfriend of a drug dealer. Audrey, like Lisa, is a young, attractive white woman. However, the fact that her boyfriend is an undocumented immigrant who will be deported after completing his prison term further casts her in a questionable light. Had a social worker placed baby James in foster care at birth—an act allowed by state law—Lisa's case might have appeared differently. We could imagine Lisa coming to court without a baby, uncertain of paternity, and as a woman who showed little concern for her young daughter in foster care. She too would have likely been seen as fungible. But as Lisa appeared with her suckling infant, she was perceived as essentially maternal, which provided her more generosity and understanding than most mothers entering the system receive. Although Lisa squandered that goodwill, she was given more chances for no other identifiable reason.

Second, both cases illustrate the subjective nature of concern for maternal drug use. Often, drug use is presented as binary: user/non-user. The actual patterns of use, quantity or timing, and impressions of use remain invisible. In reality, the meanings of drug use are more fluid. Lisa was not legally barred from breastfeeding, even though she had tested positive in the recent past. She was also largely uncooperative with drug testing requirements, and thus failed to prove her on-going abstinence from drugs. Yet, she was not perceived as presenting a risk of drug exposure to her son.

In contrast, Audrey was barred from breastfeeding. She had never tested positive for drugs, had no history of drug use, and even tested negative while complying with required tests. However, given her residence in an apartment—now seen as a drug den—and her commitment to a drug-dealing boyfriend, she was read as potentially dangerous. In these cases, we see that context and perception of a mother as potentially toxic or nurturing shape state policy and practice.

Although these cases elucidate the subjective nature of assessment of child risk, we should avoid romanticizing breastfeeding or becoming overly morose over the loss of it. In fact, in the women's own lives, breastfeeding was one issue among many. Lisa, allowed to continue breastfeeding, gave it up within a few months, as many women do. Audrey's involuntary weaning of her infant is disturbing. However, as she considered it, she identified positives. Audrey voiced disapproval of other women's extended breastfeeding, noting, "You see parents around their kids who are one or two years old and they're still breastfeeding." In citing this, she made it clear that she would not have wanted that to have been her experience, but speculated that she herself "couldn't have starved my daughter for two days so that she could get used to the bottle." As she reflected on her daughter's tough adjustment to bottle-feeding she explained, "It's kinda good [it] happened in a way, but I wish it would have happened a little later." In making sense of Audrey's experience, it is indeed her loss of the freedom to decide when that moment might have occurred that is most tragic.

THE INVISIBILITY OF THE LACTATING RESEARCHER

In conducting research, it is necessary to account for how our own embodiment affects our data. As Ruth Behar eloquently described,

> The woman who writes culture also has breasts, but she is given permission to conceal them behind her pencil and pad of paper. Yet it is at her own peril that she deludes herself into thinking her breasts do not matter, are invisible, cancer won't catch up with them, the male gaze does not take them into account. (1)

When I began this study, I was pregnant. When I completed it, I was a breastfeeding mother. As I have discussed elsewhere, my pregnancy and parenthood status affected my data in unimaginable ways (Reich, "Pregnant with Possibility"). Most poignantly, my own embodiment as a pregnant researcher revealed whose reproduction was defined as normative and whose was suspect.

In noting the differences in the reaction to the pregnancies and parenting practices of lawyers and social workers and "people like us" and those of clients of the CPS system, much was revealed. Michel Foucault explains that, "it is a normalizing gaze, a surveillance that makes it possible to qualify, to classify and to punish. It establishes over individuals a visibility through which one differentiates them and judges them" (184).

The differences between my experience as a lactating woman and those of Audrey and Lisa, even as we were in the same courtroom, are stark and revealing. Most obvious is how my breastfeeding practices remained largely invisible from the normalizing gaze of the state. I passed an electric breast pump through an x-ray machine every morning (sometimes awkwardly explaining to confused security officers what they were seeing) and snuck into conference rooms to discreetly express milk for my baby. To be clear, my practices were known. Attorneys facilitated my access to these semi-private spaces, asked frequently about my son, and usually waited for me to finish before heading to lunch. As most attorneys and social workers were middle-class professionals, my practice was unremarkable. And while it was known, it remained relatively invisible, as lactation often is (Hausman; Shaw).

The invisibility of breastfeeding may serve to undermine support for mothers and motherwork. Yet, by remaining invisible, I was free from scrutiny. In contrast, breastfeeding mothers in the child protective services system remain exposed; the state examines their personal habits, sexuality, health, presumed drug use, and aspects of their lives in search of signs of rehabilitation, remorse, or continued maternal transgression. The state interprets mothers' milk as nurturing or toxic and court orders address whether it can be provided to infants. As such, breastfeeding—even when not performed in the courtroom—remains visible.

CONCLUSION

State actors in the child welfare system are faced with complex and sometimes contradictory expectations to protect children from harm while also preserving families when possible. In identifying possible harm, illicit drugs have been identified as a source of impairment of parental ability and a form of toxicity to children. Breastfeeding can potentially deliver such toxins. As a result, state actors attempt to mitigate potential harm by specifically forbidding breastfeeding when maternal drug use is suspected.

What this article demonstrates is not the reasonableness or unreasonableness of such a policy. Rather, I suggest that judges, social workers, and attorneys are engaged in a process of reading signs of maternal worthiness and maternal behavior. Among the signs, the lactating body is simultaneously read as a sign of maternal commitment and as a source of poison. Whichever frame dominates will have potentially far-reaching effects on case outcome and thus, the families themselves, even as they may be divorced from the invisible reality of maternal drug use or sobriety.

REFERENCES

AAP Committee on Drugs. "The Transfer of Drugs and Other Chemicals into Human Milk." *Pediatrics* 108.3 (2001): 776-89.

Associated Press. "Mother Gets 6 Years for Drugs in Breast Milk." *The New York Times* October 28, 1992: B9.

Begg, Evan J., Stephen B. Duffull, L. Peter Hackett, Kenneth F. Ilett. "Studying Drugs in Human Milk: Time to Unify the Approach." *Journal of Human Lactation* 18.4 (2002): 323-32.

Behar, Ruth. "Introduction: Out of Exile." *Women Writing Culture*. Eds. Ruth Behar and Deborah Gordon. Berkeley: University of California Press, 1995. 1-29.

Center for Reproductive Law and Policy. *Punishing Women for Their Behavior During Pregnancy*. NY: Center for Reproductive Law and Policy, 2000.

Chasnoff, Ira J., Dan R. Griffith, Scott MacGregor, Kathryn Dirkes, Kayreen A. Burns "Temporal Patterns of Cocaine Use in Pregnancy: Perinatal Outcome." *The Journal of the American Medical Association* 261.12 (March 24 1989): 1741-45.

Chasnoff, Ira J., Douglas E. Lewis, and Liza Squires. "Cocaine Intoxication in a Breast-Fed Infant." *Pediatrics* 80.6 (1987): 836.

Chien, Ling-Chu, Ching-Ying Yeh, Hung-Chang Lee, Hsing Jasmine Chao, Ming-Jer Shieh, Bor-Cheng Han. "Effect of the Mother's Consumption of Traditional Chinese Herbs on Estimated Infant Daily Intake of Lead from Breast Milk." *Science of the Total Environment* 354.2-3 (2006): 120-6.

Cohen, Marc. "Environmental Toxins and Health: The Health Impact of

Pesticides." *Australian Family Physician* 36.12 (2007): 1002-4.

Das, G. "Cocaine Abuse and Reproduction." *International Journal of Clinical Pharmacology and Therapeutics* 32.1 (1994): 7-11.

Dorea, Jose G. "Exposure to Mercury During the First Six Months Via Human Milk and Vaccines: Modifying Risk Factors." *American Journal of Perinatology* 24.7 (2007): 387-400.

Food and Drug Administration (FDA). "FDA. Warning on Codeine Use by Nursing Mothers." Washington, DC, 2007. U.S. Food and Drug Administration. February 13 2008. <http://www.fda.gov/bbs/topics/NEWS/2007/NEW01685.html>.

Foucault, Michel. *Discipline and Punish: The Birth of the Prison*. Trans. Alan Sheridan. New York: Vintage Books, 1995.

Golding, Jean "Unnatural Constituents of Breast Milk: Medication, Lifestyle, Pollutants, Viruses." *Early Human Development* 49 Suppl (1997): S29-43.

Gomez, Laura E. *Misconceiving Mothers: Legislators, Prosecutors, and the Politics of Prenatal Drug Exposure*. Philadelphia: Temple University Press, 1997.

Hausman, Bernice L. "Things (Not) to Do with Breasts in Public: Maternal Embodiment and the Biocultural Politics of Infant Feeding." *New Literary History* 38.3 (2007): 479-504.

Messner, Michael. "Barbie Girls Versus Sea Monsters: Children Constructing Gender." *Gender & Society* 14.6 (2000): 765-84.

Noble, Amanda, Dorie Klein, Elaine Zahnd, and Sue Holtby. "Gender Issues in California's Perinatal Substance Abuse Policy." *Contemporary Drug Problems* 27.1 (Spring) (2000): 77-119.

Reich, Jennifer A. *Fixing Families: Parents, Power, and the Child Welfare System*. New York: Routledge, 2005.

Reich, Jennifer A. "Pregnant with Possibility: Reflections on Embodiment, Access, and Inclusion in Field Research." *Qualitative Sociology* 26.3 (2003): 351-66.

Schirm, E., M. P. Schwagermann, H. Tobi, and L. T. W. de Jong-van den Berg. "Drug Use During Breastfeeding. A Survey from the Netherlands." *European Journal of Clinical Nutrition* 58.2 (2004): 386-90.

Shaw, Rhonda. "The Virtues of Cross-Nursing and the 'Yuk Factor'." *Australian Feminist Studies* 19.45 (2004): 287-99.

Siegel, Loren. "The Pregnancy Police Fight the War on Drugs." *Crack in America: Demon Drugs and Social Justice*. Eds. Craig Reinarman and Harry G. Levine. Berkeley: California Press, 1997. 249-59.

Stowe, Zachary N. "The Use of Mood Stabilizers During Breastfeeding." *Journal of Clinical Psychiatry* 68 Suppl 9 (2007): 22-8.

Stultz, Esther E., Jennifer L. Stokes, Michele L. Shaffer, Ian M. Paul, and Cheston M. Berlin. "Extent of Medication Use in Breastfeeding Women." *Breastfeeding Medicine* 2.3 (2007): 145-51.

Vidaeff, A. C. and J. M. Mastrobattista. "In Utero Cocaine Exposure: A

Thorny Mix of Science and Mythology." *American Journal of Perinatology* 20.4 (2003): 165-72.

Washam, Cynthia. "High-Test Mothers' Milk." *Environmental Health Perspectives* 114.6 (2006): A344.

Williams, Florence. "Toxic Breast Milk?" *New York Times* January 9 2005, sec. Section 6: 21.

Young, S. L., H. J. Vosper, and S. A. Phillips. "Cocaine: Its Effects on Maternal and Child Health." *Pharmacotherapy* 12.1 (1992): 2-17.

Risk and Culture Revisited

Breastfeeding and the 2002 West Nile Virus Scare in the United States

BERNICE L. HAUSMAN

ON OCTOBER 4, 2002, I read a short article about West Nile virus and breastfeeding in my local newspaper, the *Roanoke Times*. The headline was "Infant Likely Got West Nile in Breastmilk." It reads in its entirety:

> ATLANTA—Federal health officials said Thursday that a Michigan infant has the West Nile virus and probably got it from the breastmilk of his infected mother.
>
> The child is healthy and his mother is recovering, the Centers for Disease Control and Prevention said. The CDC said it was virtually certain the virus came from breast milk, though there is no way to be completely sure.
>
> Doctors stressed that breastmilk is the healthiest food for babies and that mothers shouldn't quit breastfeeding because of West Nile fears.
>
> Last week, when the case was being investigated, the CDC urged new mothers with the virus to talk with their doctor about whether to continue breast-feeding.

The article was also published on CNN.com, from which I printed it the same day. The CNN article, indicating an Associated Press byline, is a bit longer than the one appearing in the *Roanoke Times*. According to the full article, this particular mother received a blood transfusion on the day she gave birth as well as the following day. Subsequently, the donor blood showed "signs of contamination" with West Nile virus, a fact which was confirmed on CDC web page discussing the case ("West Nile Virus [WNV] Infection and Breastfeeding: Information for Clinicians").[1]

There is a robust literature on the rhetoric of risk, including a subcategory devoted to risk discourses in medicine. Some of the contributions discuss how to better communicate risk as a method of improved management of natural and constructed dangers to human life (Powell and Leiss). Others address the rise of a "risk epidemic" in medical publications and try to ascertain both the causes and effects of such a phenomenon (Skolbekken). The research that I draw on concerns the cultural uses of risk, specifically, its relation to fundamental beliefs and institutions of a given culture.

Developing an argument first put forward by Mary Douglas and Aaron Wildavsky in 1982, Wildavsky and Karl Dake conclude that "individuals perceive a variety of risks in a manner that supports their way of life" (Douglas and Wildavsky; Wildavsky and Dake 57). The "way of life" is a reference to individuals' worldviews; according to these scholars, attitudes toward risk track both social commitments and the structures (or institutions) that those commitments rely on. This is not the same as arguing that people are only interested in risks that affect them in an objective sense. Douglas and Wildavsky argue that there is no objective perception of risk; instead, risks are always "selected for" in the context of a need to shore up and preserve not only particular social systems but the common understanding of what threatens those social systems. Risks are constructed against a backdrop of ideals, not a natural world of real risks that can be chosen over other, more illusory, dangers: "When we say, therefore, that a certain kind of society is biased toward stressing [a particular risk], we are not saying that other kinds of social organization are objective and unbiased but rather that they are biased toward finding different kinds of dangers" (Douglas and Wildavsky 8).

In the fall (i.e., autumn in America) of 2002, I was researching perceptions of HIV-positive mothers and breastfeeding; because of this, I paid attention to news and information tracking West Nile virus infection and breastfeeding. What I found is an object lesson in risk selection, American style. Fears of WNV infection through breastfeeding that emerged in fall 2002 demonstrate typically American fears of microbial dangers that threaten North America from afar. In addition, blood transfusion is perceived as more routine in the contemporary United States than breastfeeding. The double-speak that breastfeeding advocates have long noted in public discourses about infant feeding is a prominent element of the news reporting on West Nile infection and breastfeeding, as is the encouragement of mother's subservience to medical authority. These varied implications of the reporting on WNV and lactation reveal deep ambivalence about women's capacities to nourish their children outside of medical scrutiny and oversight, and a cultural tendency to select breastfeeding itself as a risky behavior.

WEST NILE VIRUS IN THE UNITED STATES

West Nile virus was originally identified in 1937 in Uganda. In 1999, residents of New York City became ill with the first West Nile infections known in the United States. A blood-borne virus, the vector for West Nile is the mosquito, with a host range of one hundred and eighty species, including birds, dogs, cats, horses, squirrels, and alligators. It is a member of a group of viruses called the Japanese Encephalitis Serocomplex of the Family Flaviridae, which exist around the globe in temperate and tropical climates. A related virus in the United States is the St. Louis encephalitis virus, "a similar flavivirus [which] caused periodic epidemics in the United States ... [which] has subsequently [after 1975] caused no large US epidemics, possibly due to herd immunity. The fact that there are only sporadic cases of WNV in the United States suggests a similar pattern" (Bartlett). Eighty percent of those infected with West Nile virus have no symptoms at all; almost twenty percent develop a fever and some neurological symptoms. Fewer than one percent of those infected develop severe West Nile fever and fewer than that die from it: "The commonly quoted mortality rate for neurologic cases is 10 percent, but for the current epidemic in the United States it is 1.6 percent" (Bartlett).

Nevertheless, some localities in the United States have returned to aerial pesticide spraying and community fogging to reduce mosquito populations. The Centers for Disease Control produced a series of prevention posters, including one with the caption "West Nile Virus Can Make You So Sick You Can Miss Work or Even Die." While technically true, the message sent with such a poster is that death is a likely or at least common result of West Nile fever. Citizens are urged to spray themselves with DEET insect repellents and to monitor their own property and their communities for likely areas of mosquito-breeding (such as standing water). Clearly, some prevention efforts are logical and health-promoting responses to the introduction of West Nile virus to the United States, but it is not at all clear that drastic measures to eradicate mosquito populations are warranted, given the nature of West Nile fever to infect most people mildly and thus to confer substantial immune advantage through natural means. But the articles on breastfeeding and West Nile virus continue the overwhelming trend of most West Nile journalism, which is to overstate the danger to individuals.

There are two vectors of contagion represented in the short article in my local newspaper: the one which constitutes the article's purported focus, breastfeeding, and the actual mechanism of infection of the mother, blood transfusion. I want to look first at how breastfeeding and its risks are represented. Initially, breastmilk figures more prominently than the activity of breastfeeding itself. Breastmilk appears in the story three times, in the first three paragraphs, while nursing is used once (third paragraph) and breastfeeding once (fourth paragraph). Breastmilk, we learn, can be a mechanism for viral transfer but is nevertheless a healthy food for babies. Thus breastmilk, generally thought of as good for babies, can also be bad for babies. This is an example of typical doublespeak concerning breastfeeding, which can be found in popular advice books on parenting and infant care (see Hausman, *Mother's Milk*). Mothers should not quit nursing "because of West Nile fears," but should consult a doctor if they actually have the West Nile virus. Breastmilk is separated from breastfeeding, conceptually, in the beginning of the article, although by the end there is the suggestion that one gets breastmilk through breastfeeding.

The baby in this instance is identified as being healthy; it is the mother who is recovering. Nothing new is really going on here, as we know that breastfeeding is one way that mothers confer important protections from illness on their infants. Further investigation of the CDC website demonstrates that the infant was never ill but did have evidence of viral antibodies in its blood. This infant may have developed the mildest form of West Nile infection, where there are no symptoms and the individual is actually not ill, because the mother passed antibodies through her breastmilk.

Since infants are usually vulnerable to the same germs with which their mothers come into contact, access to antibodies through breastfeeding is one way that infants ward off illnesses to which their mothers and families are exposed. Significantly, almost all the articles about West Nile infection in the breastfeeding baby on October 4, 2002, do not mention this common medical understanding of one mechanism through which breastfeeding helps infant immunity. Indeed, breastmilk contains antibodies to viruses that are not themselves transmitted through breastfeeding; that is, antibodies to cold and flu viruses are present in breastmilk even though those viruses are not.[2] Yet instead of stressing the immune-strengthening properties of breastfeeding and breastmilk, the articles generally focus on the potential for breastfeeding to be a vector for infection.

While the CDC was "virtually certain the virus came from breastmilk," it was actually "not clear how the mother became infected." Since there was contamination of the donor blood with West Nile virus, this was clearly a viable conclusion at the time; it has since been confirmed. Interestingly, the October 4, 2002, articles came after a month of media reporting about the possibility of West Nile spread through organ donation (Weiss, "Organ Recipients Had Virus"; Altman, "Transplants Seem Source"; Brown, "4th Organ Recipient"; Grady, "Doctors Confirm West Nile"; and Brown, "Virus's Link"). The October 4th articles are actually related to this thread in health reporting during fall 2002. The concern overall is with a new virus and its emerging modes of transmission. First, with organ transplant recipients falling ill, there is concern about the organ donation system and with blood recipients. Then, with a breastfeeding mother ill with West Nile, there is concern about what is termed "vertical transmission," from mother to baby.[3] Isolating the articles on breastfeeding obscures the more generalized fear of new vectors of West Nile infection, of which breastfeeding is only one potential route for infection.

Subsequent attention to West Nile transmission through organ donation and blood transfusion have demonstrated that infection through this route is not only possible but often lethal (Grady, "For Two Transplant Patients, a Dire Complication"; see also "CDC: Mom's milk gave baby West Nile"; "Public Health Dispatch: West Nile Virus Infection in Organ Donor and Transplant Recipients"; "Public Health Dispatch: Investigation of Blood Transfusion Recipients with West Nile Virus Infections"; "Update: Investigations of West

Nile Virus Infections in Recipients of Organ Transplantation and Blood Transfusion"; and Petersen and Hayes). When we look at breastfeeding as a possible route for transmission, we see that the potential risk to the baby emerges from the situation of modern, hospitalized childbirth and the routinization of donor blood transfusion for mothers who experience anemia post-partum or significant blood loss during delivery. The same advances in medical practice that may have saved this mother's life have made her body into a conduit for viral infection in ways unimaginable in previous historical periods. Yet in the reporting on October 4, 2002, donor blood transfusion is represented as the routine, normal behavior, while breastfeeding is not. There is an implicit alternative for mothers who wish or need to cease breastfeeding, but blood transfusions are part of an unexceptional backdrop of medical care for childbearing women.

Thus, it is the common understanding of breastfeeding as a health promoting practice but one with dangers associated with the transfer of bodily fluids that makes its representation distinctive in these media accounts. Oddly, we see no attempt to find out if breastfeeding has been identified as a route of WNV transmission in the areas of Africa where it is endemic and where breastfeeding is a widespread practice and often of long duration. Instead, breastfeeding is likened to organ donation and blood transfusion, the exchange of bodily fluids and/or tissue between two separate individuals that is mediated by medicine as a technical practice.

The analogy should give us pause, especially because breastfeeding is a sex-specific embodied function, that is, non-normative because performed only by women. The analogy between breastfeeding and organ donation or blood transfusion takes breastfeeding out of its context as a human relationship between mother and child and makes it a medical transaction presided over by a physician. Of course, this is in many ways what breastfeeding has become in modern industrialized societies, but here we see a representation that enforces this meaning at a cultural level. And not only is breastfeeding estranged from its traditional meanings by the analogy, but organ donation and blood transfusion are naturalized by their association with breastfeeding.

In addition, advances in medical research have guided us to think of breastmilk as a substance replete with important nutrients and immune factors and the necessary ratio of fats to sugars to proteins for growing human babies. As neonatologist Nancy Wight writes, "The benefits of breastfeeding in terms of species specificity, balanced, changing nutrients and enzymes, host resistance factors, immunologic protection, allergy protection and psychosocial development, make breastmilk [sic] the most important and cost effective substance we have in medicine today" (1). Thus, advances in medical research have led us to think of breastmilk as both a medicine and a food. Linked to a cultural history of lactation iconography that represents the breastfeeding mother as Madonna (the mother of Jesus, not the pop music diva), as well as to a recent history of medical breastfeeding advocacy that stresses the natural purity of breastmilk in contrast to the easy bacterial contamination of infant formulas, the medicinal and nutritional approaches to breastfeeding contribute to perceptions of it as a perfect and unadulterated food and medicine. Historical changes in the technical practice of medicine thus have encouraged us to imagine that West Nile virus would not be found in breastmilk or transmitted through breastfeeding because breastfeeding is about the transfer of a pure substance from mother to baby.

We read that mothers should not "quit nursing because of West Nile *fears*," but if they have the virus and are nursing, they should contact their doctors. This information is mentioned in each article on the topic. Mothers' actions are always under the supervision of physicians and are subject to the expert knowledge of relative risk that the physician controls. What do we think this imaginary physician would say to a mother who now understands her breastmilk may be contain and transmit an infectious virus? Some version of "Most people bitten by an infected mosquito never get sick," which is the way that the CNN.com version of this article ends? Most infants who breastfeed from mothers ill with West Nile virus will never get sick? The *Morbidity and Mortality Weekly Report* (MMWR) in 2002 about breastfeeding and West Nile virus infection states that "Because the health benefits of breastfeeding are well established and the risk for WNV transmission through breastfeeding is still unknown, these findings do not suggest a change in breast-feeding recommendations" ("Possible West Nile Virus Transmission to an Infant"). The CDC's 2002 online article on West Nile virus and breastfeeding clearly presents this message, but the public's understanding of the "unknown" risk of West Nile infection through breastfeeding—when compared to the standard of infant formula—may influence behavior toward bottle feeding. After all, what are the benefits of breastfeeding when compared to an unknown risk of infection? Ask your doctor. Mothers who are ill with West Nile Virus should do what all mothers in all instances should do: what their doctors tell them to do.

Doctors, of course, differ in their understanding of breastfeeding: their perceptions of its benefits and their knowledge of its management are notoriously unreliable, at least according to breastfeeding advocates. Nancy Wight writes, "In all cases, the risks of breastfeeding with maternal hepatitis should be weighed against the known risks of NOT breastfeeding in each individual case and environment"; similar advice concerning West Nile infection would have been appropriate and is suggested in each article about the case (Wight 4). Typical language is presented in the *Roanoke Times* article: "Doctors stressed that breastmilk is the healthiest food for babies and that mothers shouldn't quit nursing because of West Nile fears." Yet the Michigan woman whose baby and breastmilk were the focus of all this attention in fall 2002 stopped breastfeeding "on the advice of her physician when she was hospitalized" (Maugh, "Evidence of West Nile Virus Found in Breast Milk").

The Centers for Disease Control now states unequivocally that "Scientists have found no evidence that a mother's West Nile Virus infection harms her breastfeeding infant" (CDC, "Breastfeeding: Infectious Diseases and Specific Conditions"). I've never seen a newspaper article herald this information, and other websites provide more circumspect views of the potential for WNV to infect, and harm, breastfeeding infants. This lack of consistency may be one result of the longevity of some web-based information, but it also demonstrates the kind of evidentiary controversies that plague breastfeeding research and promotion strategies. Even if there is no evidence of harm through breastfeeding in the context of maternal West Nile infection, there is a theoretical risk that, for virus-phobic American citizens and their physicians, can override the common sense that no infant has been harmed yet. This is because West Nile virus is a risk that Americans see and appreciate. According to Lynn Payer, Americans see microbes, especially viruses, as primary threats to health. Yet we do not see the risks of not breastfeeding, and we demonstrate this blindness by questioning the scientific data behind breastfeeding promotion, while questionable West Nile virus risk scenarios flood the news.

WNV AND RISK

Why select West Nile virus as a particularly salient risk to breastfeeding in the United States? Anthropological approaches to risk, exemplified by Mary Douglas's work, best address this aspect of the representations of risk and breastfeeding discussed in this chapter. Pollution risks, for Douglas, exist in every culture, although they are different in each, specific to the particular context and its institutions (Douglas 35-40). Culturalist approaches to pollution avoid treating the contemporary period—or specific industrialized nations or "modernized" societies—as special with respect to how pollution risks function in cultural systems. The culturalist approach understands that "private individuals ... choose not to be aware of every danger" and "the social environment, the selection principles, and the perceiving subject [are] all one system" (Douglas and Wildavsky 72, 7). For the culturalist approach, scientific evidence concerning risk is simply one other element of a cultural system concerning the perception and experience of pollution risks, and it operates in some contexts much like the magical systems of the so-called primitive cultures, in that it provides the reason for all otherwise unaccountable phenomena. The culturalist approach helps explain individuals' decisions within communities of common practice and belief (see also Downey).

So why was breastfeeding selected as a particular risk of the West Nile virus "epidemic" in 2002 (especially since no infants at the time, or since, were harmed by breastfeeding from a mother infected with the virus)? The linkage between breastfeeding, organ transplantation, and blood transfusions—the three foci of the news media attention to WNV during the fall of 2002—shows us that breastfeeding is construed as a potentially dangerous, although generally beneficial, medical practice that involves the transfer of bodily fluids from one individual to another. It can go awry, however, when a foreign substance interferes with the (imagined) aseptic conditions necessary to insure the safety of the receiving body. This is why breastfeeding is understood to be a practice best engaged under the supervision of a physician.

How does the selection for West Nile virus and, more specifically, for specific risks attendant to breastfeeding, support a particular world view? In the terms of Douglas and Wildavsky's original 1982 analysis, viruses constitute pollutions that are singled out by American sensibilities because they have a "fear of pollution, of cancerous contamination from external intercourse" (120). A current concern in the United States has to do with the effects of globalization on the work force and economy. West Nile virus demonstrates concretely the difficulty of a truly global world in which germs, like capital, jobs, and workers, travel freely. Many of our recent (and ongoing) epidemic scares—avian flu, sudden acute respiratory syndrome (SARS), West Nile virus, even HIV/AIDS—are perceived to threaten the United States from without. That potential infection from some of these diseases involves intimate relations between people—breastfeeding, sexual relations—demonstrates the obscured intimacy and strangeness of other, technologically-mediated methods of infection—transfusion and transplantation. The threats from the outside become threats from the inside, which is another real fear—that we will not know when something gets inside us that might kill us. In the context of a society invested in risk-free living, unexpected threats to well-being are experienced as threats to the core expectations that illness can be managed successfully and that health is a right.

Organ donation and blood products can be regulated. Mothers' bodies are a different story. Some of the most common problems women have with breastfeeding involve difficulty knowing that their babies get enough milk, understanding the supply-demand system that regulates milk production, and trusting themselves to feed their babies adequately. Thus breastfeeding as an ordinary activity of motherhood involves very basic "unknowns" about whether any given mother can succeed. These uncertainties about the maternal body—felt by individual mothers and exacerbated in a cultural context in which breastfeeding is not a common public practice—constitute much of the current experience of breastfeeding in the United States. Although the fall 2002 newspaper articles consistently reiterated the "known benefits of breastfeeding" even in the context of WNV, one effect of their information was to implicitly emphasize the unknown risks. Moreover, decisions about risks are not made in a vacuum and are certainly not simply rational choices that assess competing risks in an objective, scientific sense. Douglas and Wildavsky write, "In risk perception, humans act less as individuals and more as social beings who have internalized social pressures and delegated their decision-making processes to institutions. They manage as well as they do, without knowing the risks they face, by following social rules on what to ignore: institutions are their problem-solving devices," adding, "most habits, good and bad, are rooted in community life" (80, 84).

In the United States the institution regulating mothers' decisions about infant feeding is medicine, and more specifically the specialty of pediatrics, yet mothers' experiences of risk and their initial relation to medically mediated risk decisions with respect to their babies comes largely from their experience as obstetric patients. Currently most U. S. women do not fear death when they become pregnant, although numbers for maternal and infant mortality and morbidity are stratified according to race. The represented risks of fetal injury or harm, however, continue to drive the medical management of pregnancy and childbirth, insuring women's complicity with its norms. The risk of doing damage to their babies (as well as fears of giving birth to babies already damaged) propels many women to demand or at least tolerate highly technological and interventionist management of pregnancy and childbirth. The notion that childbirth is risky overrides the commonsense idea that it is nevertheless normal and thus not, in most circumstances, deserving of intense medical scrutiny.

The idea that women can repudiate the medicalization of childbirth seems culturally anomalous. Indeed, as Robbie Davis-Floyd argues, many women "participat[ing] most fully in a society's hegemonic core value system . . . are most likely to feel empowered by and to succeed within that system" (Davis-Floyd 1137).[4] That is, many, if not most, women are likely to feel that births complying with the technological model of childbirth are appropriate and warranted, and that such births reflect well on their decision-making as (American) mothers. Any sense that there are unknown risks attendant to breastfeeding—in a cultural circumstance in which the "known benefits" are equivocated publicly—can lead to a "rational choice" to formula feed, just as the possible (but unlikely) risks of childbirth encourage women to engage in interventionist practices of unknown benefit to themselves and their infants. The representation of breastfeeding as a possible conduit for West Nile infection supports the existing social apparatus of medical regulation of pregnancy, childbirth, and infant feeding, in part by raising health risk fears about a practice that is itself culturally anomalous, but also by emphasizing mothers' subordination to the institutions that already guide maternal practice and experience.

This is an example of "life as a planning project," a paradigm regulating women into particular norms of maternal behavior and practice. If "Modern human beings take their fates in their own hands," if they "plan, they make provision, they control and optimise" and "no longer follow God and the stars," then women must consult their doctors for any activity that might endanger their offspring—that is, every activity, for certainly mothers themselves need the intervention of experts to make decisions about health and illness (Beck-Gernsheim 142). Nothing can be allowed to follow its own course in this context of intensive application of biopower to produce valuable and shaped life. Mothers are both responsible and passive in this situation, clearly a form of double jeopardy, which in turn makes practices like breastfeeding—dependent on perseverance, confidence, and the ability to proceed without direct knowledge of the child's intake of fluids—more difficult. This is an old story, familiar to lactation activists who confront a cultural context that seems to thwart breastfeeding promotion at every turn, almost without effort.

Americans experienced West Nile virus as an assault on our right to be free from unwanted, "foreign" germs, yet the media frenzy in the fall of 2002 was part of a larger assault on breastfeeding and motherhood that fits well-established patterns. Mothers' real interests are rarely paid attention to when larger debates exploit public sentiments about women and their fitness in the service of other goals. That breastfeeding is figured as a problem should come as no surprise to any feminist who has studied the politics of infant feeding and the emergence of scientific motherhood in the twentieth century. The breastfeeding body indicates and elaborates problems of the modern body more generally, acting as a site onto which other issues are displaced and then disputed. Our goal as feminists must be to return to the mother's body as a site of meanings important in their own right, analyzing those meanings with full cognizance that they are constructed in a cultural context hostile to ordinary practices of maternity and to women themselves.

[1]See also "Possible West Nile Virus Transmission to an Infant through Breast-Feeding—Michigan 2002." For other newspaper articles on the same day, see "West Nile-Tainted Breast Milk Likely Infected Baby, CDC Says," *Los Angeles Times*; "West Nile's Spread to Baby is Linked to Breast Feeding," *Wall Street Journal*; "Newborn Has West Nile Virus," *Washington Post*.

[2]A series of articles published on September 28, 2002, do a better job discussing questions concerning transmissibility of viruses through breastmilk, although even these do an inadequate job of distinguishing between blood-borne and droplet infections and the action of breastfeeding immunity (Grady, "Traces of West Nile Virus Found in Mother's Breast Milk"; Brown, "West Nile Virus is Discovered in Breast Milk of Michigan Woman"; and Maugh, "Evidence of West Nile Virus Found in Breast Milk").

[3]A subsequent article identified a possible WNV infection in a newborn, indicating that the infection occurred during gestation. The article's conclusions are speculative, however (Weiss, "Baby Had West Nile Virus").

[4]Parts of the discussion in this paragraph and the one preceding it appears in Hausman ("Risky Business" 34-35).

REFERENCES

Altman, Lawrence. "Transplants Seem Source of West Nile Virus Cases." *New York Times* 4 Sept. 2002: A12.

Bartlett, John G. "West Nile Virus." *Medscape*. 2003. Accessed 17 July 2006. <www.medscape.com/viewarticle/461720>.

Beck-Gernsheim, Elisabeth. "Life as a Planning Project." *Risk, Environment, and Modernity: Towards a New Ecology*. Ed. Scott Lash, Bronislaw Szerszynski, and Brian Wynne. London: Sage, 1996. 139-53.

Brown, David. "4th Organ Recipient Has West Nile Virus, CDC Officials Say." *Washington Post* 6 Sept. 2002: A3.

Brown, David. "Virus's Link to Transfusions Intensifies." *Washington Post* 13 Sept. 2002: A3.

Brown, David. "West Nile Virus is Discovered in Breast Milk of Michigan Woman." *Washington Post* 28 Sept. 2002: A11.

"CDC: Mom's milk gave baby West Nile." *CNN.com*. 3 Oct. 2002. Accessed 4 Oct. 2002 <cnn.health.com>.

Centers for Disease Control (CDC). "Breastfeeding: Infectious Diseases and Specific Conditions Affecting Human Milk: West Nile Virus." Department of Health and Human Services, United States Government, 28 Sept. 2005. Accessed 17 July 2006. <www.cdc.gov/breastfeeding/disease/wet_nile_virus.htm>.

Centers for Disease Control. "WNV Fact Sheet." Department of Health and Human Services, United States Government. 27 Sept. 2005. Accessed 17 July 2006. <http://www.cdc.gov/westnile>.

Davis-Floyd, Robbie. "The Technocratic Body: American Childbirth as Cultural Expression." *Social Science and Medicine* 38 (1994): 1125-40.

Douglas, Mary. *Purity and danger: An analysis of the concepts of pollution and taboo*. New York: Routledge and Kegan Paul, 1966.

Davis-Floyd, Robbie. *Risk and Blame: Essays in Cultural Theory.* London and New York: Routledge, 1992.

Douglas, Mary and Aaron Wildavsky. *Risk and Culture*. Berkeley: University of California Press, 1982.

Downey, Gary L. "Risk in Culture: The American Conflict Over Nuclear Power." *Cultural Anthropology* 1.4 (Nov. 1986): 388-412.

Grady, Denise. "Doctors Confirm West Nile in a 4th Transplant Patient." *New York Times* 6 Sept. 2002: A16.

Grady, Denise. "For Two Transplant Patients, a Dire Complication: West Nile." *New York Times*, 16 May 2006. Accessed 16 May 2006. <www.nytimes.com/2006/05/16/health/16viru.html>.

Grady, Denise. "Traces of West Nile Virus Found in Mother's Breast Milk." *New York Times* 28 Sept. 2002: A12.

Hausman, Bernice L. *Mother's Milk: Breastfeeding Controversies in American Culture*. New York: Routledge, 2003.

Hausman, Bernice L. "Risky Business: Framing Childbirth in Hospital Settings." *Journal of Medical Humanities* 26.1 (Spring 2005): 23-38.

"Infant Likely Got West Nile in Breast Milk." *Roanoke Times* 4 Oct. 2002: A9.

Lawrence, Ruth A. and Robert M. Lawrence. *Breastfeeding: A Guide for the Medical Profession*. 6th ed. Philadelphia: Elsevier Mosby, 2005.

Laws, M. Barton. Letter. *Boston Globe* 5 Sept. 2002, 3rd ed.: A14.

Maugh, Thomas H. II. "Evidence of West Nile Virus Found in Breast Milk." *Los Angeles Times* 8 Sept. 2002: A14.

"Newborn Has West Nile Virus." *Washington Post* 4 Oct. 2002: A21.

Payer, Lynn. *Medicine and Culture: Varieties of Treatment in the United States, England, West Germany, and France*. 2nd ed. New York: Henry Holt, 1996.

Petersen, Lyle R. and Edward B. Hayes. "Westward Ho?—The Spread of West Nile Virus." *New England Journal of Medicine* 351 (25 Nov. 2004): 2257-59.

"Possible West Nile Virus Transmission to an Infant through Breast-Feeding—Michigan 2002," *MMWR* 51.39 (4 Oct. 2002): 877-88. Accessed 7 July 2006. <www.cdc.gov/mmwr/preview/mmwrhtml/mm5139a1.htm>.

Powell, Douglas and William Leiss. *Mad Cows and Mother's Milk: The Perils of Poor Risk Communication*. Montreal: McGill-Queen's University Press, 1997.

"Public Health Dispatch: Investigation of Blood Transfusion Recipients with West Nile Virus Infections," *MMWR* 51.36 (13 Sept. 2002): 823. Accessed 17 July 2006. <www.cdc.gov/mmwr/preview/mmwrhtml/mm5136a5.htm>.

"Public Health Dispatch: West Nile Virus Infection in Organ Donor and Transplant Recipients—Georgia and Florida, 2002." *MMWR* 51.35 (6 Sept. 2002): 790. Accessed 17 July 2006. <www.cdc.gov/mmwr/preview/mmwrhtml/mm5135a5.htm>.

Skolbekken, John-Arne. "The Risk Epidemic in Medical Journals." Social Science and Medicine 40.3 (1995): 291-305.

"Update: Investigations of West Nile Virus Infections in Recipients of Organ Transplantation and Blood Transfusion," *MMWR* 51.37 (20 Sept. 2002): 833-36. Accessed 17 July 2006. <www.cdc.gov/mmwr/preview/mmwrhtml/mm5137a5.htm>.

Weiss, Rick. "Baby Had West Nile Virus." *Washington Post* 20 December 2002: A2.

Weiss, Rick. "Organ Recipients Had Virus." *Washington Post* 4 September 2002: A1.

"West Nile Virus (WNV) Infection and Breastfeeding: Information for Clinicians." Division of Vector-Borne Infections Diseases, Centers for Disease Control. 16 July 2003. Accessed 8 Mar. 2004. <www.cdc.gov/ncidod/dvbid/westnile/clinican_breastfeeding.htm>.

"West Nile-Tainted Breast Milk Likely Infected Baby, CDC Says." *Los Angeles Times* 4 Oct. 2002: A29.

"West Nile's Spread to Baby is Linked to Breast Feeding." *Wall Street Journal* 4 Oct. 2002: B4.

Wight, Nancy E. "Breastfeeding in High Risk Populations: The Mom with Hepatitis." *Breastfeeding Update* (San Diego County Breastfeeding Coalition) 1.4 (Dec. 2001): 1, 4. Accessed 8 Mar. 2004. <www.breastfeeding.org/newsletter/v1i4>.

Wildavsky, Aaron and Karl Dake. “Theories of Risk Perception.” *Daedalus* 119.4 (Fall 1990): 41-60.

IV. MILK THEORY

Giving Breastmilk as Being-with

KAREN MCBRIDE-HENRY AND RHONDA SHAW

IT IS ACKNOWLEDGED THAT breastfeeding is the optimum source of nutrition for infants and young children. However, research demonstrates that the majority of women wean their infants before they reach the recommended two years of age (Mozingo, Davis, Droppleman and Merideth; World Health Organisation). Research also reveals that women are well versed in the reasons why they should breastfeed their offspring (Arora, McJunkin, Wehrer, and Kuhn; Earle; Heath, Reeves Tuttle, Simons, Cleghorn, and Parnell); however, the reality of breastfeeding often leaves women questioning their decision to breastfeed (Mozingo, Davis, Droppleman and Merideth; McBride-Henry). There is therefore, a need to examine the activity of breastfeeding in greater depth so health care professionals can better understand women's embodied experience and offer appropriate support for those negotiating the transition to becoming a breastfeeding mother. This chapter presents the findings of a reflective lifeworld research project that sought to examine women's experience of breastfeeding in New Zealand in an effort to attend to this issue.

BACKGROUND

Initial experiences with breastfeeding can leave a lasting impression on a woman, and may influence future decisions about breastfeeding subsequent children (Mozingo, Davis, Droppleman and Merideth). A quantitative study (Tarkka, Paunonen and Laippala) describes how women who were provided with individualised support and education about breastfeeding in the initial postpartum period were more likely to successfully establish and maintain breastfeeding. Marja-Terttu Tarkka and colleagues interviewed women who had given birth in hospital to healthy, full-term infants. They discovered that women who feel positive about their initial breastfeeding experiences are more likely to continue breastfeeding following discharge from tertiary maternity services. For some women, initial breastfeeding experiences are described as positive and rewarding, while other women recount their experiences employing terms such as disappointing, hard, exhausting and stressful (Britton; Mozingo, Davis, Droppleman and Merideth).

The difficulties encountered during the process of initiating breastfeeding have led women to conclude that breastfeeding is not as easy as they were led to believe by others (Hauck, Langton and Coyle; Hill, Humenick and West; Mozingo, Davis, Droppleman and Merideth; Vogel and Mitchell). The gulf between idealised expectations and the reality of breastfeeding is, for some women, extremely difficult to reconcile, resulting in disillusionment and the early cessation of breastfeeding (Mozingo, Davis, Droppleman and Merideth). It is therefore, important to attend to women's experience of breastfeeding when attempting to understand ways in which women can be supported to breastfeed their infants.

METHODOLOGY

This research was informed by reflective lifeworld research, a methodology based on the philosophical work of Martin Heidegger (1962), Hans Gadamer (1989) and Maurice Merleau-Ponty (1981). In nursing studies, researchers such as Patricia Benner (1984), Karen Dalhberg, Nancy Drew, and Maria Nystrom (2001) and Pamela Ironside (1997) have shaped how the methodology is understood and called upon during the process of knowledge generation. This study draws on their work. In short, reflective lifeworld research combines existential and interpretive phenomenology to focus on describing and interpreting lived experiences. In the following discussion we have therefore endeavoured to capture the point of view of women's breastfeeding experiences by drawing on the concept of the lived body. We think this notion better explains breastfeeding relations between mothers and their infants than an ethics of care based on the sex/gender construct because the concept of the lived body refuses the distinction between sex and gender and is not biologistic. Finally, reflective lifeworld research is a methodology that aims to study the everyday world as we immediately experience it, pre-reflectively, prior to conceptualisation and categorisation. Ideally, this research approach enables the researcher to examine phenomena in their entirety and anew, initially bracketing personal and academic presuppositions where possible, and using philosophical texts as a dialogical partner to explore, elucidate, and give expression to lifeworld experiences.

METHOD

Nineteen women were recruited to participate in this study.[1] They were recruited through advertisements placed in Well Child Health clinics; potential participants responded to the advertisement by contacting the researcher, and if they met the study inclusion criteria they were included in the research. The participants were breastfeeding, or had breastfed in the last two years; many of the participants had breastfed more than one child. Each participant engaged in a single unstructured interview, which was subsequently transcribed. Analysis of the transcripts took the form of a conversation between the researcher, the text, and the writings of reflective lifeworld philosophers. This process involved paying attention to the parts and the whole of the participant's experiences; being mindful of the intricate facets of the experience, whilst also attending to the contextual-whole of the lived experience of breastfeeding. The interpretations emerged through a process of thematic analysis, constant questioning, and engaging in the dialogical conversation between the philosophy, the participant's narratives and the researcher. Finally, the process became one of writing and re-writing interpretations.

THE ONTOLOGICAL UNDERSTANDING OF CARE

For reflective lifeworld researchers, a person is a being for whom things matter. Things that have significance and value orient a person's being-in-the-world; they are the everyday activities and things that hold her focus and care. Such a being, or '*dasein*' to use Heidegger's (1962) language, exists in the world 'with-other' and this is primordially a relation of care. Things or 'others' that call out to *dasein* thus capture its concern or care. For Heidegger, "care, as a primordial structural totality, lies before every factical[2] 'attitude' and 'situation' of *dasein*, and it does so existentially *a priori*" (238): it is dasein's basic mode of being-in-the-world. Since care provides the ontological basis for approaching objects and others within-the-world it is not possible to exist without care. As Michael Inwood (2) says, "no one is wholly carefree, careless or uncaring": rather, everyone is fundamentally careful and navigates their way in the world accordingly.

Heidegger distinguishes between two types of care that are employed by *dasein*, one mode of care for objects and another mode for 'others'. *Concern* describes the care that is exhibited when one attends to objects or things that are encountered 'within-the-world', and *solicitude* describes the type of care with which we attend to others.[3] While Heidegger's notion of care is non-moral (that is, care simply *is*), both concern and solicitude have deficient as well as positive modes. Deficient solicitude typically characterises the 'everyday, average Being-with-one-another' with whom we have no familiar relationship (Heidegger 158). Heidegger describes this as 'being for, against, or without one another, passing one another by, not "mattering" to one another' (158). A characteristic feature of this deficient mode of care would be 'inconsiderateness' and 'indifference'. 'Proper' authentic care or solicitude is expressed by 'considerateness' and 'forbearance'. When one dwells 'with-Other', as Heidegger says, through the authentic mode of care or solicitude, one comes to understand the Other. In other words, when we act towards things or entities that concern us within-the-world on an everyday basis while being-with others, our concernful interactions engender understanding. The women who participated in the study this chapter draws on expressed concernful solicitude for their infants. This was evidenced by narratives that portray how they had come to care for another whilst pregnant; a call to care that became even louder following the birth of their infants, facilitating the women coming to know, and ultimately to understand, their infants.

THE CALL TO CARE

Although the care that is expressed towards other is that of solicitude, in everyday life this mode is typically deficient. To express an authentic mode of solicitude it is important to be open to 'being-with-one-another'. The example of a woman who has just given birth provides the backdrop for an interesting interpretation, and explanation, of this idea.

Newborn infants communicate primarily through non-verbal communication and crying, while a mother expresses solicitude towards her infant by striving to understand these unfamiliar communications. A crying, inconsolable infant speaks to a mother of a distressed baby. Equally, an infant that smiles in response to his or her mother's care portrays a satisfied, fulfilled child. The participants in this study engaged in a process of coming-to-know their newborn infants, and actively sought positive responses from their infants. For the women, such responses provided a visible measurement of the effectiveness of their caring. At times, their interpretations of their infant's responses to the breast and breastfeeding influenced their decisions whether or not to continue to breastfeed. The following narratives reveal how the women described their interpretations of their infant's behaviours, and the subsequent impact that had on their breastfeeding experiences.

Sue had completely weaned her son when he was three months old. She believed she had insufficient milk to satisfy her son's needs despite letting him feed for hours on end. For Sue, the most difficult aspect of her breastfeeding experience was having her young son inconsolable despite frequent feeding. As she deeply cared for her infant, watching him suffer was devastating.

> *He [my son] was a newborn baby and, particularly during the day, even from one or two days old we couldn't get him to settle during the day at all. He just wasn't contented at all—that was the most soul-destroying thing.... I thought I was doing the right thing by trying to breastfeed him and it still didn't settle him because he wasn't getting anything as we found out later. It was awful.* (Sue)

Lee questioned whether she should stop breastfeeding her son as she was in pain due to cracked nipples. Her doubt was reinforced by the perception that her son was not enjoying breastfeeding as he would constantly come on and off the nipple during a breastfeed. However, once her son was about six weeks old, he displayed behaviours that indicated to Lee that he was also enjoying the experience of breastfeeding, and Lee's decision to continue to breastfeed was validated. Lee breastfed her son until he was 15 months of age.

> *I thought I could really easily have given up [breastfeeding] because it was such a hassle and so painful and my son didn't even seem to enjoy it that much in the first six weeks. But then he definitely settled to enjoying it and being happy.... I remember, after he was six weeks old he used to do this really cute thing. That you'd fed him, he would pull his lips away from the nipple and give you a huge grin, [he would] look up at you and "ooh" and sort of smile and then he'd return to feeding. That was really sweet.* (Lee)

Jan expressed how she dealt with her son with what Heidegger calls solicitude, disclosing that through her relationship with her son, she came to understand breastfeeding as painful. She provides an example of a woman who felt forced to care through breastfeeding, believing she had no choice. The call to care through breastfeeding was strong; however, Jan's experience of breastfeeding pain drowned out the call and provided her with an overwhelming message she could not ignore.

> *[My son] he was really aggressive so it wasn't even that it was a nice experience once he got on [the breast]. He was chomping even though he had no teeth, he was like a barracuda it was awful. He was really horrible. So when I got pregnant again with my second child I was terrified of breastfeeding.* (Jan)

The experience of breastfeeding her second child, a daughter, was a very positive one for Jan. She spoke in depth during the interview about how breastfeeding facilitated authentic solicitude, leading to a close connection with her daughter. However, Jan was also cognisant of how her relationship with her son was adversely affected by her first breastfeeding experience.

> *[Breastfeeding] it's made a big difference [with my daughter]. Which is pretty hard for my son, but our relationship is fine now, it just got off to a rough start. I'm so pleased it's changed. I was so relieved because for a long time I thought I was never going to like him. That sounds awful doesn't it? It's very true, very honest when I say that I didn't like him at all. I can remember ... thinking if something happened to him I would never have had another child.... Like: 'if you were taken away tomorrow, I really wouldn't be that upset.' It's a horrible, awful, awful feeling and thing to think ... it was not a harming thing, just if I was given the opportunity I would never go through this again.* (Jan)

According to Inwood, to "will, wish or strive for anything whatsoever one must in advance already be care" (1997: 52). In this regard, the women in this study approached their infants with a stance of concernful care, and as a result wished and strove to provide them with breastmilk. Through breastfeeding, the women expressed their care; however, an important part of caring for a new infant is learning what they require to be happy. This presents a significant challenge for most women. Some of the participants decided that breastfeeding did not satisfy their infants or work for them, but those women who persevered discovered that breastfeeding was the best way to comfort their baby.

UNDERSTANDING BREASTFEEDING AS COMFORTING

According to Gadamer, a comforted person is one who is "open to new things, ready to embark on new enterprises and, forgetful of ourselves, scarcely notices the demands and strains which are put on us.... This is what health is" (112). The participants in this study understood that an aspect of coming to know and understand a new infant is being able to console and offer them comfort when they are crying. For them, comfort meant more than just a lack of crying; it was the ability to offer their infants a passage by which they could be readied to embark on life, and give themselves over to all that life had to offer. Comfort thus represented health for their infants.

For these women, breastfeeding became the tool with which they could sooth and comfort their infants. The relationships they forged through breastfeeding developed because of the solicitude the mother felt for her infant, and was facilitated by time spent, being constantly present, and working together. As the breastfeeding relationship matured into a sense of health for their infants, it also facilitated their own sense of well-being.

In the following narrative, Kay shares how breastfeeding her son comforted him like nothing else would, offering him a sense of safety, security and reassurance that he would be taken care of. Breastfeeding represented more than nutritional health—it also enabled Kay to offer her son embodied well-being.

> *It just sort of happens, if my son wants a feed he gets a feed. Sometimes at night he might want an extra one before he goes to bed, he might've had a bad dream or something - it comforts him as well. Two nights ago he woke up crying for some reason, and he wanted a comfort feed. It wasn't a feed, more of a comfort thing for him. There's no way of comforting him like a comfort feed.* (Kay).

In the following narratives, Jan contrasts her experiences in relation to comforting her son and daughter. Breastfeeding became the ultimate source of consolation for Jan's daughter when she was upset, unlike her brother, who was bottle-fed and considerably more difficult to console. Jan discussed why she believed that being at the breast furnished her daughter with a safe, secure haven; the pain, which held her daughter back from engaging actively in life, was removed through breastfeeding. She spoke of how fulfilling it was, as a mother, to be able to offer her daughter life through comfort, and satisfy her child so completely.

> *I liked bottle-feeding him [my son]; I didn't think there was much difference. But I would say that when he was beside himself, you know if he got himself really upset about something.... The bottle's not quite the same in my perception. I can snuggle close and give him his bottle but we're not quite as close and all encompassing as breastfeeding in those situations.*
>
> *Sometimes if she's [my daughter's] been distraught she's not drinking at all. She's just snuggling. She pacifies herself with my breast really, rather than having something to drink. It's not the milk, it's the being close. With my son there were a couple of occasions when I had wished I could, I would even bring out my breast and think 'Well even if you can just get close to it would that make you feel better?' But he was long gone past that stage then.... Now that she has two bottles a day it is more of a comfort than having a lot of milk and it's nice. It's usually first thing... very early in the morning, and it's just her and I, and it's very quiet, and she's having a lovely snuggle and something to eat and that's very nice. It's not just a function; it's a nice cuddly time.*
>
> *I can almost feel it mentally as well as physically; I can feel my daughter wanting to be close... And, in that crying, I'm hurt or frightened, that's what she does, she snuggles right in. She doesn't want her head out at all, she wants your arms right around her—she wants to be cocooned. And my son doesn't do that at all and he never has snuggled like that. He wants to be over your shoulder, held that way.... [To be able to comfort like that is] satisfying, really satisfying, almost like you're taking away all the pain or the fright or the hurt and you can do it so quickly. You can soothe fears and all kinds of things almost immediately.... It's great, fantastic. You can sometimes do it just by holding, but she responds so much faster and relaxes with breastfeeding, often they're tense when they've hurt themselves, and she just relaxes straight away.* (Jan)

One participant, Eva, spoke of how she experienced a sense of well-being because she could completely comfort her infant through breastfeeding. It was a method of comforting that Eva, due to the positive solicitude she felt for her daughter, was pleased to be able to provide. Breastfeeding supplied comfort and facilitated the health of both mother and child, releasing them both to engage in new enterprises and give themselves over to what life had to offer.

> *It's a really lovely feeling because you have the baby in your arms, which is a lovely feeling in itself, and you're satisfying her needs using your own body, which is a very satisfying feeling as well. If comfort is defined by having a sense of well being while doing it then, yes, absolutely. There definitely*

> *has been times when the only way we could calm her down, if she's worked herself into a frenzy, is to pop her on my breast and immediately she'll stop crying and she'll calm down completely whether she's hungry or not, she receives comfort, and I'm really happy to provide that.* (Eva)

As the women who participated in this study came to understand the ways in which their individual infants communicated, they came to understand that breastfeeding offers the ultimate source of comfort. The comfort and health that breastfeeding offered meant that both the women and infants were able to actively return to exploring and engaging with their existence. Breastfeeding offered comfort, born through relational closeness, which enabled the return to life.

BEING CLOSE

Heidegger claims that "solicitous concern is understood in terms of what we are concerned with, along with our understanding of it" (161). To express solicitude for another we must come to understand and know ourselves. In deficient modes of solicitude, such as indifference or passing each other by, it is impossible to come close to others, or know oneself, as one must come close to the 'other' to understand oneself. Hence, if *dasein* remains 'aloof' and 'hides away' it cannot come to know others, or even itself.

Contrariwise, if one dwells closely and chooses to open up to other, authentic solicitude can grow out of this closeness. As one dwells with-other in a proximal or close manner, she comes to understand the other, and also understands how to "be" with another. Being in close proximity makes 'being-toward-other' and thus, closeness, possible (Heidegger 161).

Breastfeeding requires that a woman and her infant be physically close; it also requires emotional openness to the infant, otherwise a woman will feel "tense, unhappy and uncomfortable" (Eva). In dwelling closely with their infants through breastfeeding, the women in this study were 'being-toward' their infants, thus enabling authentic solicitude for their infants. Those women who persevered with breastfeeding spoke of how it facilitated closeness between them, and through this closeness they came to understand and know themselves, as well as their infant.

Sally spoke of how she achieved solicitude in breastfeeding her son. She enjoyed breastfeeding because it was an act that excluded others, even those who were relationally close to her son, such as his father and grandparents. She relayed how she did not want to lose this privileged relationship, as it was through being close that Sally came to understand fulfilment in a different and special way.

> *[Breastfeeding] it's just something else that no one else can share with my son; my husband can't and my parents can't. I think it just makes us*

> *really, really close to each other because it's something that only ever the two of us can share.... That's part of the reason that I'm breastfeeding, you know a small part of it but it is definitely there, because as soon as I stop he's not going to need me the same... I don't want to lose that.* (Sally)

Abby also spoke of the closeness that she felt for her children as a result of breastfeeding. She had breastfed her first child, a daughter, for five months before conceiving her second child, at which point she could no longer maintain her milk supply and subsequently weaned her daughter. She went on to breastfeed her second child for 18 months. At the time of the interview, Abby was breastfeeding her third child, a boy, who was five and a half months of age. She spoke about the differences in her relationships with her daughter and her two sons, attributing these to the closeness of breastfeeding. Solicitude allowed Abby to build a close relationship with her sons. The closeness experienced through this relationship taught Abby's sons about authentic solicitude, which was expressed through their reciprocal closeness and learned ability to express solicitude for Abby.

> *I fed my son longer and I'm closer to him than I am to my daughter who I didn't feed for very long at all.... I think it's because you've spent so much time together. They're latching onto you, you're sharing a little bit more, more than you would just sticking a bottle into their mouth. My other son is quite clingy, this one [the youngest child] is fine but the other one gets quite jealous. He's forgotten what breastfeeding was but he knew that closeness.* (Abby)

Breastfeeding had opened up the opportunity for Eva to experience closeness with her daughter. She spoke about how the relationship and closeness between them existed in part because they had both worked at it together.

> *Certainly breastfeeding has made me feel closer to my baby. I'm pleased that we've been able to make it happen together. I would emphasize that it's a two-way thing, you have to learn your part but the baby also has to learn to do her part, the fact that we've managed to do that together I think makes me feel closer to her.* (Eva)

Eva had experienced a great deal of difficulty during the process of establishing breastfeeding, and had to persevere through a significant amount of pain to continue. At the time of the interview, she was still breastfeeding her daughter, who was three months of age. She expressed a stance of openness toward her daughter. This led to relational closeness with her daughter, which gave her strength to stay-the-course that was required of her to breastfeed, thereby overcoming her embodied experience of pain.

During the interview, Eva breastfed her daughter, and in the following narrative, which emerged at the end of the breastfeed, Eva expressed authentic solicitude:

> *(Laugh). You just had a lovely time didn't you? (Comment is directed to the baby). I must say this is the best moment when she comes off and her face is all pink and she can hardly hold her head up and she looks all pleased, and fat cheeked.... It's not deliberate, it just happens, you feel such wonderful feelings towards her and then she's so cute and it's just easy to do it. It just happens. You could say I don't have a choice, because I'm her sole caregiver but there's ways you could look after your baby if you didn't want to. It's just such a natural, easy thing. And, she's just so cute I can't keep my hands off her (laugh).* (Eva)

Kay also spoke about the closeness that exists between a mother and her baby when engaged in a relationship that incorporates breastfeeding. Kay was a sole parent who did not share custody with her son's father. She relayed an incident in which her young son responded to her, and discussed how breastfeeding was more than just physically providing nutrition. Breastfeeding provides many cherished intimate moments for a mother and her infant. While these moments are often asymmetrically reciprocal, they nonetheless facilitate the development of authentic solicitude. It is this mode of solicitude that cements the relationship between them.

> *Not that long ago I was sitting on the couch there feeding him and my girlfriend was sitting in here, and my son was feeding then he stopped and he was looking up at me and I was just looking at him and he went like this with his hand to my face and just touched me. My friend said 'Oh look at that that's so neat'. It was just a neat feeling, like a real bond. It's a special moment; the only way I can really explain it was through that moment. It's like the way he just looks up at you and gives a smile and touches your face like that, it's really neat.... Breastmilk is the best thing for the baby but it's also something else as well, not just feeding the baby, it's a bond.... Sometimes I look at my son and I think 'I haven't only just given birth to him, but I'm making him into who he is now. You're giving him the best possible start to life.... Sometimes you feel so much love for him when you're feeding him.... Sometimes it makes you really happy. Sometimes you get tears in your eyes; it's happiness, not sadness. One day he's going to grow too big for this (laugh).*
>
> *It's a special time while I'm breastfeeding my son. And at night before he goes to bed he knows, he sometimes looks at you and grins from ear to ear. It's for me only. No one else can share in that, which may sound a bit selfish, but I carried him for nine months, I gave birth to him, I've looked after him and no one has helped me right from day one. Right from the*

> *day I was pregnant I've had no help. So the way I see it I deserve that (laugh).* (Kay).

Women come to understand other, as well as themselves, through breastfeeding. They also come to experience authentic care in different ways because of their experience of breastfeeding.

DISCUSSION

Breastfeeding does not occur in a vacuum; it must, by necessity, involve at least two people, typically a mother and her baby. Breastfeeding is a relationship. The participants in this study discussed how a part of forging a breastfeeding relationship was learning how to respond to their infant's cues and behaviours, facilitating a positive reaction from their infants. These initial interactions provided the basis for the establishment of their breastfeeding relationship. This is particularly evident during the initial postnatal period when women dwell closely with their infants. A newborn consumes so much of a woman's time, and the focus of her thought and attention is directed accordingly. This 'being-with' an infant enables women to be concerned with, and focused on, their infant. Being-with means that the two come to know each other, defining a dynamic relationship between mother and child, which is essential if breastfeeding is to continue.

During the initial breastfeeding period, women were typically concerned with the technical function of breastfeeding; however, those women who were able to persevere with breastfeeding came to know breastfeeding as comfort for their infants. They described this comfort as 'all encompassing', illustrating the potential power of the breastfeeding act, especially in a society that values settled infants (see Beasley and Heritage; Beasley; McBride 1999). As women breastfeed over time, it becomes less about the technical act or function of breastfeeding, and increasingly about the relationship between themselves and their infants. Ultimately, the physical act of breastfeeding becomes transparent, as women came to know and understand breastfeeding as relationship.

The women in this study described how they experienced a closeness with their infants as a result of breastfeeding them. It was a closeness born from mutual physical dependence on each other—the mother for the physical comfort of releasing milk, and the infant to have their hunger satisfied. Breastfeeding closeness came from spending significant amounts of time together, which facilitated coming to know in an intimate manner. This feeling in turn strengthened the relationship between them, and the women in this study believed that the work of breastfeeding assisted in forging a relationship whose closeness extended beyond the duration of the breastfeeding period. This relationship had a transforming effect on these women. Through breastfeeding, they developed embodied knowledge that increased their confidence in their ability to mother, and experienced relational closeness in a unique way.

CONCLUSION

The women who participated in this study highlighted how they felt called to care for their infants through breastfeeding. Sometimes they struggled to respond to that call because of the difficulties they experienced whilst breastfeeding; however, for those who continued to breastfeed their children, they came to understand breastfeeding as comfort for their infants. In addition, as they dwelt with their infants through breastfeeding they experienced relational closeness, which was unique to the breastfeeding dyad and as a result highly prized.

There is a caveat to our concluding remarks about Heidegger's notion of care as a basic human way of being in the world. It may be inferred from the foregoing discussion that a mode of authentic solicitude as a relation of care is an end point for the mother-infant breastfeeding dyad. Certainly, such an interpretation can be gleaned from the narratives of the women in this study for whom being called to care by their infants is expressed as an achievement or accomplishment. However, it should be noted that Heidegger's notion of care is ontological, so we are not meant to draw moral conclusions from it (see Dreyfus; Paley). Not all women achieve the kind of solicitude we have described in this chapter when attempting to breastfeed their infants, but this does not mean that solicitude is absent from other aspects of the mother-infant relationship. Women who do not achieve or aspire to this kind of solicitude do not lack concern for the welfare of their infants; rather indifference to breastfeeding one's infant must be seen as situational and context dependent. To be absorbed and involved in an activity (such as breastfeeding), one needs to feel thoroughly at home in the world, and at home in and with one's body as it is lived and as others see it. In lieu of this homelike quality, or effortless dwelling, it is impracticable to think of giving breastmilk as being-with one's infant.

[1]Ethical approval for the study was gained through Massey University Human Ethics Committee (Ref. 99/086: 16/12/99).
[2]According to Inwood, "factical, facticity; similar to factual, factuality except that they are applied only to dasein, e.g., the sheer fact that one exists" (1997: 124).
[3]In this context, solicitude is an attempt to translate the German word *fursorge*, defined by the translators of Heidegger's work, Macquarrie and Robinson, as "the kind of care which we find in 'prenatal care' or 'taking care of the children" (157).

REFERENCES

Arora, Samir, Cheryl McJunkin, Julie Wehrer, and Phyllis Kuhn. "Major Factors Influencing Breastfeeding Rates: Mother's Perception of Father's Attitude and Milk Supply." *Pediatrics* 106.5 (2000): 67e-72.

Beasley, Annette. "*Call for action on breastfeeding promotion.*" *Public Health Association.* 2002. Accessed March 1, 2004 <http:///www.pha.org.nz/phadocs/breastfeedingjuly2002.doc>.

Beasley, Annette, Nora Chick, Marion Pybus, Janet Weber, Duncan Mackenzie and Denise Dignam. "'I Was Scared I Had Run Out of Milk!': Breastfeeding and the Perception of Insufficient Milk Among Manawatu Mothers." *Breastfeeding in New Zealand: Practice, Problems and Policy.* Ed. Annette Beasley and Andrew Trlin. Palmerston North, New Zealand: The Dunmore Press, 1998. 57-74.

Beasley, Annette, and Ann Heritage. "Breastfeeding is a Cultural Practice." *Breastfeeding Communiqué* 9 (1998/1999): 15-17.

Benner, Patricia. *Interpretive Phenomenology: Embodiment, Caring, and Ethics in Health and Illness.* London: Sage Publications, 1994.

Britton, Catherine. "'Letting it Go, Letting It Flow': Women's Experiential Accounts of the Let Down Reflex." *Social Sciences in Health* 3.3 (1997): 176-187.

Dahlberg, Karen, Nancy Drew, and Maria Nystrom. *Reflective Lifeworld Research.* Sweden: Studentlitteratur, 2001.

Dreyfus, Hubert. *Being-in-the-World: A Commentary of Heidegger's Being and Time.* New Baskerville: The Massachusetts Institute of Technology Press, 1991.

Earle, Sarah. "Factors Affecting the Initiation of Breastfeeding: Implications for Breastfeeding Promotion." *Health Promotion International* 17 (2002): 205-214.

Gadamer, Hans. *Truth and Method.* 2nd revised ed. Trans. J. Weinsheimer and D. Marshall. New York: The Continuum Publishing Company, 1989 (Original work published 1960).

Gadamer, Hans. *The Enigma of Health.* Trans. J. Gaiger and N. Walker. Stanford: Stanford University Press, 1996. (Original work published 1993).

Hauck, Yvonne, Diana Langton, and Karen Coyle. "The Path of Determination: Exploring the Lived Experience of Breastfeeding Difficulties." *Breastfeeding Review* 10.2 (2002): 50-62.

Heath, Anne-Louise, Cynthia Reeves Tuttle, Megan Simons, Christine Cleghorn and Winsome Parnell. "A Longitudinal Study of Breastfeeding and Weaning Practices During the First Year of Life in Dunedin, New Zealand." *Journal of the American Dietetic Association* 102 (2002): 937-943.

Heidegger, Martin. *Being and Time.* 7th ed. Trans. John Macquarrie and Edward Robinson. Oxford: Blackwell Publishers, 1962 (Original work published 1927).

Hill, Pamela, Sharron Humenick and B. West. "Concerns of Breastfeeding Mothers: The First Six Weeks Postpartum." *Journal of Perinatal Education* 3.4 (1994): 47-58.

Inwood, Michael. *Heidegger.* New York: Oxford University Press, 1997.

Inwood, Michael. *A Heidegger Dictionary.* Oxford: Blackwell, 1999.

Ironside, Pamela. *Preserving, Reading, Writing, Thinking and Dialogue: Rethinking Doctoral Education in Nursing.* Unpublished doctoral dissertation, University of Wisconsin, Madison, 1997.

McBride, Karen. "Breastfeeding Women's Perceptions of the Importance of Infant Care Routines." Unpublished master of nursing dissertation, Massey University, Albany, New Zealand, 1999.

McBride-Henry, Karen. *Responding to the Call to Care: New Zealand Women's Experience of Breastfeeding.* Unpublished doctoral dissertation, Massey University, Wellington, New Zealand, 2004.

Merleau-Ponty, Maurice. *Phenomenology of Perception.* Trans. Colin Smith. London: Routledge and Kegan Paul, 1981 (Original work published 1945).

Mozingo, Johnie, Mitzi Davis, Patricia Droppleman, and Amy Merideth. "It Wasn't Working": Women's Experiences with Short-term Breastfeeding. *MCN: Maternal Child Nursing* 25.3 (2000): 120-126.

Paley, John. "Heidegger and the Ethics of Care." *Nursing Philosophy* 1 (2000): 64-75.

Tarkka, Marja-Terttu, Marita Paunonen, and Paunonen Laippala. "What Contributes to Breastfeeding Success After Childbirth in a Maternity Ward in Finland?" *Birth* 25.3 (1998): 175-181.

Vogel, Alison, and Edwin Mitchell. "The establishment and duration of breastfeeding. Part one: Hospital influences." *Breastfeeding Review,* 6 (1998a): 5-9.

World Health Organisation (WHO). *Infant and Young Child Nutrition: Global Strategy on Infant and Young Child Nutrition.* Geneva: World Health Organisation, 2002.

Breastfeeding Envy

Unresolved Patriarchal Envy and the Obstruction of Physiologically-Based Nursing Patterns

KEREN EPSTEIN-GILBOA

THIS CHAPTER IS BASED on my training and experience as a psychotherapist and researcher in the field of psychology in urban Canada. I draw on object relations theory to investigate the contradictory responses of envy and obstruction of nursing patterns. I use the term 'nursing' in preference to 'breastfeeding' throughout the chapter because these two terms are not synonymous. In my view, referring to nursing as breast*feeding* erases the special physiological and emotional aspects of nursing and reinforces the association of nursing with the apparent nutritional value of breastmilk. Similar to meaning associated with the profession of the same name, nursing implies that one engages in empathetic care giving, and does not merely feed a child.

As the editors state in the Introduction to this volume, language is crucial to understandings and practices of giving breastmilk. My own research bears this out. In a study on family interaction, for instance, I observed that some fathers seem to adore breastfeeding yet, at the same time interfere with physiological nursing patterns and associated behaviours (Epstein-Gilboa *Interaction, Systemic)*. When analysing the data I wondered if unresolved envy contributed to this paradoxical pattern of simultaneous apparent love for nursing on the one hand and interference on the other.

Certainly, respect for breastfeeding is exemplified by proclamations made by health care systems lauding breastfeeding and recommending periods of exclusivity followed by breastfeeding into early childhood (WHO *International, Expert, Global*). At the same time, disdain for nursing is demonstrated by views of artificial feeding as the norm generated by medical systems and by the aggressive marketing tactics of medically-aligned artificial baby milk companies (Baumslag and Michels; Infant Feeding Action Coalition; Minchin; Palmer, *Politics*; Van Esterik). As statistics demonstrate, rates of breastfeeding exclusivity and duration veer from recommended patterns, which tend to suggest that systemic ambivalence seems to impede nursing behaviours (Australian Medical Association; CDC; Kellymom; Toronto Public Health). The similarity between this ambivalence, negative consequences for breastfeeding and envious processes at the family level prompted me to use psychological tools to examine this issue further by looking at concurring behaviours, recurring patterns and salient themes. Language, practices and narratives, including those of the historical past, provide optimal contexts for analysis.

OBJECT RELATIONS AND UNRESOLVED ENVY

The object relations model provides insights into human interaction and reviews conditions associated with simultaneous love and disdain. Humans or events are referred to as objects. One develops a worldview through interactions with objects. These perceptions contribute to behaviour (Greenberg; Klein, *Envy, Love*; Weininger). From this we understand that systemic ambiguity is likely to be influenced by feelings and interpretations, referred to as emotional processes.

The dissipation of stress is an emotional process relevant to this discussion. Terms such as attacking, destroying, obstructing, threatening and withholding are used to describe people, interactions, events or actions perceived as stressful or hurtful. Words such as tolerate and withstand are used to describe responses, and one may also use defence mechanisms to combat stress. Splitting, is a defence mechanism implying that one divides objects, including threats, into parts as a means of enhancing well being. Splitting disables one from seeing objects as whole with multiple perspectives. In summary, one might devalue a perceived threat.

Adored objects might sometimes be perceived as threats. The process associated with simultaneously loving and hating an object, and replacing respect with disgust is referred to as envy (Klein, *Envy, Love*; Weininger). The process begins with the realization that someone or something loved belongs to another and cannot be possessed. Feelings of loss may threaten well-being, resulting in splitting and reducing the value of the formerly respected object. Devaluing reduces tension by implying that the desired object is not worth envying. Disdain may lead to more anxiety and possible guilt. Emotional growth takes place when anxiety is conquered by replenishing loss and reducing guilt.

In contrast unresolved envy stifles interaction and growth. Continued anxiety may contribute to contempt for the unattainable object. This feeling may prompt the perception that hurtful actions have destroyed the object and so a sense of triumph may prevail over the envied object. However, the cyclical processes associated with unresolved envy, contempt, and triumph is complicated by additional guilt and loss, impeding resolution and relief.

Thus, it is possible to love and disdain the same object, a feeling associated with envy. That which is unresolved may lead to a series of negative consequences. Applying these unconscious processes to breastfeeding suggests that systemic social ambivalence about nursing may signify unresolved envy of breastfeeding objects, including the capacity to nurse, breastmilk, nursing infants and mothers, and the nursing relationship, which provides some insight into otherwise inexplicable contradictory messages.

AN HISTORICAL BASIS OF PATRIARCHAL ENVY AND THE OBSTRUCTION OF NURSING

A first step to understanding the simultaneous adoration and contempt for nursing associated with envy is to look at the origins of this behaviour. A review of descriptions of nursing patterns over time demonstrates that patriarchal leaders simultaneously lauded and obstructed nursing. Obstructions included interfering with the exclusivity and duration of nursing, wet-nursing and artificial feeding (Dettwyler "A Time"; Fildes; Minchin; Palmer *Politics*; Stuart-Macadam; Thurer). Interrupting exclusivity and duration implies that breastmilk and nursing are not good enough for the infant, and that women's other tasks are more important than nursing. Wet-nursing devalues nursing by fragmenting it into part objects. The breastfeeding product—breastmilk—is retained while acts of creating and ejecting breastmilk and remaining close to an infant through nursing are removed. Artificial feeding destroys all parts of nursing. These obstructive processes are contemptuous, and reduce the worth of the envied object, enabling triumph over nursing.

Next we try to understand the reasons that nursing was envied. Reports showing that nursing was obstructed most in patriarchal societies where male leaders established attitudes and practices that obstructed adored nursing (Fildes; Thurer) indicate that men, unable to nurse, envied unattainable nursing objects. This proposition is supported by theories that males envy female physiology that presumably renders women more powerful than men. Consequently, males dread women and strive to control them out of resentment and to ensure self-preservation. Male dominance is asserted by implying that males are normal and that females are the 'other' and thus, less valuable (Horney). Descriptions of maternal despondency (Blaffer Hrdy), and disgust with nursing and wet-nursing, and practices of hiring wet nurses from a lower status than mothers (Golden; Shahar; Wolf, "Mercenary," *Don't*) suggest that females also envied and belittled those who nursed when they couldn't. This view is backed by theories that women internalize male perceptions of females (De Beauvoir; Ehrenreich and English; Miedema, Stoppard and Anderson).

The likelihood that men used dominance to destroy envied female physiology is validated by a comparison of historical patterns of normal versus interrupted nursing. We note that uninterrupted maternal nursing took place in cultures where males and females owned property, and thus were considered equals. In Puritan communities, for example, nursing mothers were respected but were nevertheless seen as subordinate to their husbands and weaned early. Maternal nursing was fully interrupted and replaced by wet-nursing in aristocratic families in medieval Europe where women were considered mere male property (Fildes; Minchin; Palmer, *Politics*; Thurer). These examples verify the connection between male domination and obstructed nursing, and also indicate that the more power that men had over women, the easier it was to fragment envied nursing processes.

Women's status in comparison to other females also seemed to affect the level of obstruction. Those with the least power suffered from the most contemptuous behaviours. For example, wet nurses lived with aristocratic families of high status enabling mothers and children to have contact with one another. In comparison, children of lower status were wet nursed far away from their mothers (Golden; Ozment; Shahar; Thurer). Even though medieval aristocratic women were separated from their children during wet-nursing, their heirs received human milk and eventually rejoined their mothers. In contrast, destitute women gave up their scorned illegitimate offspring who were fed artificial milk, often culminating in their premature deaths while some of their mothers nursed the children of families of greater status (Riordan and Auerbach).

The experience of destitute mothers and offspring demonstrates the pain and devastation that vulnerable objects suffered when their natural processes were obstructed. There are other examples in the literature suggesting that obstructed nursing often concurred with additional contemptuous and painful actions. For example, infanticide and child prostitution took place in ancient Greek and Roman societies that obstructed nursing and openly scorned women, children and wet nurses (Shahar; Thurer).

The illness that women suffered when they lost the contraceptive protection associated with nursing (Blaffer Hrdy) is another example of how obstructed nursing caused pain. In this case men triumphed over females by essentially impelling women to engage in self-destruction through the abuse of their unique capacities to conceive, carry, and birth. Sickness and pregnancy likely contributed to the long-standing themes of female frailty that fortified themes of female devaluation and obstructive processes (Ehrenreich and English). Thus, men coped with their inability to birth and lactate by forcing women into a reduced status, breaking the magical and unattainable female physiological process, and by rendering the perceived powerful female weak and ill.

Views of females as weak, and men as rulers, were fortified by the attitude that the marital couple relationship preceded over the mother-child relationship. For many centuries this perspective obstructed nursing when it was combined with the myth that sexual relations tainted breastmilk (Golden; Palmer *Politics).* In the early twentieth century children were dismissed from the maternal breast when couple precedence was paired with conceptualizations of romantic love, and that breasts were male-owned sexual objects (Blum; Giles; Wolf *Don't*).

Maternal behaviours might have been a function of the conditions imposed on women, a suggestion that is congruent with theories that women may internalize male perceptions of females and exhibit them in their behaviours (De Beauvoir; Ehrenreich and English; Miedema, Stoppard, and Anderson). However, it also seems many women's actions over the ages reflected their own agendas. For example, some mothers in colonial America apparently promoted wet nursing, implying that it contributed to their well being (Benson Brown and McPherson; Golden). Mothers who suffered social costs and nursed against the grain (Benson Brown and McPherson) personify female agency. Although some women engaged in wet nursing for reasons beyond their control, this profession nevertheless required initiative in many cases and enabled some to reap economic and social benefits (Blaffer Hrdy). Agency is also most certainly demonstrated by the mothers who founded the La Leche League and by women who joined together and helped usher breastfeeding back into the lives of women and children in the later part of the twentieth century (Blum).

The initiative and strength of these women is most obvious when one notes the conditions of contempt which they faced. Contempt for nursing in the twentieth century was actualized with the help of themes of reverence for science, measurement, self-control, scheduling and distancing and reliance on expert advice versus womanly wisdom. This established physicians as the new patriarchs, women as vulnerable, and artificial feeding as the norm (Blum; Carter; Golden; Minchin; Palmer, *Politics*; Saha; Thurer; Wolf, "Mercenary," *Don't*). Physicians reinforced views of women as vulnerable through patronizing care giving behaviours (Silverman). Medical practitioners increasingly used novel and male exclusive birthing tools, replacing female healers and augmenting their control over female physiology (Cassidy; Ehrenreich and English). These controlling and debasing actions not only facilitated the destruction of maternal nursing but also the preceding birth process, which became a medical event controlled by male physicians (Arms; Harper). Thus, it seems that the destruction of nursing was part of a continuum of contempt towards females. These themes remained strong when nursing was reinstated by patriarchs who pretended to join the ranks of women demanding control of their own physiology in the 1970s (Carter; Eyer, *Mother-Infant Bonding*; Maher; Saha; Wolf, *Don't*).

In summary, historical narratives demonstrate themes indicating that unresolved patriarchal envy was probably an important variable contributing to simultaneous praise for and interference in breastfeeding. Obstructions included a break in the normal female physiology continuum and early weaning, wet nursing and artificial feeding. Concurring behaviours suggest that devalued female status and contemptuous acts facilitate obstructions.

PRESENT CONTEXT

Knowledge about themes in the past may facilitate analysis of patterns in the present. At this stage of the investigation I also refer to my own experiences of talking with women in the urban western world coping with an ambivalent patriarchal context.

ADORATION OF NURSING

Widespread patriarchal love for nursing is suggested by increasing research, novel organizations, policy statements and articles all about nursing. Medical systems proclaim their adoration for nursing by stating that it is a superior form of infant feeding (WHO, *International*). Journals, including the *Journal of Human Lactation* and *Breastfeeding Medicine*, medically-aligned professions such as lactation consultants, and professional organizations including the International Lactation Consultant Organization dedicated specifically to nursing, reinforce medical ownership of the idealized breastfeeding object. A significant measure of the idealization of nursing is the reiteration of this message in advertisements for artificial baby milk (Abbott Nutrition, Mead Johnson; Nestle). Common cultural adoration of nursing as ideal is evident in the abundant articles on breastfeeding in parenting magazines and online sources and increased breastfeeding initiation (CDC; Kellymom).

DISDAIN AND TRIUMPH

However, like in earlier times, the same society that declares its love for nursing also interferes with breastfeeding, pointing to underlying envy. Disdain is evident in practices contributing to the low rates of nursing exclusivity and duration that diverge from scientific recommendations (CDC; Kellymom). The belittling message is that exclusive nursing is not enough to sustain infants and that nursing is worthless beyond infancy.

The modern wet nurse—the breast pump—is another means of obstructing nursing. Although pumping has important functions, and some of these are canvassed by the women in Cindy Stearns' study in this volume, there are also associated risks and social consequences of using this mechanical tool. Pumping fragments nursing into less valuable part objects, thereby separating nursing, the mother and infant, and the nursing relationship from breastmilk. Milk, instead of nursing, becomes the focus, leaving the adored substance available for control and measurement by the dominant medical system. Focus on milk disembodies mothers (Blum) and obliterates maternal processes of intimacy, repair, and sensitivity associated with direct nursing (Epstein-Gilboa, *Systematic*). The unique nursing relationship is destroyed, displacing the mother and rendering the infant available for open and unspecific ownership. Triumph over nursing is suggested by the centrality of the pump in parental narratives (Epstein-Gilboa, *Systematic*), the increasing use of pumps and the proliferation and aggressive marketing tactics of companies that sell technological accessories for nursing (Heinig, "The Cost of Breastfeeding," "The 'Price' of Information"; Palmer "Give"). Today's mechanical wet nurse enables envious parties to actualize contempt by replacing the breastfeeding mother and feeding the adored breastmilk to an infant.

ENVIOUS PARTIES

The salient role that the medical system plays in the simultaneous expressions of adoration and disdain reinforces that this system is an important source of envy towards nursing. The centrality of men, and thus male envy, in this system—despite an increase in the number of female physicians—is suggested by the prominence of male terms of reference in medical discourse and by attempts to control traditionally female health care professions (Group and Roberts; Miedema, Stoppard and Anderson). Applying ecological terms (Bronfenbrenner) to this context indicates that the medical system is the patriarchal leader reflecting and influencing societal and individual views about breastfeeding practices. Views inherent to medical practice may be voiced at all levels of the system. This perspective verifies that medical systems ally with artificial milk companies, and that this alliance fortifies medical triumph by increasing the influence on cultural constructs of nursing (Minchin; Palmer *Politics*). Similarly, professionals are influenced by their individual experiences. In a culture plagued by obstructed nursing, it is likely that most professionals' personal experiences with nursing are deficient, causing envy during encounters with nursing objects. They subsequently disregard scientific evidence and hamper normal nursing patterns.

FEMALE SELF-DEBASEMENT

Supporting unattainable physiological-nursing patterns must be especially difficult for females who perceive that they deviate from this trajectory. Like their foremothers, women feel loss and envy when they are unable to nurse, have disappointing nursing experiences, or wean earlier than expected (Angier; Benson Brown and McPherson; Guttman and Zimmerman). Female envy might also reflect women's identification with patriarchal views of women. For example, descriptions of breastfeeding advocates as bullies and 'breastfeeding police' in lay female culture (e.g. Stanley) and even in feminist literature (Eyer *Motherguilt,* 72) mirror cultural vilification of nursing women or those who advocate for nursing (Minchin).

Female identification with patriarchal views is evident in feminist attempts to dismantle paradigms emphasizing biology and gender in order to promote apparent equality (Eyer, *Mother-Infant Bonding*; Firestone). Feminist models that maximize female physiology also mirror male perspectives when breastfeeding is ignored under the assumption that nursing impedes employment (Blum; Carter; Guttman and Zimmerman; Maher). Yet, using employment as a value not only reflects male terms of reference but also advances disdain for women who work at home, including mothers. Self-disdain is also demonstrated by conflicts between diverse female-oriented organizations, such as childbirth educators who ignore breastfeeding, and lactation advocates who ignore birthing issues. This is essentially a form of female fragmentation that likely provides contemptuous males with another means of sensing triumph over women. Identification with patriarchal values and the desire to succeed in a male dominated system explains why female health care providers mirror male attitudes, and contribute to perpetual disregard for the female continuum in the health care system. Hence, evidence suggests that females may join male contempt for nursing due to loss and identification with patriarchal views.

THEMES, ATTITUDES AND MYTHS UPHOLDING PATRIARCHAL ENVY OF NURSING

FRAGMENTED BREASTS

Like in the past, several themes help envious parties uphold and express their contempt for envied nursing objects. One theme is that breasts are sexual objects owned by males (Dettywler "Beauty"), and disfigured by nursing (Saha). Male contempt is demonstrated by impelling women to nurse discreetly (Bartlett; Stearns) and by punishing women who defy this rule (Benson Brown and McPherson; Maher; Saha). Alison Bartlett suggests that discreet nursing disables women from speaking proudly about nursing. In terms of envy, silencing is an attempt to reduce frustration by decreasing exposure to a desired but unattainable experience.

Discreet nursing is also essential to the contrasting theme that breasts are medically- owned objects that provide an optimal and scientific form of infant feeding, devoid of sexuality and sensuality, and female emotional connotations other than explicitly motherly thoughts (Giles; Maher; Saha). Sexless nursing apparel and the use of childish names for nursing breasts advance this view (Bartlett; Giles). Triumph is actualized through maternal disembodiment (Blum), increasing views of breasts as exclusively milk-producing and facilitating fragmentation through pumping. This view also enables contemptuous parties to punish nursing women who disclose sexual sensations, unrelated to the child, during nursing (Bartlett; Davidowitz; Maher; Saha).

Both views are contemptuous and devalue breasts by denying that they are multifunctional (Angier; Bartlett; Saha). Views of breasts as multi-faceted enable mothers to make distinct cognitive attributions about similar physical sensations associated with the secretion of oxytocin during sexual arousal and nursing (Bartlett; Saha). Data showing that parents in families nursing in tune with physiology openly acknowledge the multiple roles of the maternal breast, suggest that this mode of thinking facilitates nursing (Epstein-Gilboa *Systematic*). Nursing mothers are members of a culture that perceives breasts as sexual, and are likely to be part of couples' relationships prior to and regardless of parenting. Acknowledgement of the multiplicity of breast function might enable mothers to continue nursing when they do not have to let go of cherished aspects of their couple relationship, and when their physiologically- based sensations are normalized. This view concurs with perspectives of nursing as a whole and complex object, and contrasts perspectives of fragmentation associated envy and obstructed nursing patterns.

SCORNED FEMALE PHYSIOLOGY

Divided breasts are part of a continuum of contempt for all female physiology. The concept of a continuum of destruction of normal female processes is suggested by the rampant use of pills to prevent pregnancy, treatments to create pregnancy, psychological pressure and deception used to persuade women to donate eggs, intrusive tests during pregnancy, medically-controlled births, obstructed nursing patterns, and interference in menopause. The danger of fragmentation for women, and the likely triumph for envious parties, is illustrated by the contribution of medicated and technical interventions during birth to the alarming increase in the rate of caesarean operations (Block; Cassidy; Harper; Rabuzzi). Patriarchy's efforts to hold on to fragmenting processes is exemplified by a program claiming to improve birth outcomes by reducing hierarchy, but that actually focuses on enhancing the technical skills of medical practitioners (Society of Obstetricians and Gynaecologists of Canada). Instead of questioning the overuse of medical interventions, this program advances their use. The triumph associated with this program is especially obvious when one remembers that in the past male-owned instruments successfully enabled men to banish female midwives and women-focused birth (Ehrenreich and English).

Like in earlier times, adjunct themes and myths enable patriarchy to continue to control women. Historically, envy-powered obstruction was facilitated by demoted female status, and women of the lowest status suffered the most. Findings that women of low socio-economic status have the lowest rates of breastfeeding initiation (CDC) point to the resilience of old patterns. Medical terminology including the terms 'management' of pregnancy, labour and breastfeeding and the 'delivery' of babies implies that themes of female weakness and patriarchal control through patronizing care giving still reign. In addition, women might be enabling physiological deconstruction due to mirrored patriarchal attitudes about females. However, the degree of patriarchal power and harm that women suffer seems disproportionate to the positions females hold outside of the medical system. Hence, one cannot help but ask what causes women to accept their inferior position and the destruction of their physiology?

PATRONIZING CARING, TRICKERY AND LANGUAGE

An answer to this quandary is that patriarchy reflects past patterns and uses themes to hide envy and contempt. The relevance of this practice in present context is suggested by the assumption that physicians know that babies are not pizzas delivered to mothers, and that mothers are actually strong and able to carry, birth, and nurse babies without patriarchal managers. Male acknowledgement and fear of female power was discussed earlier in this paper and indicates that males may appease seemingly powerful women in order to control them. Appeasement is illustrated by the creation of 'Gingerbread Houses' in medical institutions that, like in the famed child's fable, use tempting treats in the form of attractive programs and enticing language to attract and hold on to clients (Epstein-Gilboa, "Gingerbread").

The deceitful use of language to abuse clients is illustrated by the use of the word 'choice'. The overuse of this word shows how patriarchy takes ownership of a client-centered and feminist term to mislead clients. The concept of choice means that one is in control of one's health and able to make decisions. However, this term is rarely offered together with real options or information. In terms of breastfeeding, choice means that nursing and artificial feeding are two interchangeable feeding choices. The term 'food', as stated at the beginning of this chapter, erases the special physiological and emotional aspects of nursing and enriches patriarchal control through the measurement of the apparent nutritional value of breastmilk. Concepts of feeding in conjunction with the term 'extended nursing' reinforces that feeding beyond a certain date is too long. A study demonstrating an association between the use of food-related terms and decreased capacity to read cues for nursing illustrates the harmful effects of this term (Epstein-Gilboa, *Systematic*).

Erroneous conceptualizations of breastfeeding also hide obstructive aims. For example, posing nursing as a superlative interferes with women's desire to be normal, hindering nursing (Wiessinger). Nursing as best is often accompanied by intricate descriptions about nursing hardships (example, Babytalk). These terms often coincide with practices of withholding information, especially about the risks of not nursing, under the guise of protecting women from guilt (Epstein-Gilboa, "Enhancing," "Psychological," *Systematic*; Newman; Walker). The guilt myth is based on themes of female weakness and patronizing care giving, and reinforces patriarchal envy and dread of the strong female.

Themes of reverence for distancing, separation, individuality and apparent independence (Bassi Zaff; McKenna; Valsiner) contradict feminist themes of connection (Gilligan) that are inherent to patterns of proximity inclusive of carrying and holding and co-sleeping associated with nursing (Ball; Epstein-Gilboa, *Systematic*; Liedloff; McKenna; Small; Valsiner). The destructive effects of normalizing separation in nursing is exemplified by the detached care of premature infants provided with pumped, or worse, artificial milk, by strangers or inanimate objects in comparison to proximity themes promoting twenty-four hour kangaroo care and direct nursing. Reverence for distancing is also evident in the term extended nursing, implying pathology.

Like in earlier times, marital closeness is encouraged instead of mother-child proximity and facilitates the obstruction of nursing. Maternal-child closeness is posed as a force negating the holy couple union, especially at night when romantic love presides (Maher; McKenna; Palmer, *Politics*; Small; Thurer; Valsiner). Melanie Klein's (*Love*) advice, that parent-child co-sleeping exposes children to sexuality, exemplifies a salient false belief that separates mothers from children.

Themes of separation, autonomy, and individualism with an emphasis on self-enhancement may also be used to interfere with the mother's ability to nurse. Myths that nursing is binding, interferes with schedules, personal freedom and employment impair mother's ability to nurse (Blaffer Hrdy; Blum; Guttman and Zimmerman; Libbus, Bush, and Hockman; Lindberg). Research demonstrates that new nursing mothers want to constantly be close to their infants. This newfound longing challenges their culturally-based conceptualizations, initially causing internal turmoil. However, the experience of physiological nursing seems to enable mothers to integrate new scripts of self that disregard cultural themes, suggesting that the process of nursing helps mothers let go of concepts of self as the 'other' (Epstein-Gilboa *Systematic*). The change that nursing induces for mothers likely frustrates envious parties and explains why myths impairing nursing are constantly repeated.

Additional themes reiterated by patriarchy and that hamper nursing are those that discredit the unique tasks associated with nursing. The message that all parenting tasks should be shared (Cowan and Cowan; Goodrich, Rampage, Ellman and Halstead) reflects feminist efforts to instill equality through sameness. However, sameness task allocation essentially provides patriarchy, under the facade of apparent respect for women, with another means of belittling and destroying the unique nursing relationship. In comparison, a study of nursing families demonstrates an association between physiological nursing, equality in the couple relationship and a system of gender-based task allocation (Epstein-Gilboa *Systematic*). This finding is not surprising in light of contrasting historical themes of reduced status and obstruction.

A significant negative repercussion of sameness paradigms in conjunction with myths of nursing as a feeding choice is that fathers should feed nursing infants. This concept enables men to actualize envious fantasies and to take over the envied object. Paternal feeding is justified by attitudes that it balances homeostasis in the couple relationship (Cowan and Cowan). The contempt inherent to this myth is that nursing can be easily replicated. The harmful effects of the myth are illustrated by psychological decrees enabling divorced fathers to separate nursing children from motherly breasts for lengthy periods of time (Lamb and Kelly). This act enables vengeful envious objects to punish both mother and child for their exclusion from their envied nursing relationship.

PATERNAL ENVY

Of course the question that begs answering is whether paternal feeding actually resolves fathers' envy. According to findings on breastfeeding families that I undertook, it does not (Epstein-Gilboa *Systematic*). This study implies instead that paternal desire to feed or to give children pacifiers is a sign of unresolved envy, reverence for cultural themes of individualism, and also signals discord between parents. The study also found that most fathers do indeed envy all, or at least parts, of the nursing relationship. Most frequently they envy the closeness between the nursing mother and child. Paternal acknowledgement of envy and ongoing validation for their feelings through open discourse contributes to the resolution of envy. In cases of compromised communication, repair is facilitated through the use of compensatory measures at the couple level, such as sexual intimacy. In addition, paternal anxiety is reduced when fathers emulate the tactile and cue-reading aspects of nursing. The likelihood that these measures resolve envy or at least make associated feelings tolerable is suggested by paternal promotion of nursing, unhampered physiologically-based nursing patterns inclusive of proximity behaviours and child-paced weaning in early childhood, and signs that fathers mirror the development of sensitive parenting styles associated with nursing. Paternal envy is therefore normal and resolvable under optimal conditions. Resolved envy supports physiological nursing patterns.

CONCLUSIONS

Unresolved envy of nursing is a salient factor with deep historical roots leading to the obstruction of physiologically-based nursing patterns. Men, as well as women, unable to experience nursing simultaneously express admiration and disdain for nursing objects. Fragmenting nursing objects enables envious parties to belittle breastfeeding and to experience contempt and triumph. Contempt for nursing is part of a continuum of contempt for female physiology.

Several themes enable the obstruction of nursing and have important implications. The association between demoted female status and obstructed nursing implies that present divergent nursing patterns signify low female status in western culture. The propensity of female ownership of obstructive processes verifies demoted female status and points to mirroring of male views of self as other, which cause women to deny that their own physiology is normal and desired. Male control over female physiology is enhanced by condescending practices, the facade of joining women through the use of language, and the proliferation of male concepts. Continued male control and centrality in female processes imply that men have not resolved their envy of female physiology. Resolved envy at the micro level suggest that repair is desirable considering that it coincides with uninterrupted nursing and the development of sensitive parenting styles, essential for normal development.

A significant illustration of maternal agency within a context of overwhelming unresolved patriarchal envy is the capacity to nurse against the grain. It is important to remember that women initiated the return to nursing, and caused a rise in initiation rates all over the world in contexts where nursing had been displaced. Women have certainly altered male and female views of nursing through their behaviours and by educating others. However, while nursing, educating and advocating for normal physiology seems to have always taken place it continues to concur with intense expressions of contempt.

Reparative processes at the micro level demonstrate that the resolution of envy includes acknowledging the pain associated with the loss of the nursing object. Like in the micro family, anxiety might be reduced at the macro level through systems promoting open, and most importantly, genuine discourse. Repair might also be facilitated by advancing means of emulating aspects of nursing that do not interfere with normal nursing patterns. For example, the cue-reading aspects of nursing may be integrated into others' interactions with children. The resolution of envy from the male perspective indicates that men will be able to more accurately see their own qualities as unique and let go of needs for dominance and destruction. This implies that women's way of healing based on intuition will return and the use of medical intervention using male-owned medical tools will disappear. Nursing and other female physiological processes will no longer be considered medical events. Most importantly, women will proudly own their processes and nurse in tune with their physiology.

REFERENCES

Abbott Nutrition. *Breastfeeding Your Baby* Booklet. 24 Nov. 2007 <http://abbottnutrition.com/resources/en-US/home/breastfeeding/BF%20Booklet.pdf>.

Angier, Natalie. *Woman: An Intimate Geography*. New York: Anchor Books, 2000.

Arms, Suzanne. *Immaculate Deception II: A Fresh Look at Childbirth.* Berkeley, California: Celestial Arts, 1994.

Australian Medical Association (AMA). AMA Position Statement on Breastfeeding, 1998. 2001. Revised 2007. 22 Sept. 2009 <http://www.ama.com.au/node/4355>.

Babytalk [online] 2008. 13 Feb. 2008 <http://www.parenting.com/article/Mom/Feeding/Yes,-you-can-use-breast-and-bottle!-21391690>.

Ball, Helen Louise. "Reasons to Bed-Share. Why Parents Sleep With Their Infants." *Journal of Reproductive and Infant Psychology* 20.4 (2002): 207-221.

Bartlett, Alison. "Thinking Through Breasts: Writing Maternity." *Feminist Theory* 1.2 (2000): 173-88.

Bassi Zaff, Laura. *Civilization and its Discontented Babies: How Growing Families International, "Babywise" and the Ezzos may be Making Psychological History.* 30 June 2000 <http://www.mamafed.com/ezzo3.html>.

Baumslag, Naomi and Dia L. Michels. *Milk, Money, and Madness: The Culture and Politics of Breastfeeding*. Westport Connecticut: Bergin & Garvey, 1998.

Becker, Dana. *The Myth of Empowerment: Women and Therapeutic Culture in America.* New York: New York UP, 2005.

Benson Brown, Amy and Katherine Read McPherson. *The Reality of Breastfeeding.* Westport Connecticut: Bergin & Garvey, 1998.

Blaffer Hrdy, Sara. *Mother Nature: Maternal Instincts and How They Shape The Human Species.* New York: Ballantine, 1999.

Block. Jennifer. *Pushed: The Painful Truth About Childbirth and Modern Maternity Care.* Cambridge: De Capo, 2007.

Blum, Linda. *At the Breast: Ideologies of Breastfeeding and Motherhood in the Contemporary United States.* Boston: Beacon Press, 1999.

Bronfenbrenner, Urie. *The Ecology of Human Development.* Cambridge: Harvard University Press, 1979.

Carter, Pam. *Feminism Breasts and Breast-feeding.* New York: St. Martins Press, 1995.

Cassidy, Tina. *Birth: A History*. London: Chatto and Windus, 2007.

Centers for Disease Control and Prevention (CDC). *Breastfeeding Practices: Results from the National Immunization Survey*. 13 Feb. 2008 from <http://www.cdc.gov/breastfeeding/data/NIS_data/data_2004.htm>.

Cowan, Carolyn Pape and Phillip A. Cowan. *When Parents Become Partners: The Big Life Change for Couples.* United States: Basic Books, 1992.

Davidowitz, Esther. "The breast-feeding taboo." *Redbook* (1992, June): 92-114.

De Beauvoir, Simone. *The Second Sex*. Trans. Howard Madison. Parshley 1953. New York: Vintage Books, 1989.

Dettwyler, Katherine Ann. "A Time to Wean: The Hominid Blueprint for the Natural Age of Weaning in Modern Human Populations." *Breastfeeding: Biocultural perspectives.* Ed. Patricia Stuart-Macadam and Katherine Ann Dettwyler. New York: Aldine De Gruyter, 1995.

Dettwyler, Katherine Ann. "Beauty and the Beast: The Cultural Context of Breastfeeding in the United States." *Breastfeeding: Biocultural Perspectives.* Ed. Patricia Stuart-Macadam and Katherine Ann Dettwyler. New York: Aldine De Gruyter, 1995. 167-216.

Ehrenreich, Barbara and Deirdre English. *For Her Own Good: Centuries of the Experts Advice to Women* (revised edition). New York: Anchor Books, 2005.

Epstein-Gilboa, Keren. *Interaction and Relationships in Breastfeeding Families: Implications for Practice.* Amarillo, Texas: Hale Publishing, 2009.

Epstein-Gilboa, Keren. *Systemic Interaction in Breastfeeding Families*. Unpublished Diss. University of Toronto, Canada, 2006.

Epstein-Gilboa, Keren. "Gingerbread House Theory." *The Journal of Perinatal Education* 12.2 (2003): v.

Epstein-Gilboa, Keren. "The Psychological Reality of Breastfeeding." *Infant Mental Health Project Print* 28 (2000): 18-21.

Epstein-Gilboa, Keren. "Enhancing Breastfeeding Education During the Prenatal Stage." *The Breastfeeding Network News* 12 (1997): 6.

Eyer, Diane. *Mother-Infant Bonding: A Scientific Myth.* New Haven: Yale University Press, 1992.

Eyer, Diane. *Motherguilt: How Our Culture Blames Mothers For What's Wrong With Society.* Toronto: Random House, 1996.

Fildes, Valerie. "The Culture and Biology of Breastfeeding." *Breastfeeding: Biocultural Perspectives.* Ed. Patricia Stuart-Macadam and Katherine Ann Dettwyler. New York: Aldine De Gruyter, 1995.

Firestone, Shulamit. *The Dialect of Sex: The Case for Feminist Revolution.* New York: Farrar, Straus & Giroux, 1970.

Giles, Fiona. *Fresh Milk: The Secret Life of the Breasts.* New York: Simon & Schuster, 2003.

Gilligan, Carol. *In a Different Voice: Psychological Theory and Women's Development.* Cambridge: Harvard University Press, 1998.

Golden, Janet. *A Social History of Wet Nursing in America: From Breast to Bottle.* Columbia: Ohio State University Press, 2001.

Goodrich, Thelma Jean, Cheryl Rampage, Barbara Ellman and Kris Halstead. *Feminist Family Therapy: A Casebook.* New York: Norton, 1988.

Greenberg, J. R. and S. A. Mitchell. *Objects Relations in Psychoanalytic Theory.* 12th printing. Cambridge: Harvard University Press, 2000.

Group, Thetis M. and Joan L. Roberts. *Nursing, Physician Control and the Medical Monopoly: Historical Perspectives on Gendered Inequality in Roles, Rights, and Range of Practice.* Bloomington: Indiana University Press, 2001.

Guttman, Nurit and Deena R. Zimmerman. "Low Income Mothers' View on Breastfeeding." *Social Science and Medicine,* 50.10 (2000):1457-1473.

Harper, Barbara. *Gentle Birth Choices.* Vermont: Healing Arts Press Inc., 2005.

Heinig, M. Jane. "The Cost of Breastfeeding Support: A Primer." *Journal of Human Lactation* 17.2 (2001): 101-102.

Heinig, M. Jane. "The 'Price' of Information." *Journal of Human Lactation,* 19.2 (2003): 133-135.

Horney, Karen. *Feminine Psychology.* New York: W. W. Norton & Company, 1967.

Infant Feeding Action Coalition. (1995, Winter). "Breastfeeding in a Bottle Feeding Culture." *INFACT Canada Newsletter* 3, 6.

Kellymom. "Breastfeeding: the Numbers. Breastfeeding Rates in the United States and Worldwide." 13 Feb. 2008 <http://www.kellymom.com/writings/bf-numbers.html#world>.

Klein, Melanie. *Envy and Gratitude and Other Works: 1946-1963.* London: Vintage, 1997.

Klein, Melanie. *Love Guilt and Reparation and other Works: 1921-1945.* London: Vintage, 1998.

Kroeger, Mary. "Restoring the Mother and Baby Continuum." *Genesis* (enewsletter of Lamaze International) 5 (2003).

Lamb, Michael E. and Joan B. Kelly. "Using Child Development Research to Make Appropriate Custody and Access Decisions for Young Children." *Family and Conciliation Courts Review,* 38.3 (2000): 306-7.

Libbus, Martha. Kay, Tamara A. Bush, and Nora Marie Hockman. "Breastfeeding Beliefs of Low-income of low-income primigravidae." *International Journal of Nursing Studies* 34.2 (1997): 144-150.

Liedloff, Jean. *The Continuum Concept: In Search of Lost Happiness.* Reading, Massachussetts: Addison-Wesley, 1985.

Lindberg, Laura Duberstein. "Women's Decisions About Breastfeeding and Maternal Employment." *Journal of Marriage and the Family* 58.1 (1996): 239-251.

Maher, Vanessa, ed. "Breastfeeding in Cross-Cultural Perspectives: Paradoxes and Proposals." *The Anthropology of Breastfeeding: Natural Law or Social Construct*. Oxford: Berg, 1995.

McKenna, James J. "Sudden Infant Death Syndrome in Cross Cultured Perspective: Is Infant Parent Co-sleeping Protective?" *Annual Review of Anthropology* 25 (1996): 201-216.

Mead Johnson Breastfeeding FAQS. [online] 2007. 23 Nov. 2007 <http://www.meadjohnson.ca/en/faq/faq_breastfeeding.html>.

Miedema, Baukje, Janet M Stoppard, and Vivienne Anderson (eds). *Women's Bodies Women's Lives: Health Well-Being and Body Image.* Toronto: Sumach Press, 2000.

Minchin, Maureen. *Breastfeeding Matters.* St. Kilda, Australia: Alma Publications, 1998.

Nestle. 24 Nov. 2007 <http://www.nestleusa.com/PubOurBrands/BrandDetails.aspx?lbid=C4485AF5-E366-4C77-BD12-7CC4D9D068B0>.

Newman, Jack. *Breastfeeding and Guilt.* [online] (2000). 8 Feb. 2008 <http://www.breastfeedingonline.com/guilt.html>.

Ozment, Steven. *When Fathers Ruled: Family Life in Reformation Europe.* Cambridge, Mass: Harvard University Press, 1983.

Palmer, Gabrielle. *The Politics of Breastfeeding.* London: Pandora, 1988.

Palmer, Gabrielle. "Give breastfeeding back to mothers." *Journal of Human Lactation*, 7.1 (1991): 1-2.

Parenting.com. 13 Feb. 2008 <http://www.parenting.com/article/Baby/Feeding/Breastfeeding-for-Beginners>.

Rabuzzi, Kathryn Allen. *Mother With Child: Transformations Through Childbirth.* Bloomington: Indiana University Press, 1994.

Riordan, Jan and Auerbach, Kathleen. *Breastfeeding and Human Lactation*. 2nd edition. Boston: Jones & Bartlett. 1999.

Saha, Prantik. "Breastfeeding and Sexuality: Professional Advice Literature from the 1970s to the Present." *Health Education & Behaviour* 29.1 (2002): 61-72.

Shahar, Shulamit. *Childhood in the Middle Ages.* London: Routledge, 1990.

Silverman, Doris K. "Mommy Nearest: Revisiting the Idea of Infantile Symbiosis and its Implications for Females." *Psychoanalytic Psychology* 20.2 (2003): 261-270.

Small, Meredith F. *Our Babies Ourselves: How Biology and Culture Shape the Way We Parent.* New York: Anchor Books, 1998.

Society of Obstetricians and Gynaecologists of Canada [online] (2008) 1 Feb. 2008 <http://www.sogc.org/more/index_e.asp>.

Stanley, Laura. *The Breastfeeding Police.* [online] 13 Feb. 2008 <http://www.parenting.com/article/Baby/Feeding/The-Breastfeeding-Police. on Feb. 13, 2008>.

Stearns, Cindy A. "Breastfeeding and the Good Maternal Body." *Gender & Society* 13.3 (1999): 308-325.

Stein, Martin T., Eyla G. Boise and David M. Snyder. "Parental Concerns

About Extended Breastfeeding in a Toddler." *Journal of Developmental and Behavioral Pediatrics* 23.6 (2002): 438-442.

Stuart-Macadam, Patricia. "Breastfeeding in Prehistory." *Breastfeeding: Biocultural Perspectives.* Ed. Patricia Stuart-Macadam and Katherine Ann Dettwyler. New York: Aldine De Gruyter, 1995. 75-99.

Thurer, Shari. *The Myths of Motherhood: How Culture Reinvents the Good Mother.* New York: Penguin, 1994.

Today's Parent [online] 2008, 13 Feb. 2008 <http://www.todaysparent.com/community/forums/?breastfeeding>.

Toronto Public Health (online) 2005. Toronto breastfeeding rates. *Health Status* 3-1, Feb. 2005, 22 Sept. 2009. <http://www.toronto.ca/health/hsi/pdf/hsn_toronto_breastfeeding_rates.pdf>.

Valsiner, Jaan. *Culture and Human Development.* Thousand Oaks: Sage Publications, 2000.

Van Esterik, Penny. "The Politics of Breastfeeding: An Advocacy Perspective." *Breastfeeding: Biocultural Perspectives.* Ed. Patricia Stuart-Macadam and Katherine Ann Dettwyler. New York: Aldine De Gruyter, 1995. 145-165.

Walker, Marsha. "The Hazards of Infant Formula: New Evidence." Paper presented at the Conference "The Cost of Not Breastfeeding: Eighth Annual National Breastfeeding Seminar Program." Toronto, Canada, 1998, June 4-5.

Weininger, Otto. *Melanie Klein: From Theory to Reality.*_London: Karnac Books, 1992.

Wiessinger, Diane. "Watch Your Language." *Journal of Human Lactation* 12.1 (1996): 1-4.

Wolf, Jacqueline H. "Mercenary Hirelings or Great Blessings?: Doctors' and Mothers Conflicted Perceptions of Wet Nurses and the Ramifications for Infant Feeding in Chicago." *Journal of Social History,* 33.1 (1999): 97- 113.

Wolf, Jacqueline H. *Don't Kill Your Baby: Public Health and the Decline of Breastfeeding in the 19th and 20th Centuries.* Columbia: The Ohio State University Press, 2001.

World Health Organization (WHO). *International Code of Marketing of Breastmilk Substitutes.* Geneva, Switzerland: WHO, 1981.

World Health Organization (WHO). *Expert Consultation on the Optimal Duration of Exclusive Breastfeeding: Conclusions and Recommendations.* March 2001. <http://.who.int/inf-pr2001/en/note2001-07.html>..

World Health Organization (WHO). *Global Strategy for Infant and Young Child Feeding.* Geneva, Switzerland: WHO, 2003.

Breastfeeding and Time

In Search of a Language for Pleasure and Agency

ALISON BARTLETT

To every thing [turn, turn, turn]
there is a season,
and a time to every
purpose under the heaven
(Ecclesiastes 3:1-8)
("Turn, Turn, Turn," Pete Seeger, 1962)

OUT SHOPPING ONE DAY ...

I RECENTLY SAW A new mum out with her baby who was quietly whimpering in the pram. The mum didn't look too concerned, but *her* mother was with them also and she responded to these little calls for attention suggesting, with all the tentativeness of a self-conscious new grandmother, the baby might want a feed. She was clearly placing the authority with the baby's mother, but offering advice and support to feed if it was needed. But the new mum was quite unconcerned, more intent on using this time for the task at hand: shopping. She offered a couple of half-hearted replies to defer the idea of a feed, but finally rejected the suggestion by concluding that anyway, it wasn't time.

This scene negotiates breastfeeding in fascinating ways, recalling the changes in breastfeeding language in recent history. The grandmother responding to the baby's call for attention is consistent with recent historical trends of breastfeeding that are baby-led, adopting the baby's needs as a priority to which we respond. The mother's defining argument mobilises a quite different conception of breastfeeding as a bodily regime which is scheduled and tracked so that the mother keeps a close watch on the baby's input and output. This regime is often associated with the period between and after the world wars in the twentieth century, when modernisation and industrialisation valued the scientification of motherhood (Reiger). But I suspect there is something else happening here, which relates to an insistence on me-time for a mum who just wanted to go shopping. Self-fulfillment, self-help, self-development have been doctrines in the western world for several decades now, as an obligation to take care of the self (which often means consuming products or services and so is closely aligned with shopping). Acquisition of goods and services is certainly something we are trained to do as mothers (Soufalis), but shopping can be a problem when our baby is with us: by drawing on an older but historically accepted idea of 'timing feeds', this mum can get on with her shopping without having to consider all the negotiations of feeding in a busy department store. Who knows why the baby was crying—she went to sleep fairly quickly—and what the 'right' response would be, but what interests me is how we assimilate such disparate understandings of time in the early—and even later—days of a new baby. Breastfeeding seems to invite a cataclysmic reassessment of the way time passes, the ways we 'use' time, or give time or even give it up: how time produces and becomes a product, and what happens when we give away or continue with the regulation of time.

LIMINAL TIME

Studies about motherhood often narrate pregnancy, birth, and the postpartum period as a time of change and adjustment, a transition to motherhood. It is a time set apart from other life, although life goes on around us and mothers participate in it at the same time as they are becoming mothers. The shift to motherhood is a shift in identity which we come to accept with the passage of time, this story implies. Often we are so accustomed to our identities as they are already formed, and time as it is already lived, however, that this 'transition' can be unexpected, sometimes disorientating, even alienating for some. Social commentator, sociologist, and satirist Susan Maushart contends that "women who succeed at breastfeeding demonstrate a heroic capacity to defer gratification, and to survive repeated violations of deeply held cultural assumptions about the proper regulation of time and space" (227-28). It's not surprising then that Camille Cronin's study of new mothers in Ireland found that time without baby was important and seen as a momentary opportunity to *return to normal*. Cronin's study examines new mothers' experiences in order to find ways to increase breastfeeding rates, so it can be seen as representative of a particular public health discourse about the 'difficulties' of motherhood. The discussion about time falls into a narrative about 'coping' with the changes involved in becoming a mother and finding 'time out' from it. Cronin describes how "mothers 'made time' or planned 'time out' in order to socialize" (265):

> Some had specific days on which to take the 'time out' and this time was almost sacred. As one said: 'Saturday is my day to myself, he is very good that way'. Some felt they had really lost their 'free time' altogether: 'The only time I really take for myself is when she is asleep' and commented on how little time they had to socialize: 'The only time I get a break is if I am going out on the weekend'. (265)

Socialising is understood to be important as a mark of *normality*, in being able to 'maintain some normality' as Cronin describes it, as if part of the transition to motherhood is being able to exempt ourself from it. Echoing the idea of me-time for shopping, Cronin cites some examples from mothers trying to incorporate their previous shopping identity into their newly maternal condition:

> 'How am I going to get into the taxi now, where am I going to put the child when I'm holding the pram?' When shopping or moving around town, negotiating the paths or finding an alternative to stairs was seen as a challenge: 'I burst out crying because I couldn't get up the stairs ... I mean even going into shops now. I never realized, like, there was a lift'. (265)

These kinds of comments are replicated in Monica Campo's study in this volume regarding bodies, and also in an earlier study by Patricia Mahon-Daly and Gavin Andrews, who are also concerned with ideas of *return* to a *normal* body and life. They use the idea of 'liminality' to account for the experience of breastfeeding as a state, space or time of transition, in which belonging to previous and particular social groups is suspended. They report that from their testimonials with new mothers, "linear time constraints made breastfeeding appear 'too time consuming' and fit poorly with a convenient model of child rearing" (71). They quote Gill saying, "I couldn't continue (breastfeeding). I mean, it was just too time consuming.... At least I'm in control" (71). The authors relate the issue of control not only to managing time but also to the impetus to measure amounts of milk being produced and consumed, which can be achieved only with bottles (71). On the topic of time, this study also cites Pera, a mother who considers the time it takes to breastfeed amidst all the other tasks involved in mothering:

> Time and breastfeeding: now that's interesting because everything is faster now. I mean I never have a minute. Breastfeeding definitely takes longer and is more of a fuss. I mean if I didn't know it was best I would have given up. He's terrible, always falls asleep. I don't know if he has had enough. I put him down and half an hour later he's at me again. (cited in Mahon-Daly and Andrews 71)

Interestingly, Pera invokes the public health promotion slogan of 'breast is best' to defend her breastfeeding practice, despite her baby's apparently bad behaviour at not separating sleeping and eating. Pera though doesn't sound really perturbed, and another interview participant, Rachel, doesn't seem to care about such disarray when she says "*We are in our own private world when I'm breastfeeding. I have no idea of time whatsoever*" (Mahon-Daly and Andrews 72). These mothers and scholars thus demonstrate a disparate range of thought and experience around time breastfeeding as a transitional or liminal state in relation to what is perceived to be normal, standard, *sans*-baby time.

HISTORICAL TIME

Many commentators have traced the way in which western cultures have inherited and interiorized an understanding of time as linear, incremental and developmental—indeed, this is the way in which history is often told: as unfolding from primitiveness to civilization, from naïveté to wisdom, crudeness to sophistication. Interestingly, this has also been applied to our current understanding of birth and breastfeeding by several critics. Emily Martin's 1987 cultural analysis of reproduction insists that since industrialization the lives and bodies of workers have been regulated, mechanised, fragmented, and alienated: in short, they have been understood as comparable to machines (16). The simultaneous rise of medical science alongside industrial capitalism has meant that women feel this alienation even more keenly than men because of the way their bodies visibly change—during menstruation, pregnancy, lactation and menopause (27-53). Due to this, women's bodies are subjected to increased scientific scrutiny and pathologisation, and this is intensified during birth and breastfeeding when time and efficiency are measures of whether—or when—technological or chemical intervention begin (54). Like Martin, Lynda Birke makes the point that medical science speaks in metaphors of machinery and technology, but with no other language readily available these metaphors come to represent our corporeal experiences metonymically—that is, in substitution. Wendy Simonds has charted the linguistic terms which rely on time to name pregnancy, birth and postpartum experiences—even postpartum is part of a suite of terms about time and birth (2002):

> This conceptualization makes pregnancy cohere with the work-week, which is what institutionalized the seven day week in the first place. (This week-based time keeping continues after birth, as the postpartum time period ticks away, as parental leaves are sparingly meted out, as developmental milestones are measured in children's lives. (564)

Simonds argues that the medical or obstetric model runs on draconian clock time while the midwifery model of care "posits a liberatory view of time as expansive (as opposed to the restrictive time keeping of medicine) because of its holistic (rather than fragmenting) world-view" (568). However this is not the experience of midwives working in hospitals which are run by the clock, as Fiona Dykes systematically outlines (2006). Taking up Martin's parallel between production and reproduction, Dykes argues that the transformation of "home-based medicine to techno-medicine in western Europe during the Enlightenment" (14) was the predecessor to hospital-based birthing in the twentieth century "in which the principles of linear time, production, control and surveillance predominated … and the clock became central to medical ideology around infant feeding" (31). This entailed a disempowerment of both mothers and midwives, as midwives feel pressured in a culture "with a production-line ethos, hierarchical structure and unpredictable, time-constrained working conditions" (72) and mothers were expected to perform maternal intimacy in a public place amongst strangers. Breastfeeding, Dykes argues, came to be seen as demanding labour rather than a relational experience, and breastmilk becomes the focused product in a culture that encourages the fragmentation of bodies into working (or not working) parts (95). She also identifies mothers' anxieties about returning to 'normal' (113), and the way this is anticipated through the use of routines, rituals and schedules as a way of feeling "in control, especially in the face of ambiguity, unpredictability and aversive situations" (131). Ironically, the desire for their baby to settle down to a routine involves the baby's passivity, while the desire for steady growth and progress requires independence and autonomy; as Dykes points out and Penny Van Esterik before her, breastfeeding babies are actively engaged in their milk consumption and constitution while bottle feeders are trained to be dependent consumers from birth (103). Dykes' analysis is searing and profoundly anchored in the operations of the hospital as an institution, advocating that this is not a suitable place for birthing mothers or midwives (179). Buried amongst all the disturbing stories and conversations, however, was one that reverberated for me. It was from a teacher named Chloe, who identified a shift in her valuing of time before birth and afterwards:

> I mean our school is being inspected in February so the last few weeks have been about action planning and statistics and that sort of thing and you know I haven't got a clue now and to be honest I couldn't care less … it's quite nice to have left all that lap top business behind and just think, oh I can actually have a bit of time where I'm in touch with what, you know, life was like in a different age. I feel like going out and reading lots of Thomas Hardy novels. It's that feeling that perhaps none of all that really matters … (Dykes 79)

Chloe's narrative expands the timeframe of life, extending past the recent consuming priorities at her work to the nineteenth century pastoral narratives of Hardy and into an expansive future of 'what really matters' from a broader perspective. Like Rachel, quoted above, Chloe doesn't seem to care about rational, linear time during her baby's early days.

POLITICAL TIME

So what's the difference between these two sets of values around normalized, efficient time regimes that need 'free time', measures, and control in motherhood, and those who relinquish these customs? And how can they be accounted for without pitting time and culture against each other, as Carol Greenhouse warns against (xii)? Greenhouse takes up anthropology's idea of 'social time' and imbues it with political agency to suggest that "time articulates people's understandings of agency: literally, what makes things happen and what makes acts relevant in relation to social experience, however conceived" (1). Theories about time that emanate from western democracies are projected onto places and cultures, Greenhouse argues, naturalising linear modernist time as the standard, much like Greenwich does for time accuracy. Greenhouse contends that this drive toward future time is predicated on the expectation and tragedy of death: death as an individual and social end is what drives western narratives of time as having a beginning and an end. What agency brings to this never-ending story is a politics of who benefits and how:

> Time is not about, or not first about, personal or collective experiences of change but about cultural formulations of agency and their compatibility or incompatibility within specific institutional forms. "Agency" names cultural propositions about how the universe works. (Greenhouse 5)

If Greenhouse's ideas are applied to breastfeeding time, then breastfeeding can not just be a liminal time or space which mother and baby occupy while waiting for 'normal' time to be returned. To understand breastfeeding as such is to devalue and constrain it to a nether-land outside of normal life. For women who breastfeed multiple children for months or years at a time, breastfeeding can be more 'normal' than not breastfeeding, not withstanding those who choose to lactate for purposes other than child nutrition (see Giles). A liminal understanding of breastfeeding imbues it as a transitional 'stage' rather than having its own lived ontology, and it eliminates the possibility of its potentially radical agency in disrupting dominant western understandings of time, as Rachel and Chloe articulate.

If we understand time the way Greenhouse does, as offering forms of agency which are compatible or incompatible with other institutions, then maternity becomes a radical alternative to standard life trajectories which revolve around transitions from school to work to retirement. In the public sphere, where men have traditionally dominated, paternity barely affects this standard trajectory. However since women's participation in the workforce has increased and been anticipated for several generations now, the 'maternity' debates have become increasingly intense in Australia at least (see Maushart; Manne; Pocock). Most of these debates focus on what to do with women while they are having children, and the solution seems to be paid maternity leave so that their skills, experience and expertise are not forsaken just because they give birth (see Goward). Paid maternity leave would be a significant gain, as Dykes argues: "if women anticipated this 'time out' without financial loss then their postnatal period might be considerably less pressured" (181). Notwithstanding the range of maternal experience, however, some women feel utterly changed by maternity, so that having 'time out' of anything, including employment, doesn't exactly address the radical intervention babies bring in terms of values, ways of living, spatial habitus, and understandings of time; it simply creates a time in which woman can indulge in maternity in between 'normal' work trajectories. In short, maternity leave understands maternity to be liminal, temporary, and transitory. In Greenhouse's terms, maternity is incompatible with most institutions of employment (and hospitals as institutions of health Dykes reminds us), and so mothers experience reduced agency. Maternity becomes the point of tension between women and work, and breastfeeding seems to exacerbate those tensions.

WORKING TIME

Philosopher Moira Gatens argues that the structural limitations of western societies are material manifestations of sexual difference—that is, that social institutions have been set up for specifically male bodies, and this historical feature is now being 'felt' by women because we are now participating in the public sphere in unprecedented numbers. She uses the example of breastfeeding to imagine a society in which the public sphere is designed around "women's historical and present capacities":

> The primary aim of such a body politic might be to foster conditions for the healthy reproduction of its members. If this were the case, then presumably some men would now be demanding that medical science provide ways for them to overcome their 'natural' or biological disadvantages, by inventing, for example, means by which they could lactate (71).

Gatens uses the reproductive differences between men and women as an example of the ways in which our social formations attribute value, and in turn how that valuing influences the development of social institutions, architecture and community design. In her example an alternative body politic looks ridiculously divided between lactators and nonlactators. And yet she is also suggesting that this happens in the reverse now: that lactation is not valued, and neither is maternity and reproduction, so women in general are not assigned the same agency as men because of this historical legacy. A revolution in the expectations of fatherhood over the last few decades has also wrought cultural changes, but not in the same league as the ongoing conundrum brought about by the material conditions of maternity. Barbara Pocock reminds us that

> The fit of *institutions* to mothers—or carers in general—with jobs is characterised by dissonance, with leave arrangements, industrial regulation and the supply of care lagging well behind demand. (240)

In her study of time and agency, Joan Tronto finds a comparable ill-fit between carers and time. Tronto outlines a discernable shift in capitalist trends from the modernist production time of factory assembly lines to the volatile, unpredictable 24/7 time of postmodern global market economies. This always-ready postmodern time might have more affinities with breastfeeding time in its fluidity and fluxing between idleness and intensity (Bartlett 2005, 186), however Tronto also notes that even when using a model of postmodern production, "time assumes a different aspect from the standpoint of care" (123):

> Time spent caring is not about mastery and control but about maintenance and nurturance … [there is] much about care that suggests that we understand in fundamental ways how time limits the capacities of humans to force their wills upon the world. (123)

Time spent caring, she argues, prevails *against* dominant understandings of time and production, and of status and success, accounting for the inadequate social valuing of the caring professions, and maternity. Time, it seems, does not work well for carers. Or perhaps we need to rework it.

ETERNAL TIME

There are other understandings of time which run concurrently to clocks and schedules. Cyclical time is often used still in relation to the cycles of the 'natural' world, like the cycle of the tides and the moon and planetary movements that are still reported in the newspapers. Cycles are often used to speak about women's bodily changes and life stages which do not rely on developmental stages but an often arbitrary passing of time. The weather provides a more fascinating example of chaos theory in which arbitrary events trigger other events in time; while chaos theory is often perceived to be abstract and difficult, it also bears uncanny resemblances to everyday life. Philosopher Julia Kristeva talks about cyclic time in an essay titled "Women's Time," suggesting that "female subjectivity seems to offer a specific concept of measurement that essentially retains repetition and eternity out of the many modalities that appear through the history of civilization" (352). She calls these two modes of temporality *cyclical* and *monumental* time, which she locates innately with the maternal body. The concept of linking to an eternal history of maternity through monumental time appeals to me and enables the emergence of a different sort of language in which to code the enormity of birth.

The 'miracle of birth' sounds like cliché, but perhaps it's a clumsy way of articulating the profound disruption to rational science and philosophy—to our very understandings of ontology—by making an 'irrational' claim to faith and the sacred. It's easy to understand women as (re)producers of the human race in the mechanistic language of capitalism, but more difficult to imagine growing another living human being inside us, and then opening ourselves to birth them, even after we've done it. How can there be 'normal' after this? In her book, Melissa Benn writes about hearing long-time birthing advocate Shiela Kitzinger talk in "a quasi-spiritual way" about the days following birth. "While this kind of language is not my own," she writes,

> I could recognize the force of Kitzinger's argument when she asserted that 'a "time of special cherishing" is at risk of being lost. Women now have to be cool and clear. They are urged to "get their figure back ... get back to normal'. (66)

Benn might feel uncomfortable with quasi-spiritual language but she titles her book *Madonna and Child*, suggesting a crucial link to one of the most enduring spiritual references of maternity. Fiona Dykes mobilises Robbier Kahn's idea of maialogical time, meaning a time of relationality, mutuality, interaction and reciprocity (Dykes 96). "If women understood the concept of maialogical time and were able to incorporate it, at least partially, into their lives, they might feel less pressured about their babies' need to take their time" Dykes argues (181). This gesture toward a mythic time which might be honoured in the everyday infuses Ina May Gaskin's 1977 book *Spiritual Midwifery.* Written in her homebirthing community in Tennessee, Gaskins instructs midwives that

> Pregnant and birthing mothers are elemental forces, in the same sense that gravity, thunderstorms, earthquakes, and hurricanes are elemental forces. In order to understand the laws of their energy flow, you have to love and respect them for their magnificence at the same time that you study them with the accuracy of a true scientist. (282)

Setting science and the divine alongside each other pervades Gaskin's writing/practice which, as Wendy Simonds notes, dispenses with the medical stopwatch altogether (564). Breastfeeding is also flexible and unpredictable Gaskin notes, as "different babies have different styles of nursing":

> Some babies latch onto the tit minutes after they're born, while others aren't interested until their mother's milk comes in ... some babies are the type that nurse for ten minutes and gulp down a bunch of milk and are full and satisfied. Other babies suck for hours at a time.... It's okay to let your baby nurse all he wants. But if you have other things to do, you can put him down for a while, if you know he's full and dry. (260-61)

Gaskin also draws on the language of holiness (which is variously Christian, Buddhist and Hindu throughout the book), claiming "Every birth is Holy. I think that a midwife must be religious, because the energy she is dealing with is Holy. She needs to know that other people's energy is sacred" (282). This might seem eccentric now, especially alongside the ecstatic language of hippie experimentalism, peaceniks and drug-induced alternative states that enable discussions of pure energy and love vibrations. But *Spiritual Midwifery* is still regularly republished and has sold continuously for thirty years. The language of the eternal and the ecstatic provides a unique tone and set of images that are unavailable elsewhere. Even if this language is not part of our regular vocabulary, it functions to set up an alternative set of narratives and timeframes around birth which offer women and their babies agency in their own time.

I feel like I have to insert a disclaimer here, that I'm not advocating heavily intoned religious tracts on motherhood, but that gesturing to a mythic, eternal or sacred element usefully figures here as a disruption to the linear clock-model of medical obstetrics. Pamela Klassen's work on the meanings of the 'sacred' in talk about motherhood demonstrates that there is an extravagant (and even contradictory) range of understandings invoked by the use of such abstract but deeply held cultural terms anyway. Gaskin's text is a product of its time and also still revered for, I believe, its rare provision of alternatives scenarios, science and stories.

TALKING TIME

The kinds of language we have available to understand time, or to re-imagine it, is crucial to the way we have interiorized a specific understanding of time. Philosopher Elizabeth Grosz maintains that temporality is all to often "elided, forgotten, or unrepresented" in many discussions and theories of the social and that this is in part a function of language itself: "The language by which we represent temporality, at last in the West from at least the time of Ancient Greece, is a language of spatiality, in which spatial terms and relations come to represent temporal movements" (215). Greenhouse also notes that while she uses ideas of postmodernity to signal a crisis in representation and legitimation, "*post*modernity is not post anything" (15). And Julia Kristeva reminds us that time is embedded in language, in the temporality of grammar, the beginning-middle-end of sentence construction, and plot narratives (353). Language/time is often counter-intuitive—it has to be learnt—therefore finding other, less 'normal' ways to imagine time is fundamental to changing the ways in which we experience it. This is to propose another way of "understanding how the universe works," as Greenhouse proposes agency asserts.

The language of work/life balance is a case in point. The slashed opposition of work/life assumes that work and life can be 'balanced', and that work is not part of life/life is not part of work. It separates our life into labour and leisure, muddling the unpaid work we do at home and the pleasures we take from work. We don't cease being mothers when we go to work, and when we become new mothers we don't simply cease being our former selves. It's rare for people to divide themselves up into separate time zones or identities; more often we operate multiple selves at the same time, as Joan Tronto explains in relation to time:

> That time is a complex subject becomes obvious if we reflect for a moment on the multiple dimensions of time that inform our lives. Time is both circular (there are repeating daily rhythms) and linear (past, present and future proceed in that order) … Each of us has had a subjective sense of time fleeting or dragging. Yet on another level, time is stubbornly resistant to human control. (120)

Too often the emphasis on the conflict between work and life—while it might describe many personal experiences—is a narrative that compels us to entertain work and life as fields of conflict, as do many breastfeeding stories and maternal subjectivities.

The critiques of the structural inadequacy of social institutions like work and health are vital, but their dismal conclusions about the ill-fit of maternity also serves to reinforce the 'problem' of working mothers, the 'difficulties' of babies, and the liminality of maternity outside of 'normal' being. I want to resist the idea that my work and my parenting are in conflict or somehow compromise each other. I want to collapse the thinking that poses our lives as a series of demands, pressures, trade-offs and debits, and restore the pleasures, reciprocity and potentials of a rounded life. And I want to claim maternity—including breastfeeding—as an expansive experience which increases our worth and skills. These provide much more enabling and energising narratives.

In fact a range of experiences, narratives, and language are needed to engage the diverse range of women and their experiences because, as Dykes notes, not all women will feel empowered by breastfeeding so social policy should not coerce women to breastfeed (181). While I might find Rachel's and Chloe's time shifting appealing, others might find it perverse or irresponsible. While I might favour an appeal to breastfeeding as a radical act of intervention in a world that values success through status and wealth, others will find more agency in breastfeeding as a normalized or even conservative activity which provides membership of a valued social group. Nevertheless, I'm going to carry on with my suggestions for radical alternatives because there are so few of them written.

What needs to be retrieved in discussions of women in work, of breastfeeding and time, I believe, is reciprocity: the ways in which our life directly nourishes our work, in which maternity expands our skills, ideas and critical enterprises rather than limiting the time we can spend on them. Philosopher Luce Irigaray argues that if our debt to maternity—to being born—were able to be socially acknowledged, then models of reciprocity and gifting would prevail (30). Rhonda Shaw uses ideas of maternal generosity and the ethics of the gift relation to think through the complexities of breastfeeding relations (see also Hird). And while Fiona Dykes argues that nothing short of a cultural revolution will change the task of breastfeeding in hospital, "if women could go beyond the one-way notion of 'giving out' to their baby and conceptualise breastfeeding in a more symmetrical relational context," she maintains, "then giving to a baby would be seen as part of a reciprocal relationship in which the mother also receives" (175). In these examples, it is a shift in cultural values and (either following or preceding) a shift in individual thinking that effects social change, but fundamentally it is a shift in language as well. The key for me in linking breastfeeding with reciprocity is finding ways to articulate what women get from it, and one thing we get is time. Another is a vast array of pleasure.

ADDI(C)TIONAL TIME

If that sounds like a conclusion, it is. But I want to finish by drawing your attention to a collection of essays called *Women Making Time*, in which Helen Keane has a chapter about young women smokers, time and addiction. She suggests that smoking (perhaps a little like breastfeeding) offers some temporal pleasures which public health campaigns mitigate against. Keane's previous work on addiction argues that the material condition and subjective experience of addiction constitutes a lived reality which is constructed as morally reprehensible by medical and social talk, and yet it often differs little from the lives of 'us', the apparently 'non-addicted'. When Keane writes of the temporal pleasures of smoking, I am reminded of the temporal pleasures of breastfeeding. "The pleasure of smoking is connected to temporal effects, the small ritual marking the passage of time as well as taking up time," she suggests (108), reminding me of the ritual breastfeed on my arrival home from work that reconnected us long after breastmilk was needed for nutrition. And the sense of repetition and anticipation is crucial to those pleasures: "addiction is not so much the terrible cost of smoking but intrinsic to its pleasure, ensuring as it does desire's predictable return" (111). The idea of addictive desire depends on the potential for endless repetition, and its anticipation. As Karleen Gribble reminds us elsewhere in this volume, babies also anticipate the pleasures of breastfeeding. The regulation of our day around such needs is commensurate with other needs like caffeine, exercise, seeing loved ones. Keane notes that "smoking creates time outside of ordinary duration, like other technologies and practices valued for their temporal otherness: reading novels, sex, listening to music" (111). Like breastfeeding, and Chloe's yearning for Thomas Hardy novels. It might seem perverse to compare breastfeeding to smoking, and yet the "temporal pleasures and plenitude available to smokers" (111) seem remarkably similar to breastfeeding the more I take the time to think about it.

Emily Martin sees women as inherently resistant capitalist subjects because we are already involved in profoundly corporeal activities which defy quantification, time-efficiency strategies and even birth plans (143). Maybe, but we are also well-trained citizens and consumers. Martin may well be optimistic but hey, there's another pleasure we can take with us shopping for ways to articulate the invaluable and intransigent pleasures of maternity and breastfeeding in their timely relations of mutuality and reciprocity. Shopping, after all, is a pleasure for many of us.

REFERENCES

Bartlett, Alison. *Breastwork: Rethinking Breastfeeding*. Sydney: UNSWPress, 2005.

Benn, Melissa. *Madonna and Child: Towards a New Politics of Motherhood*. London: Jonathon Cape, 1998.

Birke, Lynda. *Feminism and the Biological Body*. Edinburgh: Edinburgh University Press, 1999.

Cronin, Camille. "First-Time Mothers: Identifying their Needs, Perceptions and Experiences." *Journal of Clinical Nursing* 12 (2003): 260-267.

Dykes, Fiona. *Breastfeeding in Hospital: Mothers, Midwives and the Production Line*. London: Routledge, 2006.

Gaskin, Ina May. *Spiritual Midwifery*. Tennessee: The Book Publishing Co, 1977.

Gatens, Moira. *The Imaginary Bodies: Ethics, Power and Corporeality*. New York: Routledge, 1995.

Giles, Fiona. *Fresh Milk: the Secret Life of Breasts*. Sydney: Allen & Unwin, 2003.

Goward, Pru, *It's About Time: Women, Men, Work and Family*. Human Rights and Equal Opportunity Commission Final Report, 2007. <http://www.humanrights.gov.au/sex_discrimination/its_about_time/index.html>.

Greenhouse, Carol J. *A Moment's Notice: Time Politics Across Culture*. Cornell UP, 1995.

Grosz, Elizabeth. *Time Travels: Feminism, Nature, Power*. Sydney: Allen & Unwin, 2005.

Hird, Myra J. "The Corporeal Generosity of Maternity." *Body & Society* 13.1 (2007): 1-20.

Irigaray, Luce. "When our Lips Speak Together." *This Sex Which is Not One*. Trans. Catherine Porter with Carolyn Burke. Cornell University Press, 1985. *C'est Sexe* 1977.

Kahn, Robbier Pfeufer. "Women and Time in Childbirth and During Lactation." *Taking Our Time: Feminist Perspectives on Temporality*. Eds. Frieda Johles Forman and Caoran Sowton. Oxford: Pergamon, 1989. 20-36.

Keane, Helen. "Time and the Female Smoker." *Women Making Time: Contemporary Feminist Critique and Cultural Analysis*. Ed. Elizabeth McMahon and Brigitta Olubas. Crawley: UWA Press, 2006. 94-115.

Klassen, Pamela E. "Sacred Maternities and Postbiomedical Bodies: Religion and Nature in Contemporary Home Birth." *Signs* 26.3 (2001): 775-809.

Kristeva, Julia. "Women's Time." *The Portable Kristeva*, Ed Kelly Oliver. New York: Columbia University Press, 1997. 349-369.

Mahon-Daly, Patricia and Gavin J. Andrews. "Liminality and Breastfeeding: Women Negotiating Space and Two Bodies." *Health & Place* 8 (2002): 61-76.

Manne, Anne. *Motherhood: How Should We Care For Our Children?* Sydney: Allen & Unwin, 2005.

Maushart, Susan. *The Mask of Motherhood: How Mothering Changes Everything and Why We Pretend it Doesn't.* Sydney: Random House, 1997.

Martin, Emily. *The Woman in the Body: A Cultural Analysis of Reproduction.* Milton Keynes: Open University Press, 1987.

Pocock, Barbara. *The Work/Life Collision: What Work is Doing to Australians and What to Do About It.* Sydney: Federation Press, 2003.

Reiger, Kerreen. *The Disenchantment of the Home: Modernizing the Australian Family 1880-1940.* Melbourne: Oxford University Press, 1985.

Shaw, Rhonda. "Theorizing Breastfeeding: Body Ethics, Maternal Generosity and the Gift Relation." *Body and Society* 9.2 (2003): 55-73.

Simonds, Wendy. "Watching the Clock: Keeping Time During Pregnancy, Birth, and Postpartum Experiences." *Social Science & Medicine* 55.4 (2002): 559-570.

Soufalis, Zoe. "Spacing Out in the Mother Shop." *Motherlode.* Eds. Stephanie Holt and Maryanne Lynch. Melbourne: Sybylla Press, 1996. 120-128.

Tronto. Joan. "Time's place." *Feminist Theory* 4.2 (2003): 119-138.

Van Esterik, Penny. *Beyond the Breast-Bottle Controversy.* New Bruswick: Rutgers University Press, 1989.

From "Gift of Loss" to Self Care

The Significance of Induced Lactation in Takashi Miike's *Visitor Q*

FIONA GILES

"I make milk. What's your superpower?"
—T-Shirt Slogan. Australian Breastfeeding Association

I

VISITOR Q (2001) IS A black comedy by Japanese director Takashi Miike, which revolves around the motif of induced lactation. While other plot developments take place, the significance of the lactating mother is crucial to the outcome of the film; and alongside the startling and scatological comic violence, it is one of its more "freakish" components. In a film which revels in violently plundering the body and transgressing its boundaries, lactation is represented as being equally disturbing, yet in this case enlightening. Additionally, the mother's capacity to induce lactation is a pivotal plot development and marks an important process of her characterisation. It is then used at the climax of the film, influencing the behaviour of other characters, and symbolising the reunion of the family. The scene of the mother breastfeeding her husband in the garden hot house at the end of the film is also the image chosen for the film's promotion. This may be due to its being suitably eye-catching; yet it also suggests that the lactation story embedded in this complex drama is of central importance to its overall meaning.

A small number of feature films have included images of lactation and breastfeeding; and an even smaller number have to some extent explored the erotic and comic potential of lactation. For example, the European film *Les Valseuses* (1974) includes an adult nursing scene, and *La Teta y La Luna* (1994) dramatises a school-aged boy's interest in nursing. Comic nursing scenes have appeared in British and Hollywood films such as *Sunday Bloody Sunday* (1971), *Look Who's Talking* (1989), and *Me, Myself & Irene* (2000), all of which play on a male character's (or audience's) revulsion at the thought of accidentally drinking breastmilk. This interplay of the erotic and abject, desire and disgust, while sometimes split into separate narratives, implies an underlying sexual fascination with breastmilk and the capacity of women to lactate, that contemporary culture has yet to explore. One exception to this rule of separation is the Russian feature *A Place on Earth* (2001), directed by Artur Aristakisian, in which breastfeeding is part of a campaign of embodied care offered by a hippie commune to the homeless population of Moscow. Here breastfeeding is allowed to cross the border between erotic and maternal care in the context of a radical approach to the socialisation of love. The project represented in the film is based on the utopian idea that the homeless are entitled not only to food and shelter, but also to affectionate and sexual human interaction. While the film shows the social experiment to be flawed, it nevertheless allows for breastfeeding to exist along the continuum of embodied care for both adults and children—to be viewed as part of our sexuality.

Visitor Q also allows for an exploration of the maternal-sexual continuum through the motif of lactation and takes it further than *A Place on Earth* by highlighting the mother's capacity to lactate as a dramatic and transformative self-discovery. Her lactation scenes are comic and sexual, and—it could be argued—lactation is represented as spiritually redemptive. The Christian iconography of lactation in *A Place on Earth* is embedded within the ideal of charitable good works performed by members of the commune. The religious significance of lactation in *Visitor Q* may also link to Western traditions, particularly different versions during the Renaissance of *The Lactation of Saint Bernard*, in which a statue of the Virgin Mary is asked by St Bernard to prove she's a mother and she responds by spraying milk from on high at the praying saint. This idea of proof of motherhood is clearly echoed in *Visitor Q* as she proves through this means that she is a mother to her family, as much as to herself. Examples of other Renaissance images which offer milk production as spectacle include Peter Paul Rubens' *Venus, Mars and Cupid* (1540) and Tintoretto's *The Origin of the Milky Way* (c. 1575). In each of these images the manifestation of milk fountaining from the breast is central to the meaning of the painting, drawing on stories from Greco-Roman mythology in which the creation myth is linked to the act of mothering, and to female sexuality.[1]

While not a religious film as such, it is possible to find connections to Japanese Buddhism and echoes of ancestor worship and Shintoism, which in Japanese daily practice may be manifested through the custom of breastfeeding older relatives. The symbolic heritage of lactation, as saving souls and manifesting purity in its traditional Christian sense, is difficult to avoid.[2] In *Visitor Q* these references provide historical resonance to a more literal, physiological notion of sexual and maternal empowerment that the mother's lactation represents, as well as the Japanese fascination with the body *in extremis*. In a film which systematically shows the abuse, beating, rape, murder and dismemberment of the bodies of its characters, the scenes of lactation are powerfully joyful and productive. In contrast to the scattering of bodies and their parts, and the splitting of relationships, lactation represents bodily integrity, wholeness and connection.

Thus lactation in *Visitor Q* represents a bodily superpower with both religious and secular implications. These can be read in both Western and Japanese contexts of gendered power relations, and the relative disempowerment of Japanese women in the home adds to the impact of a film which suggests that lactation as a simple, though hidden capacity of the mother's body, may be a source of female emancipation. It should also be acknowledged that the extreme violence of some traditional Japanese erotica lends itself to the kind of physical extremism found in these lactation scenes: the body at its limits and beyond is a constant source of spectacle. However this is physical extremism as prowess rather than suffering. Though initiated by her visitor, the mother's enthusiastic adoption of this capacity, her control over it, and her family's interpretation of it as a benign symbol of her power and generosity means that it signifies the end of her victimisation, rather than its beginning.

II

Visitor Q concerns a dysfunctional suburban Japanese family in which the teenage daughter has left home to work as a prostitute, the mother is a heroin addict also working as a prostitute, the father has lost his job as a television reporter after being anally raped on camera by interviewees of his reality television program, and the son beats his mother while also being a victim of beatings from school bullies. The bullying of the son extends to a sense of the family as a whole being victimised in addition to each of its members, as the school bullies routinely shoot fireworks at the house once the son is inside. The implication is that the family unit is under siege, as are families in general as networks of meaningful and unmediated relations.

The film begins with the question: "Have you ever done it with your dad?" upending familial propriety together with assumptions about incest, since the daughter is seducing her father and charging him money. While the daughter persuades her father to sleep with her, they take photos of each other, she using a still camera, he a video. And as they have sex, the filming continues, as it does more or less continuously throughout the film when the father is involved. This has the effect of implicating the audience as voyeurs of dysfunction while also offering a critique of reality television and the atomisation of relationships associated with post-industrial economies and popular culture. The film suggests that while the characters obsessively record and display their lives, none of them are actually seeing each other and are therefore incapable of ethical connection.

It is into this context that Visitor Q appears as a witness. A young man in black leather jeans and a red shirt, he says little and judges nothing, and while obligingly filming any action when requested, he remains outside the drama, observing without documenting, and connecting through his silent gaze, with each family member in turn. He does however perform three acts of intervention which I will outline below.

After the father has slept with his daughter in a hotel room, he is returning home when Visitor Q, a stranger on the street, stands behind him and hits him over the head with a rock. The film then cuts to the family kitchen where the father and Visitor Q enjoy a dinner served by the mother. In Japanese style, the mother serves while her family remain seated, and they ask rudely for more food, which she provides dutifully. It is powerfully underscored that the mother is the only provider of food in this household, foreshadowing the significance of her milk production. The father, his head now bandaged, remains surly, while Visitor Q makes a show of enjoying his dinner, but he behaves as any Japanese male guest would in ignoring the servile mother. As the son begins beating his mother, the adult men continue eating, unperturbed by the mother's pain and fear, and the house falling down around them. And so Visitor Q moves in without explanation.

The next day the mother is shown tending her wounds from the beatings, injecting heroin and leaving for work as a prostitute. She has a pronounced limp, in addition to the many scars and welts from her son's beatings, and her heroin addiction, and is thus presented as a pitiful and lonely character. She dresses as conservatively as possible with pearls and a beige handbag, in an attempt to be a respectable, middle-class wife. On her return home from work, in which her sexualised body is literally the source of her labour, she finds Visitor Q reading in her daughter's abandoned bedroom, where he invites her to sit down and rest. While it seems that Visitor Q is poised to seduce the mother, instead he reveals her body to herself, showing her that she has the capacity to lactate by removing her shirt and bra, and massaging her breasts. She immediately expresses milk and is soon producing it in large quantities; and as the intensity of her flow increases, she cries out as though having an orgasm. He continues standing behind her, expressing her milk, which sprays into the hallway where her nonplussed son looks on silently. This is Visitor Q's second intervention. From this point the mother, Keiko, is named. She becomes central to the action, which begins to escalate wildly.

Having failed as a reporter, the father is attempting to sell the idea of a reality TV show to his disdainful lover who is also a colleague. His plan is to film his son being beaten and humiliated by the school bullies. While watching and filming his son being abused, the father and his lover sit in the car nearby, and Visitor Q in the back seat is instructed to film the action. The father tries to persuade his lover/colleague of his new TV show idea and begins choreographing how he'd heroically save his son—which would all be captured on film—should he become seriously endangered. In other words, any act of saving would be merely an act of self-promotion. Disgusted by his plan, the lover breaks off her relationship with the father and attempts to leave. He pursues her, still being filmed by Visitor Q, and in the process of raping her, he strangles her and she dies.

The father and Visitor Q bring the body home and the father relates his plans of dismembering the corpse in the hot house to Visitor Q, who continues to film as requested. While beginning to mark-up the corpse's body with rec pen, the father asks Visitor Q to fetch garbage bags. He enters the kitchen where he is greeted by a smiling Keiko. She asks him to stay and watch as she removes her clothes to reveal that she is herself dressed in a garbage bag, cut down especially to work as a sleeveless mini dress, with clipped openings for her breasts, for ease of lactating. Keiko begins her performance, showing Visitor Q her new skill as she begins to fountain large quantities of milk while exclaiming with pleasure. The film now alternates between images of the father in the garden having sex with his corpse, while Keiko in the kitchen showers milk, and Visitor Q watches her from under an umbrella. This becomes the transformative moment of the film. As the milk rains down and covers the floor, Keiko's parted legs reveal a deluge of another kind, the clear vaginal fluid making an explicit connection to her sexual jouissance as it blends into the pool of milk below.

Meanwhile the father discovers his penis is stuck in the corpse due to rigor mortis, and he calls out to Keiko to assist. (As she revels in the capacity of her body to give life, he remains literally stuck in death.) Keiko comes to his aid cheerfully, buoyed by her newfound skill. After soaking him and the corpse with vinegar in the bath, she injects heroin into her husband and he is freed as he comments admiringly to the still-filming visitor, "She hasn't been this competent since we got married."

Visitor Q then says to the father, in one of his very few statements, "You don't get it do you?" to which the father replies, "Get what?" And while the visitor continues to obligingly film the action as obsessively requested, it is in each of the brief unmediated exchanges between him and each character that transformation occurs. Soon after, Keiko's newfound energy and competence results in the parents joining together to fight off their son's bullies, who have again chased him home from school. After slaughtering the schoolboys in a kung fu frenzy of gardening tools and kitchen knives, the once estranged parents exchange glances and smile warmly, their first real communication since the beginning of the film. They have mutually acknowledged the needs of each other, and can now assist their son.

As the parents proceed to carve up the mistress, the rescued son lies face down in the lake of milk covering the kitchen floor. He asks the visitor why he came to their home, if he came to destroy it. Visitor Q merely smiles. The son, taking this as assent, says, "I thought so all along. Thank you." Still lying on the floor with his cheek resting in the milk, and in his black school uniform, the son repents his evil ways to the watching visitor. "From now on," he says, "I'm going to study."

The final scene occurs after the visitor makes his third intervention; and returns us to the beginning of the film in which the daughter's circumstances are addressed. On being solicited on the street by the daughter, he whacks her on the head with the same rock he used earlier on her father. She then returns home, dressed as a schoolgirl, having renounced prostitution, to find her mother in the hot house, naked but for a cloak of blue plastic sheeting, under which her father is cosily suckling from her left breast. As the film ends, the daughter joins them, crouching naked next to Keiko to suckle from her other side.

III

In *The World of the Gift*, Jacques T. Godbout makes a distinction between Mauss's conception of the gift as part of the exchange economy, and Derrida's impossibility of the gift that must be forgotten, but argues that gifting nevertheless "constitutes a system" (12). Godbout takes issue with the view that the gift no longer exists in pure form, a position based on the premise that altruism is always rewarded, even if only through one's sense of self-satisfaction. Godbout asserts instead that the reciprocity of the gift cements social relations which are not reducible to economic ones, for "The gift is the embodiment of that system of relationships that is strictly social, in that these relations cannot be reduced to factors of power or economic interest" (13). Similarly, Rosalyn Diprose moves beyond Mauss and Derrida to analyse the relationship more explicitly between sociality, identity and gifting. Insisting on the connection between bodily experience and consciousness, (22) she argues that "Generosity operates at the level of sensibility ... The openness to otherness that characterizes generosity is, I will argue, carnal and affective, and the production of identity and difference is a material production" (8). In other words, adopting Levinas' position that the subject is formed through ethical relations rather than producing them, Diprose adds to this the idea of "intercorporeal relations ... to foster social relations that generate rather than close off sexual, cultural, and stylistic differences" (15).

I would like to read Takashi Miike's film in relation to this definition of the corporeal gift and the fostering of difference which enables a balance between autonomy and care. The motif of excessive, induced lactation that the film presents, together with the figure of Visitor Q himself, can be seen to represent this ideal of the gift, based on the embodiment of social relations which are mutually beneficial. Instead of requiring no reciprocation, or the altruistic rewards of sacrifice and self-denial which are traditionally associated with maternal gifting, the film demonstrates how maternal care can co-exist with care of the self in a way that is redemptive not only for mothers, but more widely. When conceived of as a gift in Godbout's terms, as "nothing less than the embodiment of the system of interpersonal social relations," (18) it could be argued that *Visitor Q* portrays the redemptive potential of lactation, symbolizing the corporeal generosity of the maternal, whether or not the mother figure is engaged in care of her own children.[3] Godbout's theory of the gift charts a passage between the exchange model proposed by Mauss, and that of excess beyond the economy of exchange found in Irigaray and Derrida, instead arguing that reciprocation can be invoked at the level of the purely interpersonal. He writes, "Only the gift can actually—not just in the imagination or ideologically—transcend the opposition between the individual and the collectivity, making individuals part of a larger, concrete entity" (20).

My interpretation of the film is that both the act of lactation is a gift—to the mother and from the mother to the family—and that the stranger, Visitor Q, is himself a representation of the power of the gift. As Godbout puts it, "The transformation of a stranger into a familiar is what the gift is all about. It paves the way for reciprocity and the market but, first and foremost, it enables society to perpetuate itself as a society (not just a family), to renew itself in renewing the pact with every 'generation'. We therefore find the stranger where we expected him least: at the heart of personal relationships, at the core of the domestic sphere itself" (30). Thus the rescue of the family from the brink of self-destruction is dependent on recognition of an "other" beyond the family, and the embedding of the family within the social. At the same time, the visitor's role is to attend to the needs of its most victimised, othered member—the mother—dramatically revealing her value, first to herself and then to her family. That this value is based on the corporeal generosity of her body may seem problematic within the traditional maternal paradigm which equates biological determinism with enslavement. The crucial difference here though, is that the mother's plenitude is auto-erotic and something over which she exercises control. Once made aware of the pleasure of lactating, which verges on masturbatory exhibitionism, she recovers her agency. She is immediately transformed from passive victim and slave to a beacon of joyful efficiency and self-determination. As each member becomes individuated within the family structure, they also become capable of connecting, of meeting each other's gaze, of recognising their mutual needs, and of achieving ethical intersubjectivity.

I would like to propose that the act of gifting, conceived in this way, can be seen as part of the care of the self, as conceptualised by Jane Ussher in her work on the *Managing the Monstrous Feminine* as well as Michel Foucault in relation to the dual task of self-knowing and self-caring outlined in *Technologies of the Self*. Instead of something that depletes the giver, and may be recompensed either through reciprocal giving or the gratifications of altruism, lactation is in itself self-caring: it is an act of empowerment that illustrates the strength and resourcefulness of the female body; it is a renewable resource whose supply is stimulated through auto-erotic means, as well as by demand from the other; it is mutually pleasurable; and it literally connects, through suckling and ingestion, two bodies who are otherwise separate. In short, it provides an analogy for the gift of connection which benefits both parties.

At the same time it needs to be acknowledged that *Visitor Q* is macabre, and that each of the characters, especially the mother, is represented as monstrous; and that this celebration of embodied monstrosity can be viewed as a means to acknowledge the vulnerability of the self, as part of a strategy for incorporating otherness. As a physiological capacity which has come in our time to perhaps exemplify, along with menstruation and childbirth, the freakish otherness of the female body, induced lactation in particular insists on the project to reduce the distance between self and other through its spectacle of vulnerability and empowerment, and through its literal capacity for connection. As Magrit Shildrick explains in *Embodying the Monster*, the otherness of those who fall outside the normative, contained and proper body, is upheld as a means of defining normativity; it is a means of separating self from other. Like pregnancy, lactation problematises "the boundaries of self and other" (31). For, she explains, "what is at stake is not simply the status of those bodies which might be termed monstrous, but the being in the body of us all. To valorise the monster, then, is to challenge the parameters of the subject … " (3). As Jane Ussher establishes, the monster *par excellence* is the female reproductive body, which as she and others have argued (Longhurst; Hausman) is closely regulated within patriarchal culture, both in terms of the uses and behaviour of the reproductive body and the places within which it may act. Quoting Aristotle's view that, "Woman is literally a monster: a failed and botched male," Ussher goes on to argue that, "Central to this positioning of the female body as monstrous or beneficent is ambivalence associated with the power and danger perceived to be inherent in woman's fecund flesh, her seeping, leaking, bleeding womb standing as a site of pollution and source of dread" (1). The point that Ussher and Longhurst make is that the female body is marginalised as different, something to be feared, which must be contained, regulated and managed. Yet in her work in *Embodying the Monster* which looks historically at maternity as well as the idea of the freak more generally, Shildrick also sees opportunities in embracing monstrosity itself, in opening oneself to difference as a means to self-recognition and connection. She writes, "It is not simply that monsters—strangers in general—disrupt the usual rules of interaction in that their cultural instance may be offset by physical proximity, but that they may not be outside at all. Although they are always there in our conscious appraisal of the external world, they are also the other within" (4). The mother's acceptance of her own monstrous vulnerability thus enables a refusal of separation, opening out a "moment of recognition" and paving the way for connection to the needs of others. Adopting Ussher's insight into the construction of the maternal body as monstrous, and linking this to Shildrick's argument that recognition of the other within enables us to meet the needs of others (who in Diprose's view are all potentially characterised as monstrous), it is possible to interpret the scenes of lactation in *Visitor Q* as exemplifying this moment of recognition, enabling a deliberate act of corporeal generosity (since lactation is dependent for its success on the desire of the lactating subject) that is simultaneously an act of self-care.

While there are other representations in film and literature of women who lactate for reasons other than breastfeeding progeny,[4] Miike's film most dramatically and explicitly illustrates a feature of the maternal body which is, in Margrit Shildrick's terms, both monstrous and vulnerable; and the way in which this might "signal a transformation of the relation between self and other" (1). As she explains in her 2005 essay "Unreformed Bodies: Normative

Anxiety and the Denial of Pleasure," the more fearful we are of otherness, the less likely we are to accept our own vulnerability to otherness within. She writes, "The socio-cultural rejection of otherness speaks above all to a disavowed vulnerability" (329). The film then shows how the two predatory characters are also constructed as vulnerable. Their disavowed vulnerability is made manifest through the assault by the stranger (the visitor) who perhaps personifies the other within. And so in the final scene they turn away from this disavowal towards the body of the mother, to the site of her own vulnerability, where connection is most literally exemplified: her breasts.

IV

The accomplishment of *Visitor Q* is through its illustration of the process of gifting as one that is embodied, yet unlike other examples of maternal gifting, is not associated with depletion or self-sacrifice, but can be viewed as an act of self-care. The mother benefits from and experiences pleasure through this realisation as much as anyone else. Throughout the film, which is violent, erotic and funny, the gift represents various forms of the abject. The problem which, as a satire, the film seeks to oppose, is disembodiment, disconnection, disembodied representation, and—just to give it a blackly comic spin—literal dismemberment of the material body as well as metaphorical dismemberment of the family, and of subjectivity. At the start of the film, all the bodies are in crisis which, while depicted through various tropes of violence, is understood finally as an agonising separation from both self and other. As Shildrick writes, "The masculinist retreat from the body and from embodiment has denied to those others access to subjectivity itself" (1).

Yet ethical connection is based on a recognition and acceptance of difference (of both others and within oneself); and it is here that the intersection between parenting and the gift is illustrated in *Visitor Q*. Just as parenting entails a higher level of functioning as a partnership than was previously necessary, it also enables a higher level of differentiation as each parent takes on the new roles of caregiver, provider and protector. Rather than allowing these roles to undermine female sexuality by being metonymically linked to matronly stereotypes, *Visitor Q* demonstrates how they can be incorporated into a new mould of super heroism, based on sexiness in strength that is both self-serving and other-directed. As Iris Marion Young puts it in "Breasted Experience," "It means creating and affirming a kind of love in which a woman does not have to choose between pursuing her own selfish, insatiable desire and giving pleasure and sustenance to another close to her, [but allows for] *a nurturance that gives and also takes for itself*" (200, my italics).

It would be through this means that we can begin to construct the mothering subject as one which incorporates both care and autonomy. As Petra Bueskens argues in her compelling account of the motives of mothers who leave their families, such a mother would be "a creation myth of sorts for she promulgates the possibility of a mother in possession of her own desire: a desire to be a free individual and a mother. Here is the gift of loss that may just prove to catapult us out of gendered stasis and into an altogether new family history" (279). Instead of leaving the family (through drug addiction and prostitution) Keiko is free to stay, since giving and receiving have become one. And as we have seen, the image of a woman fountaining milk has been a popular representation of creation myths in the past.

The film concludes with the mother breastfeeding her teenage daughter and her husband in the glasshouse, while a song provides the soundtrack. It is a sweet, girlie song reminiscent of Japanese schoolgirl kitsch, about the oceanic quality of life, with floating bubbles as a metaphor for love and death, impermanence and eternity, and reminiscent of the Diamond Sutra, one of the best-known texts from Mahayana Buddhism which is popular in Japan. It concludes with the words:

> We should keep space between us
> And lie down for a while
> Don't say anything
> Just like this

As a concluding text for the film, the lyrics seem to suggest that a process of differentiation is inevitable in families, and in some instances slides into alienation and beyond. And this process is only encouraged by the socio-economic forces within which the family is forced to operate. The reunion of the family through contact with the mother's milk, and the return to the body as a literal source of sustenance, suggests that the differentiation, once achieved, can be accommodated. The words, "We should keep a space between us/ and lie down for a while," echoes David Schnarch's ideal of differentiation in *Passionate Marriage*, which is defined as the balancing of the "drive for individuality and the drive for togetherness" (55). This is not only a dynamic that exists in marriages, he argues, but also in relationships between parents and their children, who struggle to become "well-developed individuals while maintaining emotional contact with the family" (63).

Adult nursing is perhaps another field within which this process of differentiation is attained, since differentiation achieves, in Schnarch's words, "a 'higher order' process that involves balancing both connection and autonomy" (57). While it may be interpreted as regressive, with the male partner returning to the maternal body in his enactment of infantile dependency, it's also possible to interpret the relationship as one in which the parenting potentials of both partners, through the giving body, is equalized since it is recognised that the father is also receptive and passive and no longer the only (active) provider. Additionally, the non-genital intimacy that adult nursing provides allows it to develop the forms of communication and spiritual grace found in tantric traditions as well as maternal care: the move away from an emphasis on climax and genital stimulation and toward different forms of embodied togetherness and sensory awakening. The links between orality, nipples and arousal is commented on by Margot Anand in *The New Art of Sexual Ecstasy* (1989) where she writes:

> Oral loving can play a major role in High Sex ... When the male partner is kissing the female partner's breast, for example, he is adopting the male, or Yang, role. He is the doer, the active one, and the woman is Yin. But when the woman's breast becomes very aroused through his kissing and fondling, it sometimes produces small amounts of a thin white liquid—sweet to taste, but not the same as milk—that the man can then drink. In the sacred Taoist traditions, the mixing of love juices—such as female breast fluids and male saliva—contributes to the harmonization of Yin and Yang in both partners (314).

Anand goes on to discuss the "very pleasant form of regression" that sucking body parts, whether the breast or penis, can offer. Far from being retrograde, the links between infancy and adulthood are in this context considered a valid and enriching means of achieving bliss. She writes that fellatio in particular, offers the experience of the baby at the breast at the same time as it resembles genital penetration (since the tissue of mouth and vagina are histologically similar). "This combined feeling of being both a baby and adult," she writes, "can be an extremely erotic experience" (315). And as Shildrick points out, acceptance of vulnerability is a pre-condition for connection to the other.

Anand's reluctance to consider the "thin white liquid, sweet to taste" as breastmilk, shows that she too resists fully acknowledging the sexuality of the maternal body. In this western interpretation of an eastern tradition, there is a reluctance to view sex as anything more than a means to an end of procreation, which then desexualises the mother, rather than viewing the processes of procreation and nurturance as themselves part of the sexual continuum. That *Visitor Q* ends with the father being nursed by the mother who is also free to nurse her daughter, suggests that the power of the mother's body (of all mother's bodies) has been formerly underestimated. By the end of the film the continuity of her maternal sexuality is thus restored.

The empowerment of the mother through knowledge of her bodily plenitude in *Visitor Q* is in stark contrast to the treatment of the mother in a much earlier erotic and violent black comedy on motherhood and sexuality, *Philosophy in the Bedroom* (1795) by Sade. Here the mother figure symbolises repression, and is punished for her lack of sexual enthusiasm (and by her desire to protect her daughter's virtue) by being raped by her daughter, impregnated with syphilis and her labia sewn together. While there are many other sexual climaxes in this narrative, abuse of the mother is what the libertines have logically been aspiring to. Tellingly, the point at which the rape of the mother by her daughter and her daughter's tutors in sex, results in pleasure for the mother, is the point at which she also faints. In other words, on the brink of being forced to admit to pleasure, the Sadeian mother is better off dead. And she does of course die in the process of being assaulted by the libertines. In *Visitor Q* this is the fate of the mistress who, alongside the father and daughter, stands in for the libertines, who are punished. It is the sexualised mother who is saved, and who in turn saves her family, simply by recognising and revealing her embodied power.

Perhaps the most touching scene in *Visitor Q* is when Keiko has serviced a client and he chats to her, asking about the many cuts that cover her body as a result of beatings from her son. He is a sympathetic, though unsentimental character who in looking her over in a quietly post-coital mood says, "I wonder what you look like, I didn't get to see." With her consent, he gently proceeds to examine her genitals. The significance of his desire to see all of her body, which exceeds his desire for sexual satisfaction, is mirrored by her own attempts to care for her body, despite the beatings and the needles. The film reminds us of the importance of seeing the mother's body whole (and thus her "hole"), beyond desire, both as a physical entity unbreached by injury, and as the basis for her subjectivity. It is also a moment of unmediated recognition of difference which enables connection. That the client then asks Keiko to beat him with his belt, not only shifts the mood back to black comedy; it also implies that in the legitimated context of voyeuristic alienation which dominates, such moments of intimacy are shameful.

As Foucault explains in his historical account of the way in which care of the self has been reinterpreted from its Roman origins through Christianity and then secularisation, "'Know thyself' has obscured 'Take care of yourself' because our morality, a morality of asceticism, insists that the self is that which one can reject" (22). Yet Foucault also explains that care of the self is only possible once knowledge of the self has been attained. Thus Keiko's knowledge of her capacity to lactate precedes her interest in self-care and her ability to achieve this. Visitor Q's lesson is that self-knowledge and self-care constitute two sides of the same coin, just as recognition of self-vulnerability and the other within, accompanies ethical engagement.

There is much else that goes on in this film suggesting that Keiko's project is far from puritanical. She is not a saintly figure, she is sexually active, a prostitute and a drug addict; and in some of the most blackly funny scenes in the film, she helps her husband in his most amoral and violent moments. The film is not idealising mothering, or motherhood, or families. It merely suggests that there is something we've forgotten; and that is the body of the mother who has become the stranger within, even to mothers themselves. In being wholly restored to centre stage, armed with self-knowledge, she is no longer whipping post, workhorse, or repository of virtue, but a paragon of plenitude, connection and joy.

[1]Between the Renaissance and the twentieth century there are very few vi-

sual depictions of breastmilk at all in Western art, let alone images of milk spraying forth, with Frida Kahlo's *My Nurse and I* (1937) and *Love Embrace of the Universe* (1949) breaking the drought, as it were. A recent contemporary example of spectacular lactation is Lynn Randolph's *Contemporary Venus* (1996) which references Botticelli's *Venus* (c.1485) and is accompanied by text defending spectacular lactation as a transgressive act which resists the policing of women's bodies.

[2]For an elaboration of this connection, see Marina Warner.

[3]This is not to deny that gifts may be double-edged with both good and bad, nutritious and poisonous effects, as outlined in the work of Myra Hird and Rhonda Shaw (2003, 2004), and reinforced by recent science on microchimerism. In other words, the mother's potential to wreak havoc or to punish (or withhold) adds to her power and defends her from the matyrdom traditionally associated with maternal giving, since unlike menstruation and childbirth, lactation can be consciously controlled.

[4]One notable example is John Steinbeck's *The Grapes of Wrath* in which a nursing mother offers her breast to a starving traveller.

REFERENCES

Anand, Margot. *The New Art of Sexual Ecstasy: Following the Path of Sacred Sexuality.* London: Harper Collins, 1989.

Bueskens, Petra. "When Eve left the Garden: A Modern Tale about Mothers who Leave their Families." *Motherhood: Power and Oppression.* Eds. Andrea O'Reilly, Patricia Short and Marie Porter. Toronto: Association for Research on Mothering, 2005. 265-284.

Dharma. "The Vajra Prajna Paramita [Diamond] Sutra" Bhuddist Text Translation Society, 1997. <http://www.drba.org/dharma/vajrasutra.asp>.

Diprose, Rosalyn. *Corporeal Generosity: On Giving with Nietzsche, Merleau-Ponty, and Levinas.* Albany: State University of New York Press, 2002.

Foucault, Michel. *Technologies of the Self: A Seminar with Michel Foucault.* Eds. Luther H. Martin, Huck Gutman and Patrick H. Hutton. Amherst: University of Massachusetts Press, 1988. 16-49.

Godbout, Jacques T. *The World of The Gift.* In Collaboration with Alain Caille, Trans. Donald Winkler. Montreal: McGill-Queen's University Press, 1998.

Hausman, Bernice. *Mother's Milk: Breastfeeding Controversies in American Culture.* New York: Routledge, 2003.

Hird, Myra J. "The Corporeal Generosity of Maternity." *Body and Society* 13.1 (2007): 1-20.

Longhurst, Robyn. *Bodies: Exploring Fluid Boundaries.* London: Routledge, 2001.

Miike, Takashi. *Visitor Q.* Japan: Cinerocket and Trustech, 2001.

Randolph, Lynn M. (1996) "Cyborgs, Wonder Women and Techno-Angels:

A Series of Spectacles" Presented at the Centre for the Critical Analysis of Contemporary Culture, Rutger's University, April 23. http://lynnrandolph.com/texts/cborgs.html

Sade, Marquis de. "Philosophy in the Bedroom." *The Complete Three Novels: Justine, Philosophy in the Bedroom, Eugenie de Franval and Other Writings.* London: Arrow Books, 1965, 1st published 1795. 177-367.

Schnarch, David. *Passionate Marriage: Keeping Love and Intimacy Alive in Committed Relationships.* New York: W.W. Norton & Co., 1997.

Shaw, Rhonda. "Theorizing Breastfeeding: Body Ethics, Maternal Generosity and the Gift Relation" *Body and Society* 9.2 (2003): 55-73.

Shaw, Rhonda. "The Virtues of Cross Nursing and the 'Yuk Factor'." *Australian Feminist Studies* 19. 45 (November 2004): 287-300.

Shildrick, Margrit. *Embodying the Monster: Encounters with the Vulnerable Self.* London: Sage, 2002.

Shildrick, Margrit. "Unreformed Bodies: Normative Anxiety and the Denial of Pleasure." *Women's Studies* 34.3-4 (April-June 2005): 327-344.

Steinbeck, John. *The Grapes of Wrath.* New York: Viking Press, 1939.

Ussher, Jane. *Managing the Monstrous Feminine: Regulating the Reproductive Body.* London: Routledge, 2006.

Young, Iris Marion. "Breasted Experience: The Look and the Feeling." *Throwing Like a Girl and Other Essays in Feminist Philosophy and Social Theory.* Bloomington: Indiana University Press, 1990. 189-209.

Warner, Marina. "The Milk of Paradise." *Alone of All Her Sex: The Myth and Cult of the Virgin Mary.* London: Vintage, 2002. 1st published 1976. 192-205.

Contributor Notes

Carol Bartle has a nursing, midwifery and lactation consultant background. Her Masters thesis explores mothers' experiences of breastfeeding in a neonatal intensive care environment. Carol's current interests include the controversies in the use of donor breastmilk in neonatal intensive care, the impact of separating mothers and babies in these environments, and breastfeeding advocacy. Carol is a member of the La Leche League New Zealand Board of Consultants and a member of the New Zealand National Breastfeeding Committee. She currently works as the coordinator of the Canterbury Breastfeeding Advocacy Service for Te Puawaitanga Ki Otautahi Trust, an arm of the Maori Women's Welfare League.

Alison Bartlett is Associate Professor in Women's Studies at the University of Western Australia. Her books include *Jamming the Machinery: Contemporary Australian Women's Writing* (1998), and *Breastwork: Rethinking Breastfeeding* (2005). Her recent research has been on cultural discourses of maternity, embodiment, and breasted knowledge production. She is editor of the online journal *Outskirts: Feminisms Along the Edge.*

Annette Beasley is a medical anthropologist. Her interest in breastfeeding research grew out of her experience breastfeeding five children and involvement as a group leader with La Leche League New Zealand over many years. Annette currently maintains this link as a member of the New Zealand Board of Professional Consultants of La Leche League New Zealand. Annette is also a member of the Editorial Board of *The International Breastfeeding Journal.* Annette's publications include: *Breastfeeding in New Zealand: Practice, Problems and Policy*, (with A. Trlin, 1998), and *Breastfeeding for the First Time* (1996). Annette has also conducted research on women's experience of menopause and is currently working on a historical ethnography on the scientific investigation of the disease, kuru, which decimated the Fore people of the Eastern Highlands of Papua New Guinea during the late 1950s and early 1960s.

Naomi Bromberg Bar-Yam is trained in social work and social policy. She has been writing, teaching and researching in maternal and child health for over 20 years, including work in breastfeeding and the workplace, ethics of prenatal testing, breastfeeding and human rights, milk sharing and human milk banking. She is currently the founding executive director of the Mothers' Milk Bank of New England. Naomi is married and has four children. She lives outside Boston, Massachusetts.

Monica Campo is a doctoral student at La Trobe University Australia. Her current research examines the social production of knowledge around childbirth in popular and professional discourse and the ways this knowledge becomes embodied in women's birth experiences. Monica's publications include "Trusting the Experts, Mistrusting Birth: Women's Relationships with Private Obstetricians," *The Australian Sociological Association (TASA) 2008 Conference Proceedings*, Melbourne. Monica is also a birth activist, 'lactivist,' and mother of three.

Tanya M. Cassidy is currently an adjunct Professor with the Department of Sociology and Anthropology at the University of Windsor in Canada, and is also an affiliated researcher with the Department of Anthropology at the National University of Ireland, Maynooth. Her doctoral research, from the Department of Sociology at the University of Chicago, concerned a socio-cultural study of alcohol in Ireland. Tanya has lectured in both Sociology and Anthropology in Ireland, England, and Canada. After a career break Tanya is engaged in full-time research on issues related to infant feeding, in particular the feeding of the prematurely born.

Andrew Coco, MD, is Director of the Health Research Center in the Family and Community Medicine Department at Lancaster General Hospital. He is a graduate of the Harvard School of Public Health and the University of Massachusetts Medical School. Previously, he developed preventive health programs with the Peace Corps in Western Africa.

Denise A. Copelton, Ph.D., is Assistant Professor of Sociology at The College at Brockport, State University of New York. Her research focuses on the social experience of illness, especially the intersection of illness experience with family systems. Her current work examines the social experience of celiac disease.

Abdullahi Osman El-Tom is currently Head of the Department of Anthropology at the National University of Ireland, Maynooth. He received his doctoral training as a social anthropologist from the Department of Anthropology at St. Andrew's in the UK, prior to which he had conducted master's level work in Northern Ireland. Abdullahi is an active medical and political researcher social anthropologist who has published on topics ranging from female circumcision to genocide in Dafur. His most recent book is a creative personal narrative about growing up in the Sudan. Throughout his work, his anthropological vision recognises the value of narrative autoethnography.

Keren Epstein-Gilboa Ph.D, MEd, BSN, RN, FACCE, LCCE, IBCLC, RLC, is a psychotherapist, nurse, researcher, educator and author in private and university practice. She has been working with families in the transition to parenthood for over 25 years in several capacities, including childbirth and breastfeeding education and support, and psychotherapy. Her book on interactions and relationships in breastfeeding families explores the impact of breastfeeding unit on the family and vice versa, demonstrating how nursing facilitates the development of a sensitive family style. Her personal experience as a former nursing mother and retired La Leche League Leader contribute to her sense of the nursing experience.

Fiona Giles is a Senior Lecturer in Media and Communications at Sydney University, Australia. She has written and edited several books in the area of gender and cultural studies; and her most recent book is *Fresh Milk: The Secret Life of Breasts* (2003). Her recent academic work on breastfeeding has appeared in the *Australian Feminist Studies* thematic issue on Meanings of Breastfeeding, (2004) which she co-edited with Alison Bartlett, and the *Women's Studies* Special Issue on Body Modification (2005); and she contributed a chapter, 'The Tears of Lacteros: Integrating the Meanings of the Human Breast' to *Body Parts: Critical Explorations in Corporeality* (Eds. Christopher E. Forth and Ivan Crozier, 2005). Fiona is currently researching adult uses of human breastmilk.

Karleen Gribble is an adjunct research fellow in the School of Nursing and Midwifery at the University of Western Sydney. Her research interests include adoptive breastfeeding, long-term breastfeeding, non-nutritional aspects of breastfeeding, models of care for newly adopted post-institutionalized children, and infant feeding in emergencies. Karleen speaks and publishes widely on these subjects to lay and professional audiences and is actively involved in breastfeeding advocacy in Australia and internationally. She is the mother of two children and is an Australian Breastfeeding Association Community Educator. Karleen has published in *Early Child Development and Care, Breastfeeding Review, Maternal and Child Nutrition, International Breastfeeding Journal*, and *Birth Issues*.

Bernice L. Hausman is Professor of English at Virginia Tech, where she coordinates the undergraduate minor in Medicine and Society. She is the author of *Changing Sex: Transsexualism, Technology, and the Idea of Gender* (1995), *Mother's Milk: Breastfeeding Controversies in American Culture* (2003), and i *Viral Mothers: Breastfeeding in the Age of HIV/AIDS* (2010). Her articles have been published in the *Journal of Medical Humanities, Journal of the History of*

Sexuality, Hypatia, Feminist Studies, NWSA Journal, Technical Communicatio Quarterly, and, most recently, *New Literary History.*

Karen McBride-Henry is a Registered Nurse with a Ph.D. specializing in child and family health, who currently works in the Graduate School of Nursing, Midwifery and Health at Victoria University of Wellington, New Zealand. Karen's clinical experience in children's hospitals instilled in her a deep appreciation of the benefits that breastfeeding offers children. This led Karen to her doctoral research study, which explored how breastfeeding is experienced by New Zealand women.

Rebecca McGee, BS, is a 2007 graduate of the Sociology Program at the College at Brockport, State University of New York where she also minored in Women's and Gender Studies. She works for Monroe County Social Services in Rochester, New York, and is the mother of two children.

Tasnim Nathoo completed her graduate studies in health care and epidemiology and social work at the University of British Columbia. She currently works in the areas of reproductive health and mental health and addictions.

Aleck Ostry is a professor at the University of Victoria, British Columbia. He is an epidemiologist and historian and conducts a broad research program on the social determinants of health, with a focus on nutrition policy and food security. Nathoo and Ostry are the authors of *The One Best Way? Breastfeeding History, Politics, and Policy in Canada* (2009).

Jennifer A. Reich's research explores the intersections between the state and family. She is author of *Fixing Families: Parents, Power, and the Child Welfare System* (2005) as well as several articles and book chapters that examine reproductive decision-making, multi-racial families, families' experiences in the child welfare system, experiences of service providers and evacuees from Hurricane Katrina, and qualitative methods. She is Assistant Professor of Sociology and Criminology at the University of Denver and was formerly a fellow at the Institute for Health Policy Studies at the University of California, San Francisco. She received her Ph.D. and MA from the University of California, Davis and earned a BA from the University of California, Santa Barbara.

Timothy Riley, MD, is a physician in private practice in Lancaster, Pennsylvania, specializing in family practice.

Isis Shanbaky, MD, is Assistant Professor at the Penn State Milton S. Hershey Medical Center, where she specializes in family practice.

Rhonda Shaw is a sociologist in the School of Social and Cultural Studies at

Victoria University of Wellington, New Zealand. Since 2002 she has been researching body gifting practices including shared breastfeeding, ovarian egg donation, surrogate pregnancy arrangements, and organ donation and transplantation processes. Rhonda's work has been published in *Current Sociology*, *Social Science & Medicine*, *Sociological Research Online*, *The Sociological Review*, *Feminist Review*, *Australian Feminist Studies*, *Feminist Theory*, *Women's Studies International Forum*, and *Body & Society*.

Cindy A. Stearns has a Ph.D. in Sociology from the University of California at Davis. She joined the Sociology Department at Sonoma State University in 2007, after sixteen years as a faculty member and chair of Women's and Gender Studies at Sonoma. Her current research employs qualitative methods to study women's experiences of breastfeeding and the social context for breastfeeding and breastfeeding activism in the United States. Her past research is primarily in the areas of gender and the sociology of health and medical work.

Penny Van Esterik is Professor of Anthropology at York University, Toronto, where she teaches nutritional anthropology, advocacy anthropology and feminist theory. Past books include *Beyond the Breast-Bottle Controversy* (on infant feeding in developing countries), *Materializing Thailand* (on cultural interpretations of gender in Thailand), *Taking Refuge: Lao Buddhists in North America* (on the reintroduction of Buddhism by Lao refugees to North America),and *Food and Culture: A Reader*, edited with Carole Counihan. She is a founding member of the World Alliance for Breastfeeding Action (WABA) and has been active in developing articles and advocacy materials on breastfeeding and women's work, breastfeeding and feminism, and contemporary challenges to infant feeding such as environmental contaminants and HIV/AIDS. In 2007, she received the Weaver-Tremblay award from the Canadian Anthropology Society (CASCA) for contributions to applied anthropology in Canada.

Recycled
Supporting responsible use of forest resources
FSC
www.fsc.org Cert no. SGS-COC-003153
© 1996 Forest Stewardship Council

100%

MARQUIS
Marquis Book Printing Inc.

Québec, Canada
2010

Printed on Silva Enviro which contains 100% recycled post-consumer fibre, is EcoLogo, Processed Chlorine Free and manufactured using biogas energy.

ENVIRONMENTAL CHOICE · CHOIX ENVIRONNEMENTAL

PROCESSED CHLORINE FREE · PROCÉDÉ SANS CHLORE

100%

PERMANENT

BIO GAS ENERGY